HUMAN REPRODUCTION AND DEVELOPMENTAL BIOLOGY

Human Reproduction and Developmental Biology

D. J. BEGLEY, BSc, PhD

Lecturer in Physiology,
King's College, London

J. A. FIRTH, MA, PhD

Senior Lecturer in Structural Biology,
St George's Hospital Medical School, London,
formerly Lecturer in Anatomy,
King's College, London

J. R. S. HOULT, BA, PhD

Lecturer in Pharmacology,
King's College, London

Illustrations by Lydia Malim

First published 1980 by
THE MACMILLAN PRESS LTD
London and Basingstoke
Associated companies in Delhi Dublin
Hong Kong Johannesburg Lagos Melbourne
New York Singapore and Tokyo

Printed in Great Britain by
J. W. Arrowsmith Ltd, Bristol

British Library Cataloguing in Publication Data

Begley, D J
    Human reproduction and developmental biology.
    1. Human reproduction 2. Growth
    I. Title II. Firth, J A III. Hoult, J R S
    612.6   QP251

    ISBN 0–333–23423–5
    ISBN 0–333–23424–3 Pbk

Preface

The biology of reproduction and development forms a large and cohesive part of the scientific basis of medicine but until recently has not achieved the prominence that it deserves in medical undergraduate teaching. We think that this area of knowledge more than any other demonstrates the fundamental unity of the basic medical sciences and in writing this book we have sought to present the subject in an integrated manner, so reflecting our approach to its teaching. In our experience we have found that the traditional boundaries between the so-called preclinical 'subjects' are often arbitrary and unhelpful.

Our aim has been to explain the biological principles of human reproduction and development by tracing the process from the formation of gametes and their union, through the intrauterine development of the fetus, to birth, growth and ageing. We have also included a chapter on contraception because of its vital importance for the future, but we have excluded any discussion of classical genetics as there are already many excellent texts.

In a book of this size we have not been able to discuss all the topics as fully as we would have liked and so reluctantly we have had to leave out interesting experimental and clinical evidence for many of our statements and conclusions. In spite of this, we hope to show that reproductive and developmental biology rests on a sound experimental foundation. Indeed, the astonishingly rapid advances in this field in the past 20 years are largely due to the development of important new experimental techniques such as radio-immunoassay, electron microscopy and tissue culture.

It is our intention that this book should serve as a useful introduction for medical students and that it may provide a scientific basis for further studies in obstetrics, fertility and paediatrics. We also hope that it will interest students of mammalian biology, midwifery and nursing. We assume that readers will have an elementary working knowledge of physiology, biochemistry, cell biology and human anatomy. At the end of each chapter we have provided some limited suggestions for further reading for those who wish to explore other areas more thoroughly but these lists are not intended to be comprehensive as it is apparent that most students do not have time to use extensive bibliographies.

The task of writing this book has been exacting but enjoyable and has been made easier by the friendly tolerance of our colleagues. We offer special thanks to Lydia Malim whose excellent illustrations speak for themselves. We greatly appreciate the expert manner in which she has interpreted our crude sketches and the high quality of the results.

David Begley
Anthony Firth
Robin Hoult

King's College, November 1978

Contents

1

The Formation of Gametes

1.1 Introduction

The central event of sexual reproduction in man is the fusion of a sperm with an egg. Sperms and eggs are collectively described as *gametes*, and are specialised cells in which recombination and halving of the genetic material has taken place by a special sequence of cell division called *meiosis*.

In organisms with extremely short generation times, such as bacteria, most variation between individuals is the product of random mutation. The pool of genetic diversity thus generated acts as a substrate for natural selection which operates in favour of those few mutant genes with some survival advantage. As mutation rates are very low, very large numbers of individuals are needed to provide an adequate base for variation. In addition, most mutations are harmful; this is not too important for bacteria because their generation time is short and population growth from a single successful mutant can be explosively fast.

For more complex organisms, and above all for mammals and birds, creation of new individuals is a considerable investment of time, energy and material; it is therefore essential to produce sufficient individual variation to allow evolution to proceed without risking a very high incidence of non-viable mutants.

In higher organisms individual variation is achieved by a method known as *genetic recombination*. Each individual has two complete sets of genes, segments of which can be exchanged before passing on one set to the next generation. This gene set then pairs with a set derived from the other parent in order to provide a complete double set for the new individual. Thus there are two sources of variation: the exchange of genes between the two sets in a parental cell, and the effect of pairing of this with a set derived from another individual. This mechanism of halving and doubling keeps the total amount of genetic material per cell constant from one generation to the next.

We must now examine the production of the human gametes (the eggs and sperms) in order to understand how these changes in cellular genetic constitution can be brought about.

1.2 Mitosis and meiosis

The term *meiosis* means lessening, and refers to the halving of the total quantity of nuclear genetic material which occurs in the cell during gametogenesis. The process is similar in both male and female gamete production.

The majority of the cells in human tissues contain 46 chromosomes, arranged as 23 pairs in the female and as 22 pairs with an additional non-matching pair in the male. The sex difference in pair 23 is that the female has two chromosomes of the type designated 'X', while the male has one 'X' and one 'Y'. In gametogenesis this number is reduced so that each gamete has 23 single chromosomes, one from each pair; in the sperm there are 22 single chromosomes derived from pairs and either an X or a Y derived from the non-matching pair (figure 1.1).

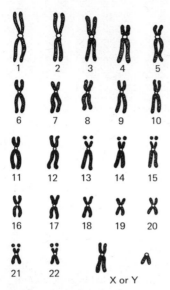

Figure 1.1   Karyotypes of X and Y sperms showing 22 autosomes and 1 sex chromosome. The sex of the offspring depends on whether the egg (always X) is fertilised by an X sperm, resulting in a female, or by a Y sperm, resulting in a male

In normal somatic cell division or *mitosis* the chromosomal DNA is duplicated before division so that each daughter cell has 23 chromosome pairs identical to those of the parent cell (figure 1.2). In meiosis DNA doubling also occurs once, but cell division occurs twice, thus achieving the required separation of the pairs into single chromosomes. During the first of these two divisions exchange of lengths of DNA between adjacent chromosomes in a pair (*crossing over* or chiasma) can take place, thus achieving gene recombination in the two chromosomes. The main features of meiosis are indicated in figure 1.3. Note that the first division resembles mitosis except that crossing over occurs, whereas the second division is not preceded by DNA doubling.

A normal somatic cell with 23 chromosome pairs is termed *diploid*, whereas a gamete with 23 single chromosomes is described as *haploid*. Under normal circumstances haploidy occurs only in gametes, but multiples of the diploid number of

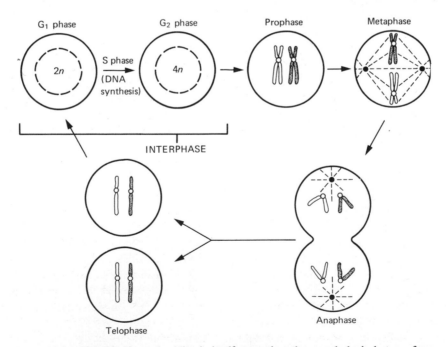

Figure 1.2   The mitotic cycle. Mitosis itself comprises the morphological stages from prophase to telophase as shown; interphase appears homogenous but can be divided into the three phases shown by tritiated thymidine labelling which is only possible during the S (DNA synthesis) phase

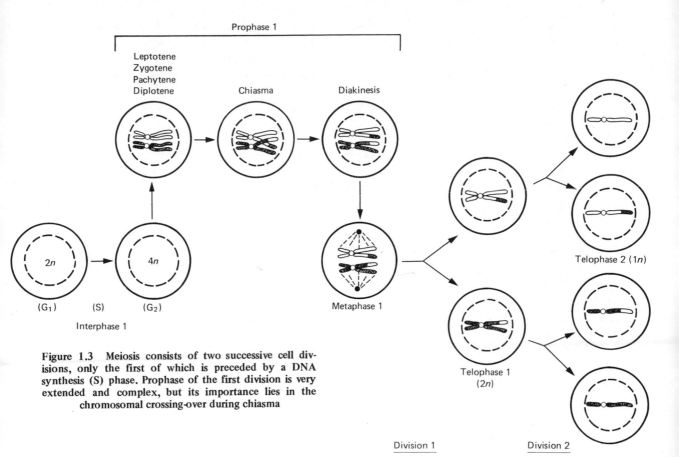

Figure 1.3 Meiosis consists of two successive cell divisions, only the first of which is preceded by a DNA synthesis (S) phase. Prophase of the first division is very extended and complex, but its importance lies in the chromosomal crossing-over during chiasma

chromosomes may be found in somatic cells in a number of tissues, for example liver parenchyma and transitional epithelium.

Although the principles and mechanisms of meiosis are similar in both sexes, its outward expression is rather different and is therefore discussed separately for each sex.

1.3 Oogenesis

The mature female gamete or *ovum* is derived by meiosis from a precursor cell type called the *oogonium*. The ovaries acquire their stock of oogonia during fetal development, and from puberty onwards draw on this stock to produce ova at regular intervals. This is very different from the process in the male described in section 1.4.

Oogenesis takes place in the cortical tissue of the ovaries, and the accompanying changes in other ovarian cell types will be examined in chapter 2.

Meiosis consists of two sequential division cycles, deriving four haploid cells from each diploid cell entering the process. The most important special feature of oogenesis is that only *one* of these haploid products is an ovum, the others being small cells called *polar bodies* to which no definite function has yet been attributed.

The oogonia are fairly large cells with a large, spherical central nucleus and voluminous cytoplasm containing the usual range of organelles found in most somatic cells. They remain in this quiescent state until puberty. Thereafter a small number enter meiosis at each menstrual cycle. They pass through the prophase of the first division, including the vital crossing-over events, but then become arrested at this stage without completing the first division (figure 1.4). Although their cytoplasmic volume increases, no further visible nuclear changes in these *primary oocytes* occur until the mid-point of the menstrual cycle when ovulation occurs. At this point the first division cycle is completed. Cytoplasmic division is unequal, producing a large diploid oocyte and a small diploid polar body (figure 1.4). The oocyte immediately enters the second (reduction) division, but becomes arrested in metaphase. This state persists during the migration of the oocyte into the uterine tube, the division only being completed in response to the penetration of the oocyte plasma membrane by a spermatozoon (see chapter 4). The completion of this second division yields a second, haploid polar body and a haploid ovum, the latter soon being converted into a *zygote* by the pairing of its single chromosomes with those of the sperm at the beginning of the first cleavage — a mitotic division.

Counting of the daughter cells mentioned earlier shows that each oogonium completing its maturation yields one haploid ovum, one haploid polar body and one diploid polar body; i.e. three cells rather than the four implied by the general description of meiosis in section 1.2. In order to preserve the symmetry of the arrangement the first (diploid) polar body should undergo a reduction division to yield two haploid polar bodies. However, it appears that this rather pointless division does not usually take place, so only two polar bodies are normally found adhering to the early zygote.

1.4   Spermatogenesis

The maturation of male gametes, like oogenesis, is centred on the process of meiosis; however, it is different in a number of important ways (figure 1.4).

First, the nature of the fertilisation mechanism makes it essential that sperms should be produced in millions per ejaculation, in marked contrast to the very low rate of gamete release which is adequate to ensure female fertility. This makes it quite impracticable to draw cells from a preformed stock, as a normal man produces many kilograms of sperms in the course of his life. Therefore the production of sperms is based on a *generator cycle*, in which multiple *mitotic* divisions of the precursor *spermatogonia* take place. One cell is returned to stock from each generator division, while the other enters the maturation sequence, thus ensuring the maintenance of a pool of spermatogonia.

Secondly, each spermatogonium entering the maturation pathway undergoes a mitotic division from which both daughter cells proceed to meiosis. Meiotic division yields four haploid gametes from each of these, so each spermatogonium entering maturation produces a total of eight gametes, in contrast with the single gamete produced from an oogonium (figure 1.4).

Thirdly, the process of sperm formation is prolonged by several events. As in the female, the first meiotic division is arrested in mid-course. An extended maturation period called *spermiogenesis* occurs after the completion of meiosis; this allows the haploid products of meiosis, the spermatids, to carry out their morphological differentiation into potentially motile spermatozoa. The sperms are then transferred to the epididymis and ductus deferens where they are stored while further functional maturation occurs. Only after this are the sperms potentially capable of fertilising an egg when deposited in the female reproductive tract.

The main features of spermatogenesis are summarised in figure 1.4.

1.5   Spermiogenesis

Since the structure of the mature spermatozoon is complex and intimately related to its functions, the way in which it differentiates will be examined in some detail.

The earliest specific changes are seen in the Golgi complex of the spermatid. The Golgi lamellae begin to package small, carbohydrate-rich particles called *acrosomal granules*. These fuse to form a large single granule contained within a membrane envelope, the *acrosomal vesicle*, which adheres to the prospective anterior end of the nucleus. The

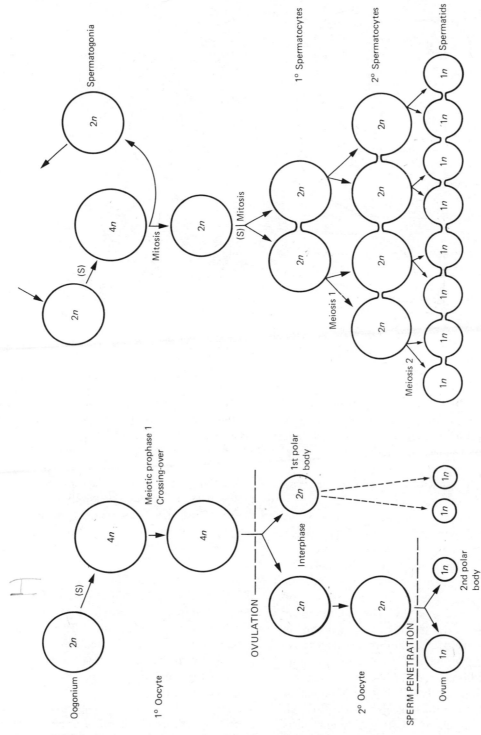

Figure 1.4   Comparison of the expression of meiosis in oogenesis and spermatogenesis. This should be compared with the general meiotic schema illustrated in figure 1.3. Note particularly the generator cycle and mitotic proliferation preceding spermatocyte meiosis, and also the number of haploid gametes produced per cell entering meiosis in each sex

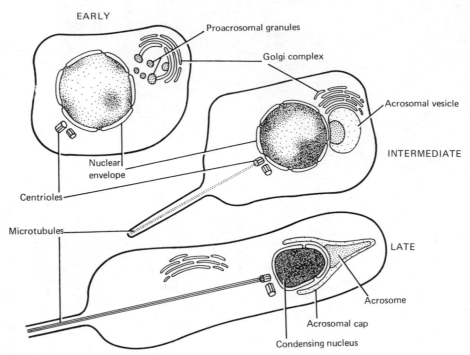

EARLY

Proacrosomal granules

Golgi complex

Acrosomal vesicle

INTERMEDIATE

Nuclear envelope

Centrioles

Microtubules

LATE

Acrosome

Acrosomal cap

Condensing nucleus

Figure 1.5   Three stages in spermiogenesis

area of attachment of the acrosomal vesicle to the nuclear envelope then increases until about the anterior two-thirds of the nucleus is enclosed. Most of the acrosomal contents remain near the anterior pole, however. The acrosome then elongates, as does the nucleus which becomes increasingly compact and dark-staining (figure 1.5).

During the period of acrosome formation the centrioles of the spermatid migrate to the posterior pole of the cell. One of these forms the initiation point for the outgrowth of the sperm tail. The core of the tail has a structure essentially similar to that of a cilium, consisting of a central pair of microtubules surrounded by nine microtubular doublets (figure 1.6). The first section of this is contained in the *middle piece* of the spermatozoon, and becomes surrounded by nine longitudinal columns of fibrous material around which are many circumferentially packed mitochondria. Posterior to this lies the *principal piece* of the tail, in which the mitochondrial array is absent but is replaced by a stack of ring-like structures — the

fibrous sheath. The longitudinal fibres progressively disappear as the posterior end of the principal piece is approached, although the microtubule arrays and the fibrous sheath remain. The final section is the *end piece*, a very slender segment in which the fibrous sheath is absent and the microtubule array becomes progressively more disorganised. During tail development a number of temporary fibrous and microtubular structures are erected and dismantled; their function is unknown.

A curious feature of sperm maturation is that all eight cells produced from a single spermatogonium entering the maturation pathway remain attached to one another until the final stages of spermiogenesis. This attachment takes the form of cytoplasmic bridges connecting the cell bodies in Siamese twin fashion; the significance of these bridges is not understood.

The process of spermatid maturation is completed by the shedding of a small membrane-limited bleb of cytoplasm called the residual body.

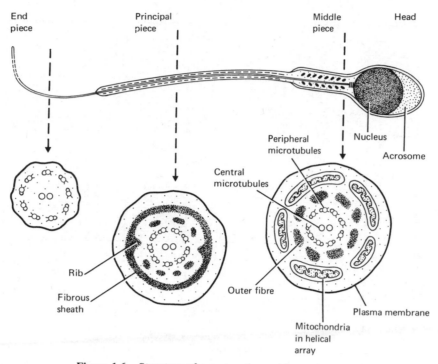

Figure 1.6   Structure of a mature human spermatozoon

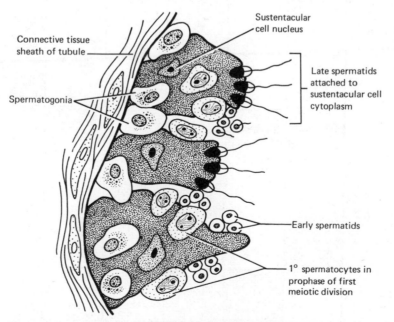

Figure 1.7   Portion of a seminiferous tubule wall showing the relationship between the germ cells and sustentacular cells

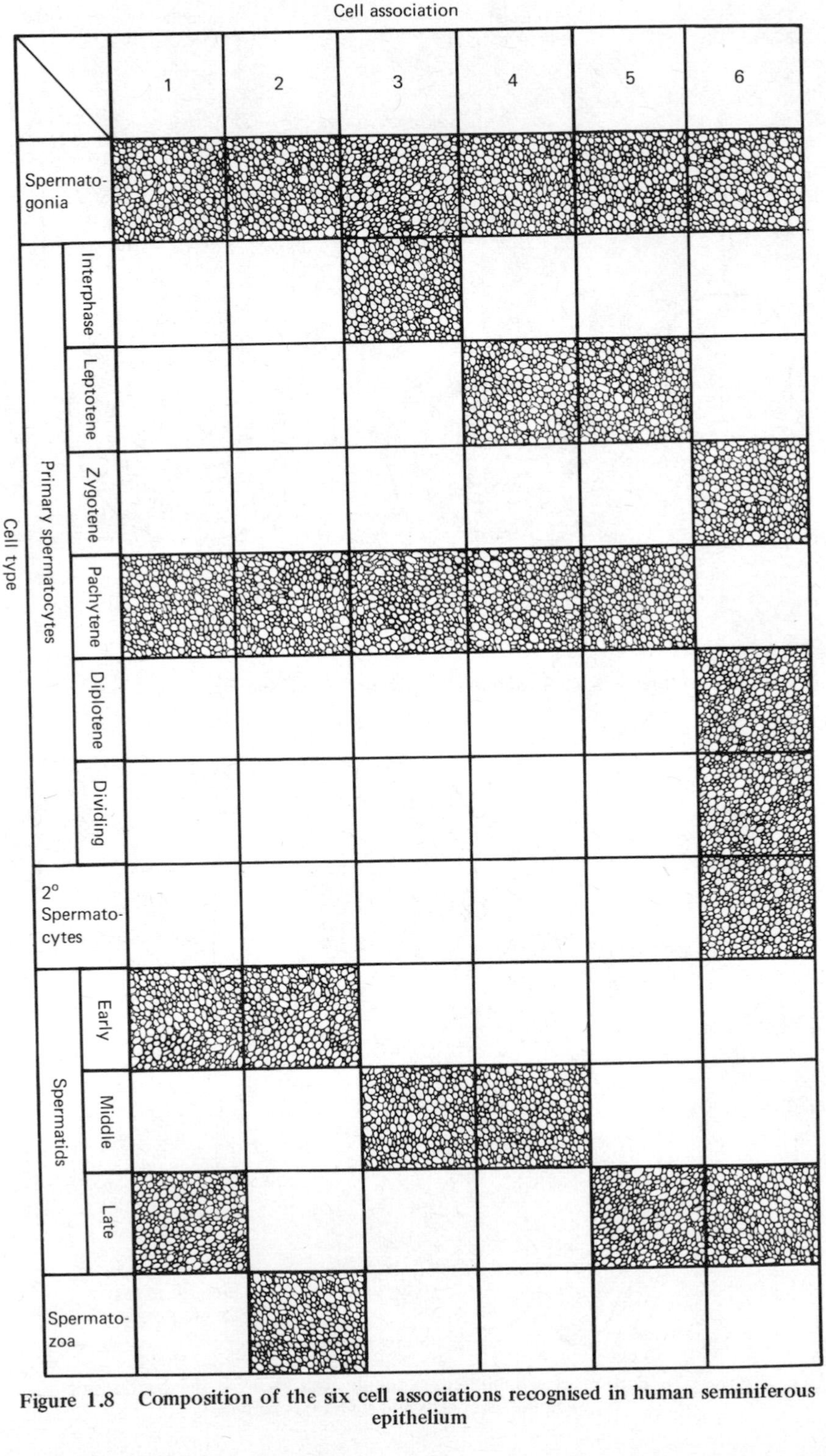

Cell association

Cell type		Cell association 1	2	3	4	5	6
Spermatogonia		▓	▓	▓	▓	▓	▓
Primary spermatocytes	Interphase			▓			
	Leptotene				▓	▓	
	Zygotene						▓
	Pachytene	▓	▓	▓	▓	▓	
	Diplotene						▓
	Dividing						▓
2° Spermatocytes							▓
Spermatids	Early	▓	▓				
	Middle			▓	▓		
	Late	▓				▓	▓
	Spermatozoa		▓				

Figure 1.8 Composition of the six cell associations recognised in human seminiferous epithelium

With this step the cytoplasmic bridges linking the spermatids into octets break down and the cells appear to be morphologically mature spermatozoa. However, further physiological maturation in the male tract is necessary before fertilisation can be accomplished (see chapters 3 and 4).

1.6   The spermatogenic cycle

So far the process of male gametogenesis has been lifted out of its histological context. This has been done in order to give a clear and uncluttered picture of the changes in the germ cells themselves, but the context of the process now needs to be considered.

The male gametogenic cells are arranged in the form of seminiferous tubules, each of which is a closed loop draining from a single point on its periphery (chapter 3). The wall of the tubule consists of developing gametes together with *sustentacular* or *Sertoli* cells (figure 1.7). The latter are elongated with characteristically wedge-shaped nuclei, into which the nuclear regions of the developing spermatids are embedded. Very little firm evidence is available regarding their functions, although they are generally thought to have protective or nutritional roles in relation to the spermatids.

Most of the apparent complexities of the histology of the seminiferous tubules may be explained by one fact: cells do not pass through the maturation cycle continuously, but in batches.

For example, if a particular batch of maturing gametes are at the early spermatid stage, the succeeding batch (lying immediately deep to them) might be primary spermatocytes in late meiotic prophase; by the time the first batch are mature spermatozoa the second batch have become early spermatids.

If batches entered the cycle synchronously along the whole tubule this would mean that certain cellular stages would not be present at a particular time. However, in reality synchrony is only maintained in small patches of seminiferous epithelium in each tubule, so the tubule wall appears as a mosaic of different cell associations. Conventionally six cell associations are described as being present in human seminiferous tubules; it will be realised that these six are merely readily recognisable moments in a continuously varying picture (figure 1.8), and the choice of six stages has no fundamental significance but is merely useful for descriptive purposes.

Further reading

Bloom, W. and Fawcett, D. W. (1968). *A Textbook of Histology*, 9th edn, Saunders, Philadelphia, pp. 685–706 and 728–736

Greep, R. O. and Koblinsky, M. A. (eds.) (1977). *Frontiers in Reproduction and Fertility Control*, MIT Press, chaps. 27 'Spermatogenesis', 28 'Ultrastructure and functions of the Sertoli cell' and 31 'The structure of the spermatozoon'

2

The Female Reproductive System

2.1 Introduction

Reproductive activity in the human female and in primates is characterised by the *menstrual cycle*. This is typified by hyperplasia of the endometrium and its subsequent partial shedding with blood loss (the *menstrual period*). Other mammals also show cyclical activity, termed the *oestrous cycle*, which although essentially similar is not marked by menstrual bleeding. The human cycle, conventionally numbered from the first day of menstruation, has an average length of 28 days and is repeated until an egg is fertilised. Ovulation occurs at mid-cycle, usually day 14, and if fertilisation occurs implantation usually begins about 7 days later.

The events of the menstrual cycle are controlled by the release from the ovaries of the steroids oestradiol-17β (henceforth referred to simply as oestradiol) and progesterone whose production in turn is controlled by the gonadotropins follicle stimulating hormone (FSH) and luteinising hormone (LH), secreted from the anterior pituitary gland. Before discussing the functional aspects of the female reproductive tract in detail it is necessary to describe its structure (figure 2.1).

2.2 Structure of the female reproductive system

The ovaries

The ovaries (figure 2.2) consist of a pair of flattened ovoid structures each measuring about 3 cm by 1 cm, and are attached to the posterior layer of the broad ligament of the uterus, below and behind the uterine tube. Their blood supply is from the ovarian artery, arising directly from the aorta, and the ovarian branch of the uterine artery. Autonomic innervation reaches the ovaries via an ovarian plexus. The peritoneal mesothelium extends over the surface of the ovaries and is modified to form a cuboidal epithelium. This used to be described as the germinal epithelium, in the mistaken belief that it gave origin to the germ cells, but it is better referred to as the *surface epithelium*. It bears areas of ciliated cells, but with increasing age these become less numerous and the whole epithelium becomes patchy and discontinuous.

The bulk of the ovary consists of vascular stroma containing spindle-shaped cells and reticular fibres. The cells superficially resemble smooth muscle but functionally are more like fibroblasts; they have the additional capacity to transform into endocrine cells secreting female sex steroids. The medullary region of the ovary contains the larger blood vessels and fibroblast-like stromal cells.

Oocyte maturation occurs in the cortical region of the ovary which in the prepubertal state contains mainly *primordial follicles*. Some follicles begin development in the fetus *in utero* due to stimulation by placental gonadotropins released during pregnancy, but these regress at birth. The oocyte of the primordial follicle is surrounded by a single layer of flattened follicular or *granulosa cells* separated from the ovarian stroma by a basement membrane (figure 2.3).

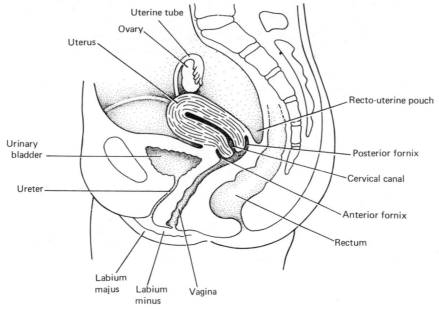

Figure 2.1   Anatomy of the female reproductive system as seen in a sagittal section of the pelvis

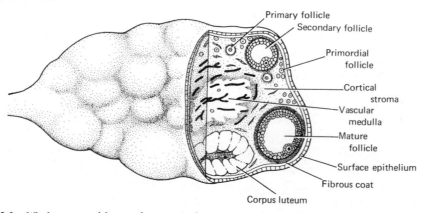

Figure 2.2   Whole ovary with a wedge removed to show the general arrangement of follicles and stroma

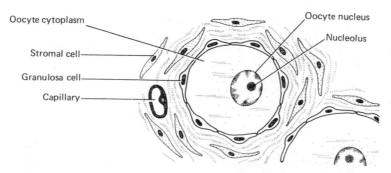

Figure 2.3   Primordial follicle

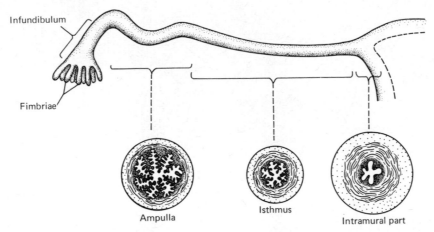

Figure 2.4   Transverse sections from three different segments of the uterine tube, illustrating the changing complexity of mucosal folding and the gradation of muscularity of the wall

The uterine (fallopian) tubes

The uterine tubes (figure 2.4) extend from each ovary to the superior angles of the uterus and run in free margins of the broad ligament. Each tube is about 10 cm long and opens into the peritoneal cavity by a funnel-shaped mouth, the *infundibulum*, which is surrounded by a ring of irregular tentacle-like *fimbriae*. The infundibulum narrows to the *ampulla*, a short sinuous and thin-walled segment leading to the *isthmus*, which is straight and thick-walled and constitutes the major length of the uterine tube. The final short *intramural* part penetrates the uterine wall to open into the uterine cavity.

The wall of the uterine tube has an outer longitudinal and an inner circular coat of smooth muscle throughout its length. The mucosa is folded longitudinally and its epithelium consists of ciliated and secretory cells; the mucosal folds are most elaborate in the ampullary region and diminish towards the body of the uterus.

The uterus and cervix

The walls of the uterus and cervix are thick and their lumina are narrow. Both organs are supplied with blood by the uterine and ovarian arteries. Innervation is supplied by sympathetic nerves from the hypogastric plexus and parasympathetic nerves from sacral segments 2, 3 and 4 which run in the pelvic splanchnic nerves.

The exact position and form of the uterus are variable. The most usual position is illustrated in figure 2.1 which shows the uterus lying between the bladder and the rectum with its long axis directed backwards and downwards. The body of the uterus is usually curved forward (anteverted), as well as being somewhat folded forward at its junction with the cervical canal (anteflexed). Deviations from this arrangement are very common, but are usually of little consequence unless the uterus fails to take up an anteverted position during pregnancy. In this case, complications of pregnancy may result.

In women who have not borne a child (*nulliparous*) the uterus is about 8 cm long but the fundus may reach as far as the costal margin in pregnancy and afterwards does not return fully to its former size. The wall of the uterus contains three smooth muscle coats, forming the *myometrium*: the fibres of the external coat are mainly longitudinal while the others have fibre tracts running in many directions. The uterus is lined with mucosa, the *endometrium*, whose surface bears patches of ciliated cells. The endometrial epithelium is secretory and forms many long, convoluted simple glands, the basal parts of which

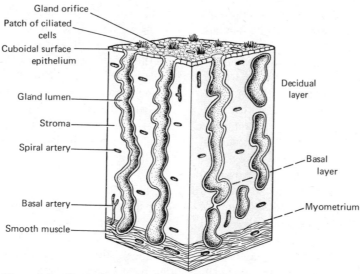

Figure 2.5   Block diagram showing the structure of the endometrium at
the end of the proliferative phase

may penetrate into the myometrium. These glands are embedded in a thick lamina propria forming the endometrial stroma (figure 2.5).

The arteries supplying the uterus branch and extend within the outer layers of the myometrium as the arcuate arteries. These in turn give rise to the basal or radial arteries which penetrate the myometrium to supply the deeper *non-deciduous* part of the endometrium. Some of these continue as *spiral arteries* through the *deciduous* endometrium towards the lumen to supply venous blood lakes in the outer part of the endometrium, and the lakes are drained by venous sinuses running down into the myometrium. At menstruation the arteries break at the junctions between the basal and spiral arteries when the deciduous endometrium is shed.

At the lower pole of the uterus a surface constriction marks the *internal os*, the junction between the body of the uterus and the cervix. The cervix is a cylindrical structure which projects through the anterior wall of the vagina at an oblique angle and opens at the *external os*, which is circular in nulliparous women but becomes a transverse slit after childbirth. The cervical canal is lined with thick folded mucosa bearing simple columnar epithelium forming numerous mucous glands, the secretions of which keep the vagina

moist. The surface of the cervix projecting into the vagina is covered with typical vaginal epithelium and the boundary between it and the cervical mucosa lies just inside the external os.

The weight of the pregnant uterus and the violence of the forces involved in parturition make firm support of the uterus and cervix essential if prolapse and other injuries are to be avoided.

The uterus itself is attached to the sheet-like *broad ligaments* and the cord-like *round ligaments*; both are fairly slack and non-supportive in the non-pregnant state but in late pregnancy restrain the uterus from retroversion and twisting. However, they can do little to prevent prolapse through the pelvic floor. The uterine weight is mainly supported from below by tone in the levator ani muscle and by three pairs of thickenings of the pelvic fascia: the *pubocervical, lateral cervical* and *sacrocervical ligaments*. These anchor the cervix very firmly to the pelvis so that it cannot be forced down into the perineum but instead forms a fixed ring through which the fetus can be expelled.

The vagina

The vagina (figure 2.1) is 7—9 cm long and is longer on the posterior wall than the anterior as a result of the oblique entry of the cervix; it runs upwards and backwards from the *vestibule* to its junction with the cervix.

The external surface of the cervix is surrounded by the vaginal *fornices*, its angled entry resulting in the posterior fornix being deeper than the anterior. The vaginal wall is thin with a muscular coat comprising interlaced longitudinal and circular bundles of smooth muscle, and a sphincter of skeletal muscle surrounds the vaginal orifice at its point of entry into the vestibule. It is lined by stratified squamous non-keratinising epithelium folded into transverse rugae which are studded with conical papillae. The underlying lamina propria is vascular and contains many elastic fibres. Thus the structure of the vagina is well suited to its function as a distensible organ able to accept and stimulate the penis. In its resting state the anterior and posterior walls of the vagina collapse to oppose each other, and thus the lumen in cross-section forms an H shape. The walls of the upper and middle parts of the vagina are poorly innervated and have few sensory receptors, unlike the sensitive lower third.

The vulva

This is the collective term for the female external genitalia. The vagina opens into the vestibule formed by the cleft between two longitudinal folds, the *labia minora*. The lateral walls of the vestibule contain the *greater vestibular glands* (Bartholin's glands) which secrete lubricant mucus. This is expelled from ducts opening on to the medial surfaces of the labia minora. Numerous smaller glands also open into the vestibule. Mucus secretion from all of these glands is greatly increased during sexual arousal (see chapter 4). The labia minora fuse anteriorly to form a hood or prepuce to the *clitoris*, which is the female homologue of the penis. The clitoris has a diminutive glans and, like the vestibule, it is well supplied with sensory nerve endings; unlike the penis it does not contain the urethra, which opens between it and the vestibule. Spongy erectile tissue is present both in the clitoris and in the vestibular

bulbs which are paired masses lying on either side of the vaginal orifice.

The lateral boundaries of the vulva are formed by the *labia majora*. These are large longitudinal folds which run back from the mons pubis to form a commissure posterior to the vestibule. Their medial surfaces resemble the labia minora in that they are hairless and well supplied with sebaceous glands, whereas the lateral surfaces are pigmented and hairy.

2.3 Function in the female reproductive system

Although the most important cyclical changes during the menstrual cycle concern the ovaries and endometrium, other organs also show cyclical variations in activity as the result of changes in plasma levels of ovarian steroids.

The ovarian cycle

The ovarian cycle is divided into two parts. The pre-ovulatory phase in which the follicles develop is called the *follicular phase*. Following ovulation at approximately mid-cycle the ovary enters the *luteal phase*, distinguished by the presence of a functional corpus luteum. The first 4–6 days of the follicular phase coincide with menstruation.

There are over 2 million primordial follicles in the fetal ovary prior to birth, but by the beginning of reproductive life the number has declined to about 250 000. This is because more than 80 per cent of the follicles regress during early life to form *corpora atretica* in the stroma. Despite this, a woman is supplied with a more than adequate number of primordial follicles for her reproductive life, since she will only ovulate some 300–400 times. This number would be reduced further through pregnancies or the use of oral contraceptives.

The first histological sign of follicular maturation is the differentiation of the follicular epithelium to cuboidal *granulosa cells*. This occurs in a small number of primordial follicles in each ovary during the late luteal phase of the preceding

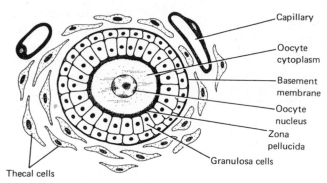

Figure 2.6 **Primary follicle**

cycle, and mitotic division in the epithelium produces a multilayered follicle. At the same time a refractile, basement membrane-like *zona pellucida* is laid down between the oocyte and the follicular epithelium. These changes are accompanied by conversion of the stromal cells surrounding the developing follicles to active endocrine cells. This sheath of cells is called the *theca*, and it subsequently differentiates into an outer layer of poorly vascularised tissue, the *theca externa*, and a well-vascularised inner layer, the *theca interna*. The whole of this spherical mass of cells constitutes a *primary follicle* (figure 2.6).

When the diameter of the follicles reaches about 200 µm, irregular fluid-filled spaces appear among the granulosa cells. Further enlargement causes these spaces to coalesce to form a single cup-shaped cavity, the *antrum*, which incompletely surrounds the oocyte and its attached *cumulus* of

follicular cells, giving the *secondary follicle*. From this point onwards the main change is simply an increase in follicular diameter up to about 1 cm, reached just before ovulation (figure 2.7).

The developing follicles and the corpus luteum formed after ovulation are the sites of synthesis of the principal ovarian steroid hormones, oestradiol and progesterone. These are the active forms of the hormones in the body but in practice are often measured indirectly in urine in terms of the excretory products produced by metabolism outside the ovaries. These metabolites are oestriol and oestrone, which are often measured together with oestradiol to give total urinary oestrogen, and pregnanediol, the excretory product of progesterone. Figure 2.8 shows typical urinary levels of these substances during the menstrual cycle.

There is some controversy concerning the steroid-secreting ability of the various cellular

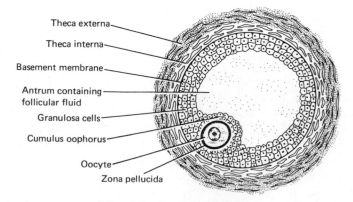

Figure 2.7 **Secondary follicle**

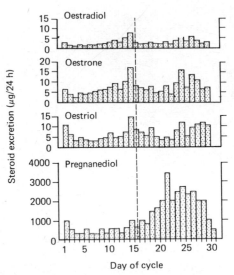

Figure 2.8   Urinary levels of pregnanediol and the three oestrogens during the menstrual cycle (Modified from Catt, K. J. (1971). *An ABC of Endocrinology,* **Lancet Publications, London)**

components of the developing follicle. Certainly we know that the only route by which ovarian steroids can enter the blood is from the vascular theca interna. Experiments on horses suggest that in the first instance the granulosa cells elaborate progesterone which is then converted to the intermediate 17α-hydroxyprogesterone. This accumulates in high concentrations in the antral fluid and a limited amount escapes into the blood but has little hormonal activity. Plasma 17α-hydroxyprogesterone reaches a peak level just before ovulation and can therefore be used as an index of follicular maturation. Most of the 17α-hydroxyprogesterone produced by the granulosa cells is then metabolised by the theca interna cells to oestradiol which enters the blood as the active hormone. Small amounts of oestrone are also released by the ovary and so are low concentrations of androgens, principally androstenedione and dehydroepiandrosterone, which are produced by stromal cells. Steroids released into the blood stream bind reversibly to carrier proteins: oestradiol binds to the same carrier protein as testosterone (testosterone/oestradiol binding globulin), whereas progesterone shares the same carrier as cortisol, i.e. transcortin.

As development of the follicle continues, the oocyte, now surrounded by the zona pellucida and a *corona* of granulosa cells, becomes detached from the cumulus and floats free in the follicular fluid. By this time the entire follicle has migrated to the surface of the ovary and it begins to bulge out because the patch of surface epithelium and stroma overlying it becomes thin. At ovulation this thin spot ruptures and the oocyte with its surrounding cumulus is expelled into the peritoneal cavity with a gush of follicular fluid. Shortly before ovulation, the oocyte, which was arrested in the extended prophase of the first meiotic division (chapter 1), completes this division with the expulsion of a polar body. It thus becomes a secondary oocyte. Immediately after this the second meiotic division starts, only to be arrested in metaphase, and is not completed until fertilisation. The expelled secondary oocyte is now free to enter the uterine tube. In many mammals there is a periovarian sac which prevents the oocytes becoming lost in the peritoneal cavity, but this is absent in the human and indeed oocytes do occasionally lose their way between the ovary and uterine tube although they are generally efficiently retrieved. If they get lost, this is of clinical significance as it may lead to ectopic pregnancy (chapter 5).

After the loss of the oocyte and much of the follicular fluid, the follicle collapses with some bleeding into the lumen. The theca interna and granulosa cell layers differentiate into luteal cells to form the *corpus luteum* which sinks slightly into the stroma but still leaves a small bulge on the surface of the ovary. The ruptured area in the theca interna heals to reform a complete sphere and the luteal cell layers become vascularised (figure 2.9). The cells derived from the theca interna remain distinguishable from the granulosa cells by virtue of their smaller size but it is not known whether the two cell types retain separate functions. Morphologically both cell types look like steroid-secreting cells since they contain abundant smooth endoplasmic reticulum, mitochondria and lipid droplets. The distinction between theca interna and granulosa cells becomes blurred as the luteal tissue develops further and

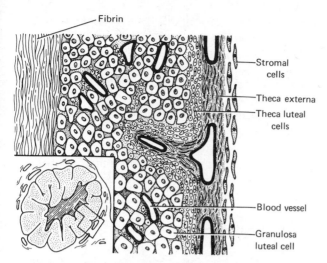

Figure 2.9 Section of corpus luteum depicting the smaller theca luteal cells and the larger granulosa luteal cells. The inset shows the relationship of this section to the whole corpus luteum which lies just below the surface of the ovary

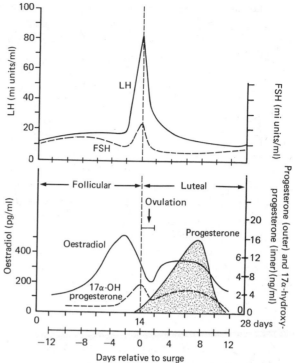

Figure 2.10 Plasma hormone levels during the ovarian cycle. Note that the cycle is divided into follicular and luteal phases on both histological and endocrine criteria (see also section 2.3 of the text)

the central blood clot is vascularised. The cells acquire the yellow pigment lutein, responsible for the characteristic colour of the corpus luteum, and they also secrete large amounts of both oestradiol and 17α-hydroxyprogesterone as well as of progesterone, all of which enter the blood from the vascular corpus luteum.

This produces the typical plasma profiles of the ovarian steroids seen during the ovarian cycle (figure 2.10). Oestradiol levels rise as the follicular phase proceeds and reach peak levels of 400–500 pg/ml plasma prior to ovulation. 17α-Hydroxyprogesterone concentrations also rise at ovulation to a peak of about 3 ng/ml plasma, then decline somewhat but show another rise during the luteal phase. During the follicular phase progesterone levels are extremely low. At ovulation the plasma levels of oestradiol and 17α-hydroxyprogesterone decline briefly until full corpus luteum function is established. Within 36 hours the corpus luteum starts to secrete large quantities of progesterone which reach maximal levels of about 15 ng/ml plasma during the luteal phase. As mentioned, oestradiol and 17α-hydroxyprogesterone are produced by the corpus luteum and the plasma levels

of these steroids rise again. It should be emphasised that the concentrations of progesterone and 17α-hydroxyprogesterone are much higher than those of oestradiol. The plasma levels of all the steroids decline when the corpus luteum begins to regress at the end of the menstrual cycle.

2.4   Control of the ovarian cycle

In the idealised ovarian cycle of 28 days, ovulation occurs at day 14. However, in reality the timing of ovulation as well as the length of the cycle itself often show a considerable variation, even from cycle to cycle in the same woman, and may vary some 2–3 days on either side of day 14. Generally speaking, the length of the follicular phase is more variable than that of the luteal phase and it is the duration of the former that determines the time of ovulation. This uncertainty about the precise timing of ovulation is one reason why the rhythm method of contraception is unreliable (see section 6.3).

The ovarian cycle is controlled by the secretion of the gonadotropins FSH and LH from the anterior pituitary gland. The pattern of gonadotropin secretion in the female differs greatly from that of the male, and is cyclic rather than tonic. The cycle of secretion is repeated every 28 days and thus determines the duration of the ovarian cycle and thereby the ovarian steroid-dependent endometrial cycle (see later). Just before ovulation there is a large surge of LH release superimposed on the cyclic secretion of gonadotropins. Thus gonadotropin secretion in the female is a dynamic phenomenon and the entire functional activity of the reproductive tract reflects this pattern.

The initial growth of the primary follicles appears to be independent of gonadotropin influence since the first stages of follicle development occur late in the preceding luteal phase when plasma gonadotropin levels are low. In addition, some development of primary follicles occurs before puberty and apparently also in hypophysectomised women. On the other hand, secondary follicular growth from antrum formation onwards is dependent upon both FSH and LH secretion from the pituitary. After regression of the corpus luteum, FSH and LH levels begin to rise on day 1 of the cycle, or possibly even earlier, and steadily increase towards the late follicular phase (figure 2.10). FSH levels, and possibly levels of LH, decline in the late follicular phase as a result of negative feedback inhibition by oestradiol on the adenohypophysis and hypothalamus (see section 2.7). During the follicular phase the plasma level of oestradiol increases as a result of continued secretion and accumulation of the steroid in plasma. This is due to an increase in the number of steroid-secreting cells formed as the follicles enlarge.

The induction of ovulation is dependent upon the mid-cycle surge of LH and FSH. If both gonadotropins are administered to a woman deficient in these hormones in amounts sufficient to produce typical follicular phase plasma hormone profiles, she shows normal follicle development

but does not ovulate. However, ovulation may usually be induced by injection of a large dose of LH after approximately 14 days. Although both FSH and LH are released by the pituitary in an episodic manner at mid-cycle, plasma levels of LH reach a higher peak. Indeed, this hormone appears to be the more important of the two since FSH injected alone does not induce ovulation.

The precise manner in which ovulation is induced by LH is not known but it may be caused by a sudden rise in intrafollicular pressure resulting from the swelling of the granulosa and theca interna cells during their differentiation into luteal cells. A sufficient rise in pressure might cause rupture of the follicle, now at the surface of the ovary. Follicle rupture may stimulate sensory nerve endings in the ovary, and this may be the reason for the painful abdominal sensation experienced by some women at ovulation. Ovulation usually follows after a delay of some 18 to 36 hours following the gonadotropin surge, rather than immediately as is often supposed.

It is interesting that although a number of primordial follicles in each ovary begin to develop during each cycle, generally only a single oocyte is released. The other follicles regress to form *corpora atretica*. Follicles which become atretic are probably those which do not become sufficiently differentiated to ovulate in response to the gonadotropin surge. Perhaps there is also some mechanism whereby one follicle takes the lead to suppress the further development of the others. Post-mortem evidence shows that one follicle is usually well in advance of the others when the late follicular phase is reached. If correct, this idea of inhibition implies the involvement of a systemic hormone so that regression of follicles in the contralateral ovary can be explained. Possibly the most advanced follicle ovulates, forming an active corpus luteum, so that the plasma levels of oestradiol and progesterone rise sufficiently to cause negative feedback inhibition on the pituitary and consequent fall in plasma levels of FSH and LH. Thus gonadotropin support of the less advanced follicles would be withdrawn so that they become atretic.

Atresia of follicles can occur at any stage of their development. If the follicle is small, as is always the case in the prepubertal ovary, the oocyte shrinks and degenerates first, followed by the follicular cells. If the follicle is close to maturity, the follicular cells usually show the first signs of degeneration. In either case the granulosa and cumulus cells become invaded by vascular connective tissue and granulosa cells are shed into the antrum. Eventually the follicle collapses and the antrum disappears. The basal lamella separating the follicular cells from the theca interna thickens, forming the *glassy membrane*, and the theca interna proliferates and its cells adopt a radial arrangement. Lipid droplets accumulate and the atretic follicle now somewhat resembles a late corpus luteum, from which it can be distinguished by the presence of the remains of the oocyte and zona pellucida. Finally the atretic follicle becomes completely invaded by vascular connective tissue which disrupts the theca interna, forming a small mass of scar tissue which gradually disappears.

If two follicles reach exactly the same stage of development simultaneously, a double ovulation may occur and dizygotic twinning is therefore a possibility. Note that double and multiple ovulations must occur more often than is suggested by the frequency of dizygotic twinning (1 birth in 138) because even if coitus occurs at the optimal time the chance of fertilising both oocytes is not 100 per cent. Furthermore, some oocytes are probably able to survive longer than others and thus one may remain viable after the other has died. The frequency of double or multiple ovulations increases with age. There are also racial differences: for example, the frequency of dizygotic twinning is greatest amongst negroes, intermediate in caucasians (the incidence quoted above) and least in mongolians. However, the incidence for monozygotic twinning is the same for all races and is 1 in 276 births.

The corpus luteum formed after ovulation has a life of approximately 14 days and then involutes to form a *corpus albicans*. In the degenerating corpus luteum the luteal cells become heavily loaded with lipid and begin to regress together with the connective tissue cells of the theca externa. The extracellular spaces become filled with hyaline material and the corpus albicans

organises as a fibrous scar which sinks into the stroma and gradually disappears. During involution luteal steroid production declines rapidly. Plasma levels of progesterone decline more rapidly because it has a much shorter half-life than oestradiol (30 minutes compared to about 2 days).

The maintenance of the corpus luteum depends in many species upon continued secretion of LH from the anterior pituitary gland, and until recently this was thought to be the case in the human. However, a normal corpus luteum forms in a hypophysectomised woman after ovulation has been induced as described above. Furthermore, exogenous LH administered to normal women does not significantly extend the life of the corpus luteum. Thus in the human the life of the corpus luteum appears to be largely self-determined.

In some species, regression of the corpus luteum is brought about by specific *luteolysins*. For example, there is good evidence in sheep and guinea-pigs that prostaglandin $F_{2\alpha}$ released from the uterus reaches the ovaries and causes luteolysis by suppressing progesterone synthesis. However, there is no evidence that uterine factors influence ovarian function in the human although the possibility remains that the ovary might produce its own locally acting luteolysin. There is no indication that prostaglandin $F_{2\alpha}$ causes luteolysis in the human, even though it is found in the uterus, but it may have roles in menstruation or parturition.

When the corpus luteum regresses, plasma levels of ovarian steroids fall, thus releasing the hypothalamo–pituitary axis from negative feedback inhibition. FSH and LH levels begin to rise and a new cycle is initiated.

2.5 The endometrial cycle

During the ovarian cycle the changing levels and balance of oestradiol and progesterone produce extensive alterations in the morphology of the endometrium and to a lesser extent of tissues elsewhere. The endometrial cycle may be divided into proliferative, secretory and menstrual phases: of these, the menstrual and proliferative phases coincide with the follicular phase of the ovarian

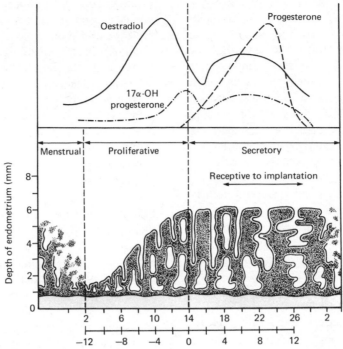

Figure 2.11 The endometrial cycle in relation to plasma levels of ovarian steroid hormones. The upper time scale shows the cycle dated from the first day of menstruation, and the lower scale is dated using ovulation as day 0

cycle and the secretory phase with the luteal (figures 2.10 and 2.11).

The proliferative phase

The proliferative phase begins immediately after menstruation has ceased, that is on about day 6 of the cycle. During this phase the rising oestradiol levels induce the outgrowth of endometrial epithelium from the surviving portions of the glands in the basal endometrium. The epithelial cells divide mitotically and migrate outward from the glands to cover the areas of bare stroma. The repair is complete within 2 days of the end of menstruation. There is rapid proliferation of cells in the epithelium and stroma so that the endometrium thickens and the glands lengthen. The overall depth of the endometrium increases from about 1 mm in the early proliferative phase to 5–6 mm by the time of ovulation. It is important

to realise that the endometrial epithelium itself remains one cell thick throughout the cycle. The increased thickness of the endometrium results from a combination of proliferation of the stromal cells, increased gland length and oedema of the stroma. As the endometrium regrows, its blood flow increases and the arteries begin to show a spiral form. The glands are initially long and straight with narrow lumina but later become more tortuous. The epithelial cells and the cells of the glands begin to synthesise glycogen; during the proliferative phase this is stored within the cells but is not secreted. The structure of the endometrium at the end of the proliferative phase is illustrated in figure 2.5.

The secretory phase

After ovulation the corpus luteum secretes large amounts of progesterone. This hormone acts synergistically with oestradiol on the oestrogen-primed endometrium to convert it to a secretory tissue. The endometrium becomes highly vascular with pronounced spiralling of the arteries and the formation of venous lakes. The stromal tissue becomes oedematous and the cells themselves also swell, causing the endometrial thickness to increase still further to 6–8 mm. The endometrial glands now become highly convoluted and begin to secrete glycogen into the uterine lumen. The surface of the endometrium at this stage becomes characteristically folded and is now fully prepared for implantation. Should fertilisation be achieved, implantation begins about 7 days after ovulation (day 21 of the cycle) and is completed by 14 days after ovulation. As long as progesterone and oestradiol levels remain high the endometrium can support implantation.

The menstrual phase

If fertilisation is not achieved the corpus luteum begins to degenerate towards the end of its 14-day life span and its steroid output falls. The ratio of plasma progesterone to oestradiol changes in favour of oestradiol because of the shorter half-life of progesterone mentioned earlier, and this change in the steroid ratio causes the endometrium to become unstable. It initially shrinks due to water loss and this tends to compress the spiral arteries and encourage endometrial anoxia. The increase in resistance of the spiral arteries reduces the perfusion pressure of the tissue which in turn reduces the oedema still further, thus potentiating shrinkage and anoxia. The basal arteries become intensely excitable, perhaps due to the dominance of oestradiol over progesterone. Thus tissue autolysis begins and the upper endometrium breaks down and separates from the deeper layers; there is no clearly marked shear zone but the upper two-thirds of the tissue sloughs away roughly at the junction of the basal and spiral arteries. As a result of tissue breakdown there is considerable bleeding into the stroma. The change in the steroid ratio also increases the excitability of the myometrium and this undergoes spontaneous contractions

which increase the anoxia and help to dislodge the dying decidual tissue. The anoxia also encourages the release of lysosomal enzymes which assist autolysis.

An important characteristic of menstrual blood is that it normally does not clot due to the presence in the endometrium of large quantities of plasmin which breaks down fibrin as it forms. In women who bleed heavily, clot formation may occur due to dilution of the plasmin. This is not harmful itself, but the excessive blood loss may be a cause for concern, particularly with regard to possible iron deficiency. Blood loss between 10 and 80 mℓ is usual, with a mean value of about 35 mℓ and implying a mean total menstrual iron loss of about 0.5 mg. Since the average daily absorption of iron from the gut is only just higher than the average daily loss, heavy menstruation can easily lead to iron deficiency.

After menstruation the endometrium is thin and poorly vascularised and only the bases of the endometrial glands remain. The menstrual phase ends when oestradiol levels start rising as a result of development of new primary follicles in the ovary. As mentioned before, the initial growth of the follicles is pituitary-independent and may simply begin at a fixed time after ovulation.

2.6 Non-endometrial sites of action of the ovarian steroids

The fluctuations in the plasma levels of the ovarian steroids during the menstrual cycle exert hormonal influences on tissues throughout the body.

The myometrium

The excitability of the myometrium is critically dependent upon the balance between progesterone and oestradiol; thus oestradiol tends to increase excitability of the smooth muscle, whereas progesterone reduces it. Both hormones have direct effects on the resting membrane potential. The myometrium usually shows least contractile activity during the lureal phase of the cycle when both steroids, particularly progesterone, are present in large amounts. At the end of the luteal phase, when progesterone levels fall rapidly leaving oestradiol unopposed, the myometrium is at its most active and spontaneous contractions occur. At this time the myometrium is also more responsive to oxytocin, whereas during the follicular phase it shows only moderate contractility and low sensitivity to oxytocin. Steroid-dependent changes in myometrial excitability are of significance in pregnancy and for the onset of parturition and will be discussed further in chapter 12. Contractile activity of the myometrium at the end of the menstrual cycle may lead to transient uterine ischaemia and pain before and during menstruation.

The cervix

The mucus secreted by the cervical glands during the follicular phase is watery and turbid but after ovulation large quantities of a thicker, clear mucus are produced. Mucus secreted at about the time of ovulation crystallises in a typical fern-like pattern if left to dry on a glass slide and this can be used as a crude index of ovulation.

The vagina

During the follicular phase the superficial layers of the vaginal epithelium consist of large flat cells with acidophilic cytoplasm. During the luteal phase these cells become polygonal with pyknotic nuclei and more basophilic cytoplasm. There is an increase in the glycogen content of the vagina resulting from the secretory activity of the endometrium and to a lesser extent of the vaginal epithelium itself. Lactobacilli present in the vagina metabolise the glycogen to lactic acid and this is largely responsible for the characteristic low pH of the vagina during this phase. The pH in the vaginal lumen is about 6.5 during the follicular phase but drops to about 4.5 during the luteal phase.

The uterine tubes

During the follicular phase there is an increase in the number of ciliated cells and in the frequency and coordination of the peristaltic contractions of the tubes. The contractions reach a maximum at about the time of ovulation. During the luteal and menstrual phases the tubes are relatively quiescent. The ciliary and peristaltic movements aid fertilisation (chapter 4).

Other actions of ovarian steroids

Oestradiol and progesterone also have important actions outside the genital tract. Oestradiol is largely responsible for the development and maintenance of the female secondary sexual characteristics, including the female pattern of subcutaneous fat, and axillary and pubic hair distribution. It is ideally suited to this role because it is always present in significant quantities throughout the cycle and unlike progesterone does not show very large fluctuations in plasma levels.

In the human, oestradiol and progesterone act synergistically to induce the secondary sexual characteristics at puberty, although oestradiol is without doubt the more important of the two (chapter 15). Oestradiol also maintains the female reproductive tract in the adult condition. However, the secondary sexual characteristics in the female seem to be less reversible than those in the male, so the drastic regression of these characteristics that occurs after male castration is not seen after ovariectomy or the menopause. However, ovariectomy as well as hypophysectomy abolishes all the cyclical changes in the female tract discussed above.

The ovarian steroids also exert an influence on the breasts. The development of adult mammary tissue is largely oestradiol-dependent and thus the rising plasma levels of this hormone in the follicular phase may cause a small degree of hyperplasia of the ducts and alveolar tissue. Progesterone acting synergistically with oestradiol during the luteal phase enhances the proliferation of alveolar tissue. Slight breast enlargement is often evident during the luteal phase and some women experience a degree of discomfort or tenderness which contributes to premenstrual tension.

Progesterone favours salt and water retention by interfering with the action of aldosterone in the kidney (see chapter 11). Thus urine production falls slightly during the luteal phase and rebounds to reach a maximum on the first day of menstruation. Progesterone also causes a small increase in basal body temperature but the mechanism is controversial. The temperature rise may be due to the metabolic effects of pregnanediol (the principal metabolite of progesterone), or result from interaction of progesterone with receptors in the hypothalamus, resetting the hypothalamic thermostat. The rise in basal body temperature coincides with and provides a marker for ovulation.

2.7 Hypothalamic and pituitary control of the menstrual cycle

The complex integrated sequence of events of the menstrual cycle is regulated by endocrine interactions between the hypothalamus, anterior pituitary gland and ovaries.

Control of the release of hormones from the adenohypophysis is achieved by means of *releasing hormones* synthesised in neurosecretory neurones of the hypothalamus and stored in their terminals in the median eminence. After secretion, these releasing hormones are transported in the hypophyseal portal blood to the anterior pituitary where they interact with specific receptors to cause release of pituitary hormones. Although it was widely expected that separate releasing hormones might control the release of FSH and LH, it has recently become clear that release of these two gonadotropins is in fact controlled by a single peptide hormone which is now designated as *gonadotropin releasing hormone* (GnRH). An identical decapeptide has been purified from huge numbers of hypothalami from both pig and sheep and minute amounts of this material, as well as the same decapeptide prepared synthetically, release both FSH and LH from pituitary explants and *in vivo*.

As might be expected, the actions of GnRH on the pituitary *in vivo* are complicated, not least because they are modified by effects of circulating ovarian steroids. The existence of a single GnRH might explain why the anterior pituitary releases a surge of both LH and FSH just before ovulation and why the gland appears to have difficulty in effecting a perfect differential release of the two hormones. The fluctuating ratios of FSH to LH released during the menstrual cycle might reflect a change in the responsiveness of FSH- and LH-producing adenohypophyseal cells to a single releasing hormone, with the change induced principally by alterations in the plasma levels of the ovarian steroids.

Oestradiol and progesterone modulate the release of gonadotropins by actions on both the hypothalamus and pituitary and this negative feedback is critical to the control of the menstrual cycle. It appears from experiments that oestradiol has a greater feedback potency than progesterone on a weight basis, and this is also true for the peripheral effects of these hormones. Increases in the plasma concentrations of oestradiol and progesterone increase the sensitivity of the adenohypophyseal cells to a given amount of the releasing hormone, but also exert negative feedback effects on the hypothalamus as well, thus reducing basal GnRH release. The net effect is the pattern of gonadotropin secretion shown in figure 2.10. The increase in pituitary response to GnRH can be shown by injecting given amounts of the hormone at different points in the follicular phase.

In contrast to these examples of negative feedback, there is evidence that the mid-cycle surge of LH and FSH release is triggered by positive feedback of steroids on the hypothalamus. It is thought that there are neurones in an anterior hypophysiotropic area of the hypothalamus bearing receptors for oestradiol which have a set threshold. When the rising oestradiol levels exceed this threshold the neurones are activated and stimulate neurosecretory neurones containing gonadotropin releasing hormone. This causes a rapid release of GnRH into the hypophyseal portal system, followed by a surge of LH and FSH release from the pituitary. Indeed, the gonadotropin surge can be produced experimentally in women by administering oestradiol just before the natural surge is expected. If this hypothesis is correct, the rate at which oestradiol levels build up in the plasma during the follicular phase and the set point of the threshold will together determine the time of ovulation and the length of the follicular phase. The feedback effects of the ovarian steroids on the hypothalamus and pituitary are summarised in a conceptual scheme shown in figure 2.12.

Therefore at the present time we have a general explanation of how gonadotropin secretion is

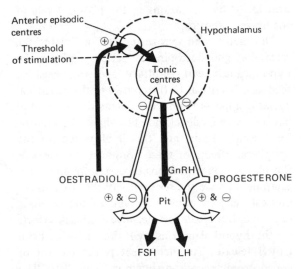

Figure 2.12 **Schematic diagram of the hypothalamus and anterior pituitary showing the feedback relationships of the ovarian steroids with gonadotropin releasing hormone. Both oestradiol and progesterone feed back on the pituitary to increase its sensitivity to GnRH. Rising oestradiol favours LH release in response to GnRH and rising progesterone may have the opposite effect but in the normal cycle the influence of oestradiol predominates. Thus the ratio of the two gonadotropins released in response to GnRH changes during the mestrual cycle, depending on the relative amounts of the two sex steroids in the plasma. Both oestradiol and progesterone also feed back on the tonic hypophysiotropic centres to reduce the amount of GnRH released, thus largely offsetting the increase in pituitary sensitivity to the releasing hormone that occurs during the follicular phase. In the anterior hypothalamus the episodic hypophysiotropic centres respond to levels of oestradiol above a certain threshold by inducing a surge of GnRH release which produces a much magnified surge of LH and FSH from the sensitised pituitary. Feedback sites are indicated by ringed + and− signs; positive feedback arrows are shaded and negative feedback arrows unshaded**

mediated and of how ovarian activity is controlled. However, there remains great difficulty in explaining the remarkable regularity of the menstrual cycle. There is good reason to suppose that there must be some form of hypothalamic clock which regulates the cycle and preserves its inherent rhythmicity. If so, the hypothalamic clock is probably driven by a complex interaction of structural, hormonal and environmental influences acting at the hypothalamic level, which might be susceptible to further influence from higher brain centres. For instance, it is well known that emotional upset can cause variations in the duration of the menstrual cycle and in some cases can impair fertility. Stress may prolong or suppress the menstrual cycle and therefore delay the anxiously awaited menstrual period by retarding ovulation through block of GnRH release and the gonadotropin surge.

In certain species, for example the cat and the rabbit, ovulation only occurs after coitus (*induced ovulation*). In these species hypothalamic neuronal mechanisms linked to and reflexly stimulated by sensory receptors in the genitalia induce the gonadotropin surge. It is generally believed that the human is a spontaneous ovulator, but there is some scanty evidence to suggest that the precise timing of ovulation can be affected by coital activity.

It should be stressed that although input drive and timing of ovulation in the menstrual cycle are mediated by the hypothalamus, the overall cyclical rhythmicity and sequencing of the cycle is the product of the whole hypothalamo—pituitary—ovarian axis, and that normal function is vitally dependent upon suitable dynamic interaction of the various components of the system in the correct manner and order.

The regularity of the menstrual cycle in the average woman of today is remarkable if one considers that regular menstruation throughout reproductive life is historically a relatively recent phenomenon. It is supposed that pregnancy was far more frequent amongst our ancestors, although there is little decisive evidence on this point.

In the female, sexual drive or *libido* is produced, as in the male, by the action of androgens on higher centres. However, in the female plasma levels of testosterone are very low and neither oestradiol nor progesterone have this action. Libido in the female may be stimulated by adrenal androgens, principally dehydroepiandrosterone and andros- tenedione, but if so the brain must be very sensitive to them as their plasma levels are low. Control of libido by the adrenal glands may explain why the female sex drive does not vary consistently with the other fluctuations of the menstrual cycle and also why adrenalectomy often reduces libido without affecting the cycle. However, the metabolic conversion of other steroids to form significant quantities of potent androgens cannot be ruled out, and nor can the direct synthesis of other androgens by the ovaries be totally excluded. For example, small amounts of androgens are synthesised by the ovary (see section 2.3) and some androstenedione is converted to testosterone by metabolism outside the ovary. This route is the major source of the small amounts of plasma testosterone found in the female, and a similar conversion may occur within the hypothalamus itself.

2.8 Hormonal treatment of female infertility

Most cases of female infertility not due to structural defects of the reproductive system are caused by the failure of the normal function of the hypo- thalamo—pituitary—ovarian axis. For example, the following three defects have been observed: absence of hypothalamic GnRH, insensitivity of anterior pituitary cells to GnRH, and absence of pituitary gonadotropins or defects in their release mechan- ism. Synthetic GnRH has been used successfully to release gonadotropins in infertile women because

it reaches the hypothalamus in sufficient amounts after injection. Purified gonadotropin preparations have been used for some time to treat infertility caused by pituitary failure; however, multiple ovulations and a painful and dangerous 'hyper- stimulation' of the ovary often occur. The syn- thetic anti-oestrogen clomiphene has also been widely used to treat infertility due to failure of the gonadotropin surge. It appears to act by occupying but not stimulating the negative feed- back oestrogen receptors, thus freeing the hypo- thalamus and pituitary from inhibition, thereby triggering GnRH release and the gonadotropin surge.

Further reading

Glenister, T. W., Hytten, F. E. and Kerr, M. G. (1976). 'Human reproduction', in *Companion to Medical Studies*, vol. 1, Blackwell, Oxford

Greep, R. O. (ed.) (1973). 'Female reproductive system', in *American Handbook of Physiology*, sec. 7, Endocrinology, vol. II, pts. 1 and 2, American Physiological Society, Washington

Greep, R. O. and Koblinsky, M. A. (eds.) (1977). *Frontiers in Reproduction and Fertility Control*, MIT Press, chaps. 1 'Gonadotropins', 6 'Endo- crinology of ovulation and corpus luteum formation', 7 'Induction of ovulation', 9 and 10 'Gonadotropin secretion and its control', 13 'The oviduct' and 14 'The uterus'

McCann, S. M. (1977). 'Luteinising hormone releasing hormone', *New England Journal of Medicine*, **296**, 797

Shearman, R. P. (1972). *Human Reproductive Physiology*, Blackwell, Oxford

Wilson, E. W. and Rennie, P. I. C. (1976). *The Menstrual Cycle*, Lloyd-Luke, London

3

The Male Reproductive System

3.1 Introduction

Reproductive function in the male differs from that of the female because fertility and reproductive activity are continuously maintained from puberty onwards. There are no cyclic variations in the plasma levels of pituitary gonadotropins or of testosterone secreted from the interstitial cells of the testis. The formation of male gametes, spermatogenesis, within the seminiferous tubules is also continuous and their maturation proceeds as they move through the different regions of the testis and epididymis.

3.2 Structure of the male reproductive tract

The gross structure of the male reproductive system is shown in figure 3.1.

The testis

The testes (figure 3.2) are paired ovoid structures of about 5 cm in length and 3 cm in diameter. They are enclosed by a thick, fibrous capsule, the *tunica albuginea*, and are surrounded by a serosal cavity except at the posterior margin where the tunica is thickened to form the mediastinum. Each testis is divided into 200–300 lobules by thin fibrous partitions which are continuous with the tunica and extend into the body of the testis.

Blood is supplied to each lobule by a branch of the testicular artery and drains via the pampiniform plexus into the testicular vein. The testes are well supplied by sensory and autonomic nerves.

Each testicular lobule contains up to four seminiferous tubules. These are highly convoluted loops, both ends of which drain into the mediastinum. The histology of these tubules was described in chapter 1. The interstitial tissue packed between the seminiferous tubules has an endocrine function and contains blood vessels and connective tissue elements. The endocrine cells lie in well-vascularised clusters and have features characteristic of steroid-secreting cells, such as abundant smooth endoplasmic reticulum and moderate numbers of mitochondria, but have relatively few cytoplasmic lipid droplets. Large crystalline structures, called the crystals of Reinke, may also sometimes be seen in the cytoplasm of the interstitial cells, but their significance is obscure.

The rete and epididymis

Spermatozoa develop in the seminiferous tubules (see chapter 1) and pass into a system of anastomosing channels in the mediastinum, known as the *rete*, in which mixing of the products of the individual lobules occurs. A dozen short *efferent ducts*, about 5 mm long, arise from the upper part of the mediastinum and lead to coiled ducts called the *vascular cones*. These are packed together to form the upper pole of the *epididymis* (figure 3.2), a

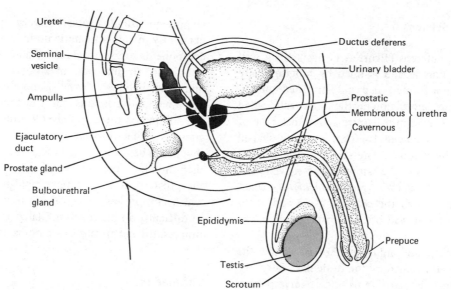

Figure 3.1   The male reproductive system showing midline and left side structures

mass of duct tissue running down the posterior aspect of each testis. The vascular cones join to form a single highly coiled epididymal duct in which maturation of the spermatozoa takes place. This epididymal duct forms the middle and lower parts of the epididymis. Macrophages are found in the epididymal lumen and are responsible for the phagocytosis of dead spermatozoa. Their activity is much increased when spermatozoa accumulate in the epididymis after vasectomy.

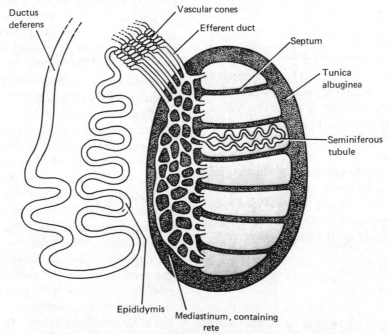

Figure 3.2   The testis and epididymis. For clarity, the numbers of small ducts and the length and tortuosity of the epididymis have been reduced

The ductus deferens

The ductus deferens (figure 3.1) has a thick wall of smooth muscle and is lined by longitudinally ridged mucosa formed of pseudostratified epithelium carrying large, non-motile microvilli called *stereocilia*. The terminal, intra-abdominal part of the ductus is enlarged to form a spindle-shaped structure, the *ampulla*. The seminal vesicles enter the ductus below the ampulla, after which it continues as the short, straight *ejaculatory duct*. This passes through the prostate gland and opens into the posterior wall of the prostatic part of the urethra.

In the extra-abdominal part of its course the ductus is accompanied by the testicular artery, the pampiniform plexus of veins and a nerve plexus. Also running with these is the *cremaster muscle*, composed of bundles of skeletal muscle fibres derived from the anterior abdominal wall. This bundle of structures is termed the *spermatic cord*. Contraction of the cremaster muscles, for example in response to erotic, tactile or thermal stimulation, shortens the cord thus raising the testes in the scrotum.

The seminal vesicles

The seminal vesicles (figure 3.1) are elongated sacs which arise from each ductus deferens between the ampulla and the ejaculatory duct. The wall of the seminal vesicle contains smooth muscle and is elaborately infolded into the body of the gland to divide the lumen into numerous small pockets. The epithelium lining the vesicles is pseudostratified low columnar. From puberty onwards the seminal vesicles secrete a thick viscous fluid and the height of the lining epithelium and the level of secretory activity are dependent on the circulating levels of testosterone.

The prostate gland

The prostate (figure 3.1) is a single spheroidal gland surrounding the initial or prostatic part of the urethra. It consists of 40 or more irregular compound tubuloalveolar glands opening independently into the prostatic urethra. The glandular components are surrounded by abundant connective tissue stroma rich in smooth muscle. The lining epithelium of the gland is cuboidal to columnar and contains many secretory granules. The lumina of the gland alveoli often contain oval granules called *prostatic concretions* which are thought to be formed from the prostatic secretions; their number increases with age. In elderly men the prostate often undergoes benign hypertrophy which compresses the prostatic urethra and leads to difficulty in micturition. Malignant transformation resulting in prostatic carcinoma can also occur.

The urethra

The male urethra (figure 3.3), unlike that of the female, is shared by both the urinary and reproductive tracts. In the male the urethra is much longer and more tortuous than in the female and this explains why ascending infections which reach the urinary bladder to cause cystitis are much less common in men than in women.

The urethra has three anatomically distinct segments: the *prostatic urethra*, the very short *membranous urethra* passing through the pelvic diaphragm, and the *cavernous urethra* which passes along the length of the corpus cavernosum urethrae to the tip of the penis. There are also three principal histological divisions of the urethra but these do not correspond exactly with the anatomical divisions. The prostatic urethra is lined by transitional epithelium which is continuous with that of the urinary bladder and contains the twin openings of the ejaculatory ducts and the multiple prostatic orifices. The membranous part of the urethra and most of the cavernous part are lined by pseudostratified columnar epithelium, whilst the *navicular fossa*, the expanded terminal part of the urethra within the glans penis, is lined with stratified squamous epithelium which gives way to the keratinising epithelium of the epidermis at the lips of the urethral meatus.

Numerous glands open into the urethra. The majority of these are small tubuloacinar mucus-

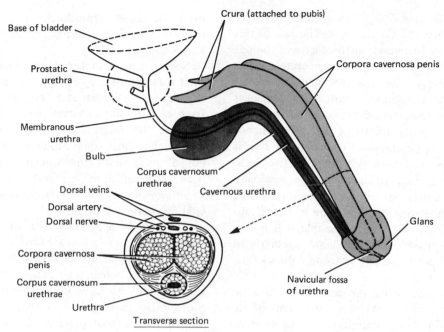

Figure 3.3   Structure of the penis. Skin, fascia, nerves and vessels are shown in the transverse section

secreting glands which empty into the dorsal part of the cavernous urethra. There is also a pair of small lobular *bulbourethral glands* which lie in the perineum and open via short ducts into the posterior part of the cavernous urethra. All these glands produce mucus which helps to lubricate the head of the penis during coitus. The secretion of the bulbourethral glands may also form a minor part of the ejaculate.

The penis

The main structural features of the penis (figure 3.3) are determined by its three masses of erectile tissue: the paired dorsal *corpora cavernosa penis*, and the single ventral *corpus cavernosum urethrae*. The navicular fossa passes through the terminal *glans penis*, which is formed by an expansion of the corpus cavernosum urethrae.

The corpora cavernosa form the erectile tissue of the penis and consist of a mass of connective tissue through which ramify many cleft-like vessels. When the spaces fill with blood, considerable

hydrostatic pressure is built up producing turgor and erection of the penis (chapter 4). The glans penis is very well supplied with sensory nerve endings and is the main erogenous zone in the male.

The glans penis in the resting state is covered by a folded cylinder of skin, the *prepuce* or foreskin, which normally retracts when erection takes place or intromission is attempted. This fully exposes the sensitive glans. The foreskin may commonly be removed by circumcision of the infant, either for religious or social reasons or because it is too tight.

The scrotum

The testes are carried outside the abdominal cavity in the scrotum (figure 3.1). This is a thin-walled sac covered with hairy, rugose skin well supplied with sebaceous glands. An incomplete layer of smooth muscle, the *dartos*, and connective tissue underlie the skin. The scrotal skin has a large surface area and is well vascularised, so that under most circumstances the temperature of the testes is maintained some 2–3°C below that of the body core. Although the functional significance of this is not fully understood, spermatogenesis cannot proceed normally at body temperature. The testicular artery and the pampiniform plexus function as a countercurrent heat exchanger reducing the temperature of the blood perfusing the testis. Sterility results if the testes do not descend during development or sometimes even if they become overheated by tight, restrictive clothing worn over long periods. In some seasonally breeding animals in which the inguinal canal remains fully patent, the testes are retracted into the abdominal cavity when the animal is not in the breeding season. This mechanism together with cessation of gonadotropin secretion halts spermatogenesis.

The temperature of the testes may also be regulated to a certain extent by the activity of the cremaster and dartos muscles which contract to pull the testes against the body for warmth or relax to allow them to hang pendulously. The testes are anchored to the lower border of the scrotum by a ligament called the *gubernaculum* (see chapter 9).

3.3   The origins and composition of the ejaculate

The fluid ejaculated at orgasm comprises spermatozoa suspended in seminal plasma.

After the formation of spermatozoa, a period of maturation must take place in the male reproductive tract before they are capable of fertilisation. This process consists of maturational changes in the sperms themselves as well as changes in the composition of the fluid in which they are suspended. The processes required for full sperm viability and motility are not in fact ever completed within the male and the final stages of activation, called *capacitation*, occur after the sperms are deposited in the vagina. Although spermatozoa may sometimes reach the oocyte within 15–30 minutes after coitus, fertilisation does not occur for at least 2–3 hours. Sperm are more likely to fertilise an oocyte *in vitro* if they are retrieved

from the female reproductive tract after coitus than if they are collected by masturbation or electroejaculation.

Spermatozoa comprise about 10 per cent of the total volume of the ejaculate. The seminal plasma is produced by the glands of the male reproductive tract, each forming a characteristic secretion which modifies the medium in which the sperm are bathed. The final composition of the ejaculate is not achieved until the moment of ejaculation itself, as described in chapter 4. The combination of different components of the ejaculate is probably vital for sperm activation.

It should be appreciated that the two cardinal aspects of sperm function are fertility and motility. Non-motile sperm are obviously not capable of fertilisation although their heads may be normal. Likewise motility alone is no criterion of fertility. Since these two aspects of sperm function are related to different parts of the spermatozoon, they can vary independently. Spermatozoa are motile in the female tract for between 48 and 60 hours but are only capable of fertilisation for some 24–48 hours. Their maximum rate of swimming by flagellate motion is about 8 mm/h.

The normal ejaculate volume ranges from 2 to 6 ml and contains about 100 million spermatozoa per millilitre; sperm counts of below 35 million per millilitre are invariably associated with impaired fertility. The precise volume of the ejaculate and its composition vary somewhat in the same individual and depend to a large extent on sexual activity patterns. It is normally a flocculent, viscous liquid with a colour varying from opalescent white to yellow; the yellowish tinge increases with sexual abstinence. The ejaculate has a characteristic bitter-sweet odour; this smell is largely due to the prostatic component of the seminal plasma, and may be altered in prostatic disease.

Following spermatogenesis and spermiogenesis, which take about 64 days in man, sperm pass through the rete into the epididymis. This movement results from fluid secretion in the seminiferous tubules, probably from the sustentacular cells. Spermatozoa removed from the tubules, rete or epididymis are non-motile and cannot be induced to fertilise an oocyte. The spermatozoa show an increasing capacity for motility as they pass through the epididymis, and after a period of 10–12 days they become potentially capable of fertilisation.

Later on, the sperm pass into the tail of the epididymis, the ductus and its ampulla where they are stored to await ejaculation. They are now capable of intense metabolic activity but paradoxically this limits their motility. This is because their oxidative metabolism produces a very high partial pressure of carbon dioxide in the lumina of these storage structures. The resulting acidity inhibits further metabolic activity; thus sperm withdrawn from these areas are fertile but immobile. The sperm may be stored in this dormant state without loss of viability for up to six months prior to ejaculation.

A complex process of sperm maturation takes place in the epididymis. Considerable concentration of the spermatozoa occurs in the epididymis, as plasma collected from the seminiferous tubules contains far fewer sperm per unit volume than in samples from the ductus or in the final ejaculate. As the sperm mature in the epididymis, their specific gravity increases due to dehydration, probably as a result of changes in the deoxyribonucleoprotein content of the head. There is rearrangement of chromatin and the number of disulphide bridges increases so that the DNA becomes less susceptible to thermal denaturation. The histone content of the nucleus also increases and the net result of these changes is that the chromatin becomes less hydrophilic.

During transit through the epididymis a bleb of cytoplasm, the *kinoplasmic droplet*, migrates along the midpiece of the sperm and is shed at its distal end. If this does not occur the spermatozoon remains infertile.

The composition of epididymal fluid is of some interest. The potassium concentration is very high compared with extracellular fluid and may equal or exceed that of sodium. Micropuncture studies show that the ratio of potassium to sodium rises as the fluid moves along the lumen of the epididymis. This may be caused by potassium secretion or by movement of water out of the tubule together with sodium during active transport. The resulting high potassium levels appear to suppress sperm motility.

Epididymal fluid also contains high concentrations of glycerylphosphorylcholine which may be hydrolysed by a diesterase to choline and glycerylphosphate (α-glycerophosphate). This is oxidised by the spermatozoa through the glycolytic pathways and the tricarboxylic acid cycle. The diesterase is also present in the uterine secretions of several species. Epididymal fluid contains small amounts of certain enzymes such as hyaluronidase and other carbohydrate-cleaving enzymes, but these are probably released from dead or disrupted spermatozoa rather than from the epididymis itself. For example, hyaluronidase is present in normal seminal plasma but is absent in azoospermic individuals lacking spermatozoa. It is unlikely that spermatozoa are themselves capable of enzyme synthesis; it is more probable that they acquire these enzymes during spermiogenesis in the sustentacular cells.

The ductus deferens contributes little to the fluid bathing the spermatozoa except in the ampulla which secretes small amounts of ergothionine and fructose. The major function of the ampulla is as a storage organ and it contains as many sperms as the ductus and the epididymal tail combined.

In spite of their name, the seminal vesicles of the human do not store spermatozoa but secrete a major component of the ejaculate. Their secretion is a viscous fluid and contains a globular sialomucoprotein, large amounts of fructose, ergothionine, prostaglandins, inositol, phosphorylcholine and amino acids. The most important ions are potassium and citrate.

The secretions of the prostate gland form about 30 per cent of the volume of the ejaculate. The prostatic secretion is alkaline and serves to neutralise the acid medium in which sperm are bathed in the ductus. It contains bicarbonate, citrate, magnesium, zinc, acid phosphatases and plasmin and is watery and opalescent. Sodium is the major cation and there is also much calcium and potassium. The citrate concentration is high but very variable.

At ejaculation the contents of the ducti, ampullae and seminal vesicles are combined with that of the prostate to produce the ejaculate or semen. The final composition of fresh ejaculate is given in table 3.1.

It is only when the sperm find themselves in this environment that they become intensely motile and show considerable metabolic activity. The primary factor initiating motility in the sperm appears to be the neutralisation of the contents of the ductus by the large volume of prostatic secretion. Fresh ejaculate has a pH of 7.5 although the optimum pH for sperm motility is 6.5, and at first sight it would thus appear that the acid contents of the ductus have been overneutralised. However, an optimum pH is reached when the semen is deposited in the vagina because vaginal fluid is acid.

Active sperm need a freely available energy source and this is provided by the fructose secreted from the seminal vesicles. Fructose concentrations in the seminal fluid decrease with age and this may contribute to the decline of fertility. Spermatozoa

metabolise fructose very actively by anaerobic glycolysis, but not by the pentose phosphate pathway. Oxidative phosphorylation appears to be limited and the oxygen consumption of sperm is always low. Since fructose utilisation does not vary with oxygen partial pressure it seems that the rate of glycolysis is already maximal, and pyruvate is produced faster than it can be removed by oxidative phosphorylation. Thus sperm fructolysis is characterised by a rapid conversion of fructose to lactate in the ejaculate.

Although metabolism of fructose is undoubtedly the major energy source for spermatozoa, oxidative phosphorylation in the mitochondria provides an additional source of ATP for the contractile proteins of the flagellum. After fructose depletion excess lactate formed from it, as well as that already present in the vagina, may be utilised by the sperm mitochondria. Glycogen in the uterus and vagina may also be utilised by the sperm. The partial pressure of oxygen in the uterine lumen is 24–45

Table 3.1   The major components of fresh ejaculate

General		Solutes	
Total volume:	3 ml (range 2–6)	Sodium:	100–135 mmol/l
pH:	7.5	Chloride:	28–57 mmol/l
		Potassium:	17–27 mmol/l
Spermatozoa:	100 million/ml	Calcium:	5–7 mmol/l
	Highly motile, 40–50%		
	Moderately motile, 20–30%		
	Non-motile, 30%		
	Morphologically abnormal, 40%	Total protein: 58 mg/ml	

Prostate-derived components	Seminal vesicle-derived components
Bicarbonate	Fructose
Citrate	Prostaglandins
Acid phosphatase	Phosphorylcholine
Plasmin	Ergothionine
Magnesium	Inositol
Zinc	Amino acids
Spermine	Sialomucoprotein*

* Also secreted by the bulbourethral glands.

mmHg which is sufficient to support aerobic metabolism.

The high concentrations of magnesium and zinc ions in prostatic fluid are also vital for sperm motility; sperm suspended in artificial media from which these ions are omitted soon become non-motile.

Immediately after ejaculation the semen coagulates due to reaction of the sialomucoprotein with other components of the ejaculate. In man the sialomucoprotein comes from the seminal vesicles but in many other animals it derives from the bulbourethral glands. The sperm can only move with great difficulty in coagulated semen, but after a few minutes it liquefies again due to the action of plasmin and citrate.

Seminal plasma contains large amounts of prostaglandins, especially of the E series, and human semen is one of the richest known sources of these substances. Although the role of prostaglandins in seminal plasma is still uncertain, it is possible that they may alter the motility of the female reproductive tract so as to facilitate the transport of spermatozoa into the uterine tubes.

Prostaglandins stimulate uterine smooth muscle contraction *in vivo* and *in vitro*.

3.4 Seminal analysis and male fertility

Most of the information about the composition of the ejaculate and the contributions from the different glands discussed above comes from seminal analysis by the *split ejaculation technique*. This method involves collection of at least six serial fractions of a single ejaculation and requires cooperative volunteers with a good deal of practice. The technique relies on the fact that the composition of the ejaculate varies with time because the different components do not enter the prostatic urethra simultaneously at emission. There is an orderly sequence of contractions, first of the capsule of the prostate followed by the ampullae and the ducti and finally the seminal vesicles, so that the contributions of the various parts of the male reproductive tract can therefore be assessed. A typical result of a series of seminal analyses is shown in figure 3.4.

One important feature illustrated by this figure

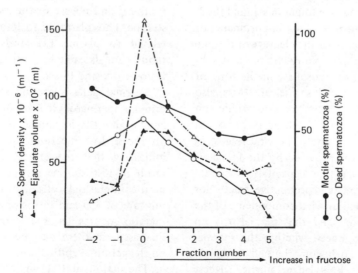

Figure 3.4 Analysis of ejaculates split into eight fractions showing variations in volume, sperm count and proportions of motile and non-motile spermatozoa (Redrawn from Eliasson, R. *et al.* (1974). *Male Fertility and Sterility* (Eds. Mancini, R. E. and Martini, L.), Academic Press, London)

is the very large number of non-motile sperm found mainly in the early fractions of the ejaculate. These spermatozoa have probably been in the reproductive tract for some time and have become senescent. The non-motile sperm and those which are morphologically abnormal amount to about 60 per cent of ejaculated spermatozoa in the normal individual (table 3.1), and all of them would probably be incapable of fertilising an egg. This very high proportion of infertile spermatozoa is characteristic of apes and man and on this basis puts them among the most infertile mammals known. If the average man were a stud dairy bull he would have been 'retired' long before his seminal analysis reached this state of degeneracy.

Men that are judged infertile on the grounds that they appear to be incapable of fathering a child show either a much reduced sperm count (*oligospermia*) or even higher proportions of non-motile or morphologically abnormal spermatozoa in the ejaculate. The lower the absolute sperm count the more crucial to a man's fertility becomes the proportion of viable sperm.

Other substances which influence male fertility by altering motility of spermatozoa or by affecting their ability to fertilise the egg or to promote early embryonic development are found in seminal fluid, but it is often hard to assess their importance. For example, the significance of the cleavage of choline and phosphate from phosphorylcholine and subsequent precipitation of phosphate in the form of spermine phosphate remains unclear. It is also difficult to extrapolate from *in vitro* studies on seminal fluid to the events which occur *in vivo* in the female reproductive tract. The vital role of as yet unidentified factors provided by the female is indicated by the fact that capacitation is only completed in the female reproductive tract. Nor is it known how much or what components of the seminal plasma accompany the spermatozoa up the female tract, or indeed whether the spermatozoa soon escape and become bathed in female secretions. Further knowledge might suggest treatments for certain types of infertility resulting from poor sperm viability and also permit development of new male-orientated contraceptive measures.

3.5 The hormonal control of male reproductive function

Gonadal function in the male is controlled by the plasma levels of the gonadotropins LH and FSH. In the male the secretion of gonadotropins is tonic rather than cyclic and there is no evidence of any circadian or other regular fluctuation in plasma levels. However, small fluctuations may occur as these hormones are released from the anterior pituitary gland in a pulsatile manner.

In the male the plasma levels of LH are usually about three times higher than those of FSH. Typical values in the male would be: LH, 13 milli-International Units (miu); FSH, 4 miu per millilitre of plasma.

LH and FSH are released from the anterior pituitary by a single gonadotropin releasing hormone as in the female. The ratio of the two gonadotropins is determined by the pituitary response to the releasing hormone.

3.6 Actions of the gonadotropins

LH acts on the interstitial tissue to promote the synthesis and release of the male sex steroid testosterone. Thus plasma testosterone levels are directly related to plasma LH levels. The seminiferous tubules are also able to synthesise and release some testosterone and this activity is also LH-dependent.

Spermatogenesis can be supported up to the primary spermatocyte stage in hypophysectomised animals by LH injections. Similar effects can be produced by injections of testosterone alone, indicating that the effects are produced as the result of testosterone synthesis stimulated by LH in the interstitial cells. However, with LH or a mixture of LH and testosterone the frequency of meiotic figures in the germinal epithelium is increased, so there may be a direct action of LH on the germinal epithelium.

The action of FSH in the seminiferous tubule seems to be principally on the later stages of spermatogenesis and on spermiogenesis. FSH acts on the sustentacular cells to maintain their morphology and thus their supportive role in sperm maturation. On its own, FSH is unable to initiate or maintain spermatogenesis; it has no action on the prepubertal testis unless the germinal epithelium has been primed with an androgen. The actions of both FSH and LH are very probably mediated through a cyclic AMP-sensitive mechanism and both gonadotropins raise cyclic AMP levels in testicular tissue.

Prolactin may also have a role in gonadal function by exerting a tropic effect on the sustentacular cells. Prolactin receptors have been identified in the testis. High plasma prolactin levels in men are often associated with poor gonadal function and loss of fertility and libido even when gonadotropin levels are normal. High concentrations of prolactin probably antagonise the actions of the gonadotropins at the gonads. In many experimental hypophysectomised animals prolactin as well as LH and FSH must be injected to restore spermatogenesis to its former level.

3.7   The control of gonadotropin secretion

Figure 3.5 shows that injection of a large dose of testosterone in man inhibits LH secretion by a negative feedback effect on the pituitary but has no effect on FSH secretion. This illustrates that feedback control of LH and FSH secretion in the male differ. Testosterone feeds back to the hypothalamus and pituitary in a classical negative feedback manner thus maintaining plasma LH and testosterone levels relatively constant. Plasma levels of FSH are regulated by a different mechanism. They correlate closely with the rate of spermatogenesis assessed histologically. For example, in Klinefelter's syndrome in which the seminiferous tubules are rudimentary and there is no germinal epithelium, the plasma levels of FSH are very high whilst LH levels may be normal or only slightly elevated. This is also the case in individuals with azoospermia or oligospermia where the defect lies in the germinal epithelium and not in the ability of the pituitary to produce gonadotropin.

It is not known how information regarding the rate of spermatogenesis is communicated to the hypothalamus and pituitary, but obviously a

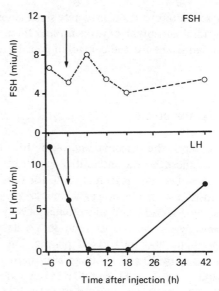

Figure 3.5   Suppression in the male of LH secretion but not FSH secretion by a single intramuscular injection of 50 mg of testosterone propionate at the time indicated by the arrow (Redrawn from Franchimont, P. (1970). *Reproductive Endocrinology* **(Ed. Irvine, W. J.), E. and S. Livingstone, Edinburgh)**

mechanism maintaining the sperm count relatively constant in the face of a varying frequency of ejaculation is advantageous to the species. A polypeptide called *inhibin*, extracted from bull testis, depresses FSH release but does not affect LH secretion significantly. Inhibin may regulate FSH secretion physiologically, and it is thought that it is secreted by the sustentacular cells or by some other component of the germinal epithelium of the seminiferous tubules. However, inhibin has not been demonstrated in some mammals studied.

The control of gonadotropin secretion in the male can be summarised as follows. There is a single gonadotropin releasing hormone which releases both LH and FSH from the pituitary. Feedback control of gonadotropin secretion is principally at the level of the pituitary, and testosterone and inhibin respectively reduce the amounts of LH and FSH released in response to gonadotropin releasing hormone. Inhibin and testosterone may both feed back at the hypothalamic level, as do oestradiol and progesterone in the female, so as to reduce the synthesis and release of gonadotropin releasing hormone.

The seminiferous tubules secrete small amounts of oestradiol and other oestrogens, and these may also be significant for the control of gonadotropin secretion.

3.8   Testosterone

Testosterone is the principal androgen of the male and is produced by the interstitial cells at the rate of 6–7 mg/day. The principal route for synthesis of testosterone from pregnenelone is via 17α-hydroxyprogesterone and androstenedione.

Plasma levels of testosterone in fertile men average about 500 ng/100 ml plasma, but vary between about 200 and 2000 ng. Testosterone has a half-life of between 60 and 80 minutes and most is carried in plasma in association with the testosterone–oestrogen binding globulin. Like the adrenal, the testis also releases small amounts of the androgens androstenedione and dehydroepiandrosterone. Conversely the adrenal secretes a little testosterone. Small concentrations of circulating oestrogens, namely oestradiol and oestrone, are also found in the male. Some is secreted directly by the gonad but the rest is produced by testosterone metabolism in adipose and other peripheral tissues.

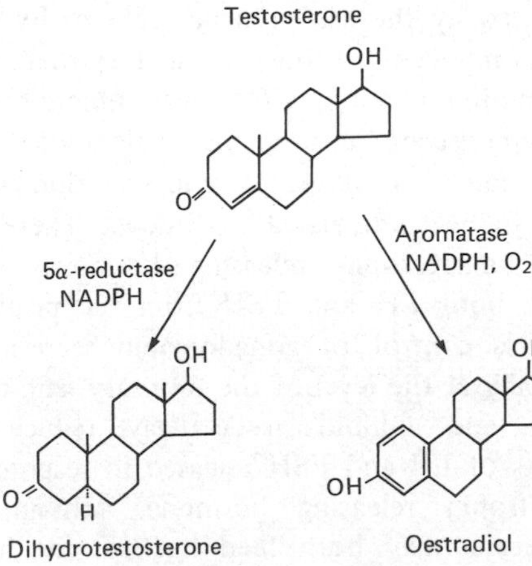

Figure 3.6 **Two important routes of testosterone metabolism in the testis and peripheral tissues**

The two principal metabolites of testosterone are dihydrotestosterone and oestradiol (figure 3.6). Most of the circulating dihydrotestosterone and half of the oestradiol originate from testosterone, but of these dihydrotestosterone occurs in plasma in much higher quantities, at about one-tenth of circulating testosterone levels. This is of importance as testosterone must be converted to dihydrotestosterone in order to act on target tissues. In the testicular feminisation syndrome, genetic males with normal testosterone secretion fail to develop male secondary sexual characteristics because this conversion of testosterone to dihydrotestosterone cannot be made due to a lack of the necessary enzyme. The fact that their secondary sexual characteristics are principally female is due to the unopposed action of circulating oestrogens. At the cellular level, all of the changes in the male at puberty are the result of the action of dihydrotestosterone. However, for the sake of simplicity the actions of testosterone will be discussed as if they were direct.

Testosterone causes enlargement of the male accessory organs and stimulates their secretory activity. The penis and scrotum enlarge and folds appear in the scrotal skin. Testosterone causes development of hair on the face, chest and abdomen. However, the observed variation in male hairiness is not related to the amount of testosterone secretion but is due to genetically determined differences in the sensitivity to testosterone of the target hair follicles. Any genetic predisposition to baldness is also unmasked by the presence of circulating testosterone.

Testosterone is a powerful anabolic hormone which promotes protein synthesis and growth. This largely accounts for the greater body mass of the male, principally due to muscle. Testosterone also promotes the fusion of the epiphyses of the long bones, and this ultimately halts growth in stature. Finally it acts centrally to produce libido or sexual drive.

The significance of the peripheral conversion of testosterone to oestrogens is not understood, but the conversion to oestradiol is of considerable importance for feedback control of the pituitary and hypothalamus, both of which can aromatise testosterone to oestradiol. It is in this form that testosterone is thought to exert its negative feedback action. By contrast dihydrotestosterone cannot be aromatised to oestradiol and has no effect on gonadotropin secretion.

Further reading

Glenister, T. W., Hytten, F. E. and Kerr, M. G. (1976). 'Human reproduction', in *Companion to Medical Studies*, vol. 1, Blackwell, Oxford

Greep, R. O. and Koblinsky, M. A. (eds.) (1977). *Frontiers in Reproduction and Fertility Control* MIT Press, chaps. 26 'The control of testicular function', 29 'Leydig cells', 32 'The metabolism of mammalian spermatozoa', 34 'The epididymis', 35 'Semen', and 37 'Sperm motility'

Hamilton, D. W. and Greep, R. O. (eds.) (1975). 'Male reproductive system', in *American Handbook of Physiology*, sect. 7, Endocrinology, vol. V, American Physiological Society, Washington

Setchell, B. P. (1978). *The Mammalian Testis*, Elek, London

Shearman, R. P. (1972). *Human Reproductive Physiology*, Blackwell, Oxford

4

Coitus and Fertilisation

4.1 The role of coitus

It is unrealistic to discuss reproductive phenomena in man as if the desire to perpetuate the species were the sole motivation for coitus. The human being differs from most mammals in that sexual intercourse not only satisfies a basic drive but also produces pleasure and gratification of a character and intensity unequalled by any other activity. Although many other mammals show signs of extreme sexual excitement before coitus, the observer does not often obtain the impression that coitus itself is a particularly momentous or enjoyable event for the participants. Neither is there much evidence that the strength of pair bonding in animals is related to the quality of their sexual experience.

Several observations justify this distinction between human and animal sexuality. For example, man shows a high coital frequency at all seasons of the year and has devoted enormous energy and much ingenuity to devising ways of enjoying copulation without breeding children. Much of his leisure time is spent in pursuit or appreciation of sexual matters. In addition, it has been suggested that the stability of marriage is better correlated with the frequency of sexual intercourse than with any other single measurable variable. One idea is that the enduring pair bonding in humans may have been necessary to maintain the integrity of the child-rearing partnership of mother and father in primitive hunter-gatherer societies in which the parents were separated for long periods.

Pair bonding is particularly important for man in view of the extended period of parental dependence required by the offspring. Whatever the explanation for the great importance of coitus to human beings, it is true to say that our interest in it has moulded many of our social institutions and customs.

4.2 Male sexual arousal and coitus

Arousal in both sexes can be narrowly defined as a series of physiological responses which prepare the body for coitus. At its simplest, sexual arousal is a spinal reflex activity and can occur even in the presence of spinal cord transection above the lumbar region. Such purely reflex arousal may be produced by stimulation of the skin in and around the genital regions, and in the male this may culminate in ejaculation. However, arousal can also be triggered by inputs from the special sense organs via inhibitory and facilitatory pathways from the higher centres. For example, visual and olfactory stimulation and anticipation or imagination of sexual activity may all cause sexual excitement and arousal. Similarly arousal can often be inhibited or suppressed by changes of mood or in certain social contexts.

The most conspicuous feature of sexual arousal in the male is erection of the penis. Erection is initiated by increased cholinergic activity in the parasympathetic fibres reaching the penis through the pudendal nerves. This causes vasodilatation of the central artery of the penis, increasing the pressure in this blood vessel and causing engorgement of the corpora cavernosa. This in turn compresses the penile veins, thus restricting blood outflow, and leads to further engorgement of the erectile tissue. It is perhaps assisted by compression of the veins as a result of contraction of the skeletal muscles of the perineum. Erection is maintained as long as vasodilatation and venous compression persist. The cremaster muscles contract so as to pull the testes closer to the perineum, and this is assisted by contraction of the dartos muscle which reduces the size of the scrotum by corrugating its skin. The bulbourethral and other urethral glands produce a mucoid secretion which is released on to the glans and assists in both retraction of the prepuce and initial penetration into the vagina. These genital changes are accompanied by nipple erection, flushing of the face and trunk due to cutaneous vasodilatation, and increased systemic blood pressure, heart rate and respiratory rate.

After the penis is inserted into the vagina, mechanical stimulation of the glans by to-and-fro movement against the vaginal walls maintains and heightens arousal and finally triggers *emission*. This is achieved by contraction of the smooth muscle of the ducti deferentes, prostate and seminal vesicles, and the products of all of these organs are expelled into the urethra. The resulting urethral dilation stimulates *ejaculation*, which is produced by rhythmic contractions of the perineal skeletal muscles, especially the bulbocavernosus. These contractions occur at intervals of about 0.8 s, and the first five or six expel the bulk of the urethral contents. During ejaculation other generalised responses occur: skeletal muscle tone increases during arousal, and at ejaculation this reaches a peak and may result in involuntary contractions in many parts of the body, followed by a period of reduced tone and relaxation. Transient sweating usually occurs over most of the body surface. The events described above are accompanied by intense sensations referred to as orgasm; the nature of these is highly subjective and varies greatly from one occasion to another.

Emission, ejaculation and orgasm are followed by a phase of reversal of arousal known as detumescence. Muscle tone decreases, cardiovascular and respiratory activity falls, penile vasodilatation ceases and erection is lost; there usually follows a refractory period during which the male cannot again be sexually aroused. Sometimes, more especially in young men, erection may be maintained and the sequence recommenced without a refractory period. The relationship between neural activity and the events described is shown in figure 4.1.

The sequence of events in the female preceding and during coitus is in many respects similar to that in the male, apart from the absence of emission and ejaculation. Parasympathetic stimulation through the pudendal nerves produces erection of the clitoris and vestibular bulbs by a mechanism similar to that described for the male. The clitoris becomes erect and moves away from the vaginal introitus, so that although it is the principal erogenous structure it is not readily stimulated by direct contact with the penis. Rather it is stimulated by pressure of the male pubis on the mons veneris, but this bony contact is sometimes inadequate or uncomfortable and other means of stimulation of the clitoris may be used. Bulbar erection forms the so-called orgasmic platform around the vaginal orifice, the penis being gripped most firmly at this region. This part of the vagina is well supplied with sensory nerves, which are relatively sparse in the middle and upper parts.

Most of the vulval and vaginal lubrication facilitating intromission and coitus is provided by the female. The vulva are locally lubricated by secretion from the bulbourethral glands, while both vagina and vulva are lubricated by cervical mucus and by a serous transudate produced by the very well-vascularised vaginal mucosa. At maximal arousal during coitus the upper vagina becomes elongated and dilated, perhaps due to reduced intra-abdominal pressure.

Nipple erection occurs early in female arousal, but later it is somewhat obscured by vascular engorgement of the areolae and general breast enlargement. Flushing of the skin occurs in the same areas as in the male. Orgasm in women occurs after a period of full sexual arousal and stimula-

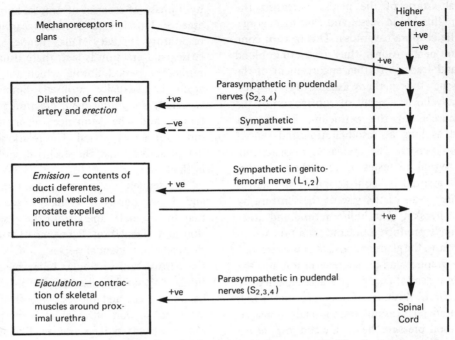

Figure 4.1   Nervous mechanisms in the male sexual response. Positive (+ve) and negative (−ve) effects are indicated

tion. It closely resembles male orgasm in that there are contractions of the perineal muscles at intervals of about 0.8 s, together with more generalised skeletal muscle contractions as well as localised and general sensory excitation. However, female orgasm differs in two respects apart from the absence of ejaculation. First, there is no female equivalent of the male refractory period, and thus in principle several orgasms separated by fairly brief plateaux of arousal can occur, although this is not very common. Secondly, achievement of orgasm has an important learned component and may become progressively easier after a successful experience. Sometimes this learning process does not occur because female arousal generally follows a slower time course than that of the male, and so a woman may not achieve orgasm by the time the male ejaculates. Another difference between the sexes is that women can be passive partners in coitus even if not aroused, whereas a man cannot achieve intromission without sufficient arousal. However, if erection and intromission are achieved male orgasm usually follows. From an evolutionary

point of view female orgasm is not necessary for fertilisation, so the selection pressure for its attainment at every coital event must be small.

Detumescence in the female follows a similar course to the male, with loss of erection, muscular relaxation and return to normal of blood pressure and respiration. Nipple erection is most conspicuous in early detumescence as the areolar engorgement subsides before loss of nipple erection itself.

The pattern of neural control of arousal and orgasm is similar to that in the male, and can be inferred from figure 4.1.

4.3 Gamete transport

It is believed that the motility of spermatozoa probably plays little part in their transport up the female genital tract because dead sperm and other inert particles are transported as fast as living ones. The main propulsive force is provided by contraction of the muscle of the uterus and uterine tubes which may be stimulated by prostaglandins present in the seminal plasma and by circulating oxytocin released from the pituitary during coitus. Sperm released into the vagina will only remain there for any length of time if the woman remains lying down after coitus so that the superior end of the vagina is lowest. During detumescence the extension and dilation of the superior end of the vagina is reversed so that the cervix may dip into the pool of seminal fluid. This provides a good chance for bulk quantities of spermatozoa to be transported through the cervical canal towards the upper parts of the reproductive tract. Sperms are propelled through the slit-like uterine lumen into the uterine tubes and accumulate in the isthmus of the tubes, being slowly released into the ampullae where fertilisation usually takes place.

Although oocytes are released into the peritoneal cavity they are retrieved with surprising efficiency by the fimbriae on the mouths of the uterine tubes. This is accomplished even if only one tube and the contralateral ovary are present.

Upward sperm movement and downward egg movement must both take place within the ampullae. This apparently contradictory manoeuvre is probably achieved by ciliary transport, and discrete areas of tubal epithelium carrying cilia beating in either upward or downward directions have been identified. There is presumably a selection mechanism to ensure that each type of gamete makes contact with cilia beating in the correct direction. The tubal cilia are hormone-dependent, growth being stimulated by oestrogens and activity by progesterone. Thus the cilia are at their most active during the early luteal phase when the oocyte is released.

4.4   Gamete preparation and capacitation

The freshly ovulated egg is arrested in metaphase of the second meiotic division; it is surrounded by the non-cellular zona pellucida, outside which are the adherent follicular cells from the cumulus, the *corona radiata.*

Although the spermatozoa have undergone 'maturation' in the epididymis, they are still far from competent to fertilise the egg. Transport of

sperms up the female reproductive tract may take up to 5 hours in man, during which time the spermatozoa undergo *capacitation.* Studies on rabbits show that capacitation consists of two main steps: first the sperm is stripped of adherent epididymal and seminal plasma proteins, after which its own surface glycoproteins are modified by attack by carbohydrate-splitting enzymes. The hydrolytic step reduces the number of negatively charged groups on the plasma membrane of the sperm head, perhaps in readiness for the acrosome reaction described below. Although capacitation is of vital functional importance, only small ultrastructural changes of the spermatozoon are discernible at this stage.

Capacitation can occur at several sites in the female reproductive tract, and in different species the uterus or uterine tubes or both may be effective. The precise site of capacitation in the human is not known. In the hamster the cells of the corona radiata seem to provide the most potent stimulus for capacitation, so in this species it occurs at the last possible moment before the commencement of fertilisation itself. Capacitated sperm may be decapacitated experimentally by treatment with seminal plasma glycoproteins, or may be inhibited by membrane stabilising agents such as steroid sulphates.

4.5   The acrosome reaction

A series of changes in the plasma membrane and acrosomal membrane of the spermatozoon is initiated as it burrows actively between the cells of the corona radiata. The end result of this *acrosome reaction* is the release of acrosomal hyaluronidase. This enzyme aids sperm penetration through the extracellular material of the corona. In addition a portion of the acrosomal membrane is exposed at the sperm surface in preparation for penetration of the zona pellucida.

Fusion between the plasma membrane and the underlying outer acrosomal membrane takes place at many points within the sperm head, resulting in the progressive disintegration of both of these membranes into small vesicles and the intercalation

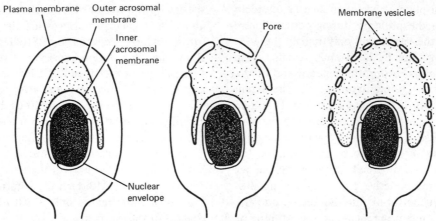

Figure 4.2   **The acrosome reaction. Three stages of focal fusion between the sperm head plasma membrane and the outer acrosomal membrane are shown. The resulting vesicles forming the acrosomal cap remain adherent to each other and to the spermatozoon until binding to the zona pellucida occurs**

of the inner acrosomal membrane into the plasma membrane of the sperm head (figure 4.2). The vesiculated areas of membrane remain attached to the sperm in the form of the *acrosomal cap* until contact is made with the zona pellucida, at which time separation of the cap takes place. An apparently normal acrosome reaction can be induced *in vitro* by treatment with serum proteins. Pyruvate and lactate are required for a normal acrosome reaction. The reaction is produced by the activation of a trypsin-like enzyme which is probably the acrosomal enzyme *acrosin* itself. If so, this must involve conversion of the proenzyme proacrosin to the active form. Calcium is essential for the acrosome reaction, probably because it is needed for membrane fusion. Calcium entry into the cell begins at capacitation and reaches a peak during the acrosome reaction; its influx is necessary to produce the altered sperm motility pattern needed for zona penetration.

4.6   Penetration of the zona pellucida

Spermatozoa which have penetrated the corona radiata and undergone the acrosome reaction bind strongly to the external surface of the zona pellucida. The strength of the binding reaction increases with time, and sperms or eggs which have already participated in binding show an accelerated binding reaction if tested a second time. Attachment takes place at the acrosomal cap region of the sperm, and is probably translated from a loose attachment to a firm binding by changes produced in the zona by acrosin activity. However, prior incubation of eggs in acrosin inhibits sperm binding. Neuraminidase, glucosidases and other carbohydrate-splitting enzymes do not affect the binding reaction which therefore probably depends on a polypeptide in the zona pellucida rather than on a glycoprotein or polysaccharide. These zonal polypeptides do not appear to be species-specific, since zona pellucida extracts from one species may be used experimentally to inhibit the binding of sperms to eggs in another species.

Acrosin is the most important factor concerned in the creation of a pathway for sperm through the zona pellucida. Inhibitors of acrosin and trypsin strongly inhibit fertilisation, and incubation of eggs in acrosin leads to dissolution of their zonae. Acrosin is not free within the acrosome, but is firmly bound to the inner acrosomal membrane. Since the presence of free acrosin could lead to destruction of zona binding sites, it is logical that the enzyme should be bound and that there are acrosin inhibitors in seminal plasma.

The path taken by the sperm through the zona pellucida is usually oblique and slightly curved

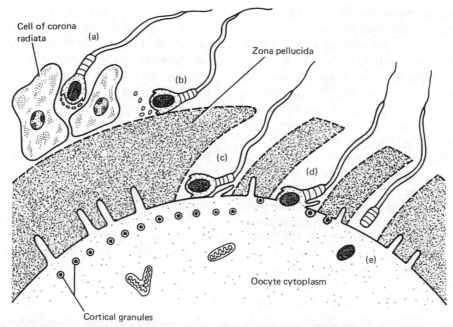

Figure 4.3 Fertilisation: (a) the acrosome reaction has occurred but the acrosomal cap remains during penetration of the corona; (b) binding to the zona pellucida and dissolution of the acrosomal cap; (c) penetration of the zona pellucida and adhesion to the oocyte plasma membrane; (d) membrane fusion between oocyte and sperm, and degranulation of cortical granules; (e) enclosure of sperm nucleus within oocyte and shedding of sperm tail

(figure 4.3); penetration of the weakened zona is assisted by the pattern of sperm swimming movements, which after capacitation and the acrosome reaction are oscillatory rather than progressive. Penetration of the zona pellucida in the hamster takes anything from a few minutes to nearly half an hour, and the corresponding time for man is probably of the same order.

4.7 Gamete fusion

Fusion of cells is a carefully controlled event in nature which only occurs under very special conditions, even between genetically identical cells of a single organism. Resistance to fusion between genetically different cells is strong and fusion of gametes is the only important natural example. Factors which normally oppose cell fusion include repulsion between the negatively charged groups on cell surfaces and incompatibility of the distribution of integral proteins in the two plasma membranes.

Gamete fusion is initiated by wrapping of egg surface microvilli round the sperm head; the slender, elongated shape of the microvilli allows contact to be achieved without very much mutual repulsion between the egg and sperm due to the negative charge on both surfaces. The plasma membrane of the egg shows high fluidity over most of its surface, thus reducing spatial interference between membrane macromolecules at fusion by allowing them to move in the plane of the membrane. The most fluid region of the sperm plasma membrane lies in the part of the head just behind the acrosome, and it is here that fusion with the oocyte usually occurs.

4.8 Polyspermy and its avoidance

Production of a diploid zygote requires the fusion of one egg and one sperm. Fusion of more than one sperm with the egg is called *polyspermy*, and in mammals does not often occur. There are two principal mechanisms which prevent polyspermy, one involving the plasma membrane of the egg and the other acting on the zona pellucida.

Fusion of a sperm with the egg evokes a rapid rise in the free calcium level in the cytoplasm; this is probably released from bound intracellular stores rather than admitted from outside. The rise in calcium concentration triggers the fusion with the plasma membrane of numerous membrane-bounded *cortical granules* in the egg cytoplasm. The granule contents are released by exocytosis.

The first mechanism blocking polyspermy is called the *vitelline reaction* and depends on the incorporation of cortical granule membranes into the plasma membrane which occurs during granule exocytosis. Studies with cell surface labels show that complete mixing of the two types of membranes occurs, resulting in changes in the cell's surface properties. An important change is that the charge on the cell surface becomes more negative because of the increase in density on the surface of glycoproteins rich in sialic acid. This increases the resistance to further membrane fusion. It is not only the cortical granule membranes that are incorporated into the egg surface; the plasma membrane of the sperm head suffers a similar fate during cell fusion. However, the membrane area involved is smaller and it is not clear to what extent this incorporated sperm membrane contributes to the vitelline reaction.

The second mechanism preventing polyspermy is due to the actions of substances formed within the cortical granules. They affect the zona pellucida so as to reduce both its sperm binding properties and the ease with which sperm can penetrate it. The most important of these components is heat-labile and is neutralised by trypsin inhibitors but has not yet been characterised. These properties are reminiscent of those of acrosin, except that acrosin remains firmly attached to the acrosomal membrane whereas the cortical granule factor is released as a free enzyme. As mentioned earlier, free acrosin destroys sperm binding sites in the zona pellucida; likewise this is probably the basis of the action of the enzyme released from the cortical granules. The material in the granules is in the form of a proenzyme which is activated by calcium, and this too is similar to acrosin.

The efficiency of these protective mechanisms is dependent on the age of the egg and the properties of the extracellular medium. Eggs which are experimentally exposed to sperm before they are ripe for ovulation are incapable of the cortical granule reaction and undergo polyspermy readily. The efficiency of the response also declines with increasing postovulatory age. Furthermore, the surrounding medium must have the correct composition; eggs exposed to sperm in physiological salt solutions undergo polyspermy, whereas in full tissue culture media a normal polyspermy block is developed.

Prevention of polyspermy thus depends upon the cortical granule reaction, which itself depends upon a signal, triggered by sperm fusion, which is propagated across the plasma membrane. In the very large eggs of birds this propagation cannot occur and multiple sperm penetration results. This 'physiological' polyspermy does not lead to abnormal development because only one sperm nucleus associates with the egg nucleus and undergoes further development. The mechanism by which only one sperm nucleus is selected is not known.

4.9 Formation of pronuclei and of the zygote nucleus

The fusion of egg and sperm triggers changes in both nuclei in preparation for formation of the zygote nucleus. The egg chromosomes, which until fusion are suspended in metaphase of the second meiotic division, complete the division with expulsion of the second polar body (see chapter 1). The haploid ovum nucleus becomes surrounded by an irregularly shaped nuclear envelope, and at this stage is known as the *female pronucleus*. At the same time the envelope of the sperm nucleus breaks up into vesicles and loses its identity. The chromatin becomes much more dispersed and euchromatic. A new envelope forms around the sperm chromosomes, and the reformed structure is called the *male pronucleus*.

Pronucleus formation is followed by fusion of the pronuclei and entry into the first cleavage division. The envelopes of both pronuclei develop protrusions which interdigitate with each other. The interlocked membranes break down to give a single nucleus, while at the same time the chromosomes of both pronuclei condense. The nuclear envelopes disappear completely, a spindle is formed and the chromosomes of both pronuclei come together to form a single metaphase plate. Labelling of DNA with tritiated thymidine shows that the DNA in each pronucleus is replicated before the formation of the zygote nucleus, so the daughter cells from the first cleavage are normal diploid cells.

4.10 Other events occurring at fertilisation

Fusion of a sperm with the egg induces a rapid and short-lived action potential which initiates the rise in intracellular free calcium already mentioned. In addition to triggering the cortical granule reaction, the rise in intracellular free calcium stimulates a large increase in cellular respiration. After this the rates of entry of amino acids, phosphate and nucleosides are increased and rapid protein synthesis begins.

During zygote formation only the sperm head becomes integrated into the egg cytoplasm and the rest of the body and tail components remain outside and are lost. It is significant that no sperm mitochondria persist in the zygote, because this means that all the mitochondrial genes in the embryo are of maternal origin.

The large numbers of sperms which do not participate in fertilisation are rapidly removed from the female reproductive tract. Those that do not leak out of the vagina are destroyed by phagocytosis; this is mainly carried out by leukocytes entering the uterine tubes, uterus and cervix, but the endometrial epithelium also shows a significant phagocytic capacity for degenerating spermatozoa.

4.11 Parthenogenesis

Various types of physical and chemical stimulation may evoke a cortical granule response in an unfertilised egg and thus set in train embryonic development. These eggs can sometimes develop as far as the blastocyst stage, but are unable to implant in the uterus. However, the capacity for differentiation of their cells is quite substantial, as recognisable tissues are produced if cells from these *parthenogenetic* embryos are transplanted to immunologically sheltered sites in an adult animal. Parthenogenetic embryos may be haploid or diploid, depending on whether extrusion of a second polar body has taken place.

4.12 Fertilisation *in vitro*

One cause of female infertility is obstruction of the uterine tubes, and sometimes this cannot be corrected surgically. In theory pregnancy could be achieved by removal of mature oocytes from the mother followed by fertilisation *in vitro* with the male partner's sperms and introduction of the resulting pre-implantation embryo into the uterus. However, this is very difficult technically owing to the stringent environmental conditions required for sperm capacitation, fertilisation and implantation. Many of these technical problems have now been overcome after much painstaking research in experimental animals and in humans, and the goal of delivery of a healthy baby after *in vitro* fertilisation has been achieved. It remains to be seen whether this technique is reliable enough to become an established treatment for this type of infertility, but the outlook currently seems hopeful.

Further reading

Cauthery, P. and Cole, M. (1971). *The Fundamentals of Sex*, W. H. Allen, London

Cohen, J. (1977). *Reproduction*, Butterworths, London, pp. 64–72 and 128–143

Greep, R. O. and Koblinksy, M. A. (eds.) (1977). *Frontiers in Reproduction and Fertility Control*, MIT Press, chap. 36 'Capacitation of spermatozoa and fertilisation in mammals'

Hopkins, C. R. (1978). *Structure and Function of Cells*, Saunders, Philadelphia, pp. 57–94

Masters, W. H. and Johnson, V. E. (1966). *Human Sexual Response*, Little, Brown & Co., Boston

Myerscough, P. R. (1976). 'Adam and Eve (normal human sexual behaviour)', in *Companion to Medical Studies*, vol. 1. Blackwell, Oxford

5

Implantation and Establishment of the Conceptus

5.1 Gene expression in the zygote

Strictly defined, the conception of a new individual occurs at the moment when chromosomes from the male and female pronuclei associate to form the mitotic figure of the first cleavage. Despite the fact that each gamete contributes 23 chromosomes to the zygote, the contributions of egg and sperm to the development of the embryo are not equal in practice. Because the zygote cytoplasm is almost entirely derived from the egg (see section 4.7), all of the embryo's mitochondrial DNA is therefore maternal. This condition persists for the entire life span of the new individual. In addition other molecules of shorter life such as some RNA and proteins are derived from the egg. Thus much of the metabolic activity and initial behaviour of the zygote depends entirely on molecules of maternal origin.

5.2 Cleavage

The union of the male and female pronuclei leads without pause into the early cleavage divisions of the zygote. These cleavages result in the segmentation of the zygote cytoplasm into somewhat less than 100 cells. These divisions are mitotic and generally occur alternately in the polar and equatorial planes so that the resulting cells are roughly cuboidal. One frequently sees references to cleavage embryos at the 4-cell, 16-cell or 32-cell stages, implying that the divisions are synchronised so that the cell number at any given moment is a power of two. In fact the degree of mitotic synchrony is very small, so embryos at, for example, 3-cell or 7-cell stages are readily found.

Cleavage results in the formation of a ball of cells, the *morula*. The cells forming this appear to be identical structurally, but transplantation studies on early mouse blastocysts have demonstrated that 'inside—outside' pattern formation has occurred (see section 8.3) so that the cells on the morula surface may not be interchangeable with those from the interior.

The cleavage process has two unusual characteristics. First, no growth in the size of the conceptus takes place during this entire phase; in fact a slight loss of mass occurs due to metabolism of its food reserves. Secondly, the early part of this phase is dependent purely upon maternal gene products; for example, maternal messenger RNA present in the egg supports protein synthesis for the first few divisions.

5.3 Blastocyst formation

Cleavage takes about 3—4 days, in which time a morula consisting of about 60 cells is generated. During this period the conceptus is transported down the uterine tube to the uterus, probably mainly by the action of the tubal cilia. The adherent granulosa cells forming the corona radiata are lost over this period but the zona pellucida remains intact.

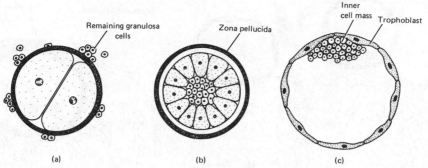

Figure 5.1   Pre-implantation stages of the conceptus: (a) early cleavage; (b) morula; (c) blastocyst showing inner cell mass

After entry into the uterus the radial symmetry of the conceptus is lost; fluid is secreted into the intercellular spaces of the morula to form cavities which coalesce to make a single large *blastocyst cavity* or *primary yolk sac* (figure 5.1). The surface cells of the morula have by now formed junctional complexes with one another and so form a cohesive surface layer, the *trophoblast*. The interior cells, however, are displaced to one side to form the *inner cell mass*, from which the embryo proper develops. This hollow fluid-filled conceptus is called the *blastocyst*. The zona pellucida is weakened by enzymatic digestion during blastocyst formation so that the trophoblast comes into direct contact with the endometrium.

5.4   Nutrition before implantation

The conceptus floats free in the fluid film on the walls of the uterine tube and uterus during cleavage and the early blastocyst phase. Its nutritional needs must be met by whatever it can obtain by diffusion from this fluid and from its stored reserves. However, mammalian eggs, unlike the yolky eggs of the other classes of vertebrates, contain little stored food. During cleavage some of the structural macromolecules of the egg are broken down, thus accounting for the slight reduction in mass that occurs at this time. The conceptus is probably especially dependent on its own reserves during passage down the uterine tube; once it reaches the uterus it has access to the

glycogen-rich secretions of the endometrial glands. The conceptus breaks down glycogen to pyruvate through the glycolytic pathway and this then enters the tricarboxylic acid cycle; the oxygen tension in the uterine lumen is adequate for the complete oxidation of carbohydrate. At blastocyst formation the rate of glycolysis increases sharply. Although the mechanism of this increase is unknown, it is one of several signs of increased biochemical activity at the start of embryogenesis.

Distribution of nutrients and gases through the conceptus is by diffusion alone. Since the morula has a diameter of over 100 μm the distances involved are large compared with those for diffusion in vascularised tissues and the rates of transfer must be correspondingly low. Although the size of the conceptus increases at blastocyst formation the diffusion problem may not in fact worsen as solutes may be transported by bulk movements of fluid in the primary yolk sac. However, the transport potential of simple diffusion is strained to its limit and the need for early acquisition of a blood vascular system is evident.

5.5   Conditions for implantation

Further development of the blastocyst is dependent upon the occurrence of *implantation* which takes place at approximately day 21 of the menstrual cycle or 7 days after ovulation. This is the process by which the blastocyst becomes embedded in the connective tissue stroma of the endometrium and establishes contact with the maternal circulation.

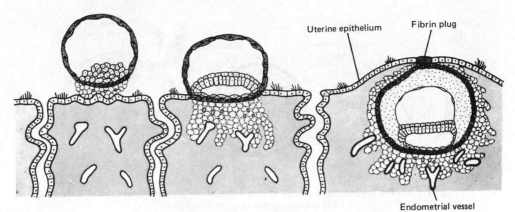

Figure 5.2   Three phases of implantation. Note the expansion of the syncytiotrophoblast (shaded) from the embryonic pole to cover the entire surface, eroding maternal vessels as it grows

Implantation in the uterus can only take place at the correct phase of the menstrual cycle. Such conditions are achieved by about the third day after ovulation, in the secretory phase of the uterine cycle (see chapter 2), principally through the action of progesterone secreted from the corpus luteum. Similarly the stage of embryonic development is critical; it must be in the early blastocyst stage. Excessively slow or rapid transport of the conceptus down the uterine tube may result in a failure of implantation. Since there is no evidence for any mechanism synchronising embryonic with endometrial development it is probable that implantation failure due to mistiming is common, as suggested in chapter 10.

This timing problem is particularly relevant to the successful achievement of implantation of human embryos obtained by fertilisation of eggs *in vitro* (see chapter 4). Synchronisation in this case is achieved by culturing the embryo for a few days after fertilisation to allow the uterus to reach the secretory phase before implantation is attempted.

5.6   The mechanism of implantation

The shedding of the zona pellucida exposes the trophoblast at the surface of the conceptus, thus preparing the way for trophoblastic invasion of maternal tissues. Initially the trophoblast consists of an epithelium-like layer of rather flattened cells

joined by junctional complexes. In preparation for implantation (figure 5.2) the outer cells at the embryonic pole of the blastocyst (adjacent to the inner cell mass) start to fuse with their neighbours to form multinucleate giant cells. These in turn fuse until the outer trophoblast is converted into a multinucleate cytoplasmic mass not subdivided into cells (a *syncytium*). Invasion of maternal tissue can take place as soon as the embryonic pole of the blastocyst is covered by this *syncytiotrophoblast*. Embryonic invasiveness appears to be characteristic only of syncytiotrophoblast. Little is known about the mechanism of trophoblastic cell fusion, but it seems to differ from the types of pathological cell fusion produced by certain viruses and chemical agents.

Contact between the microvilli on the surface of the syncytiotrophoblast and those on the endometrial epithelial cells leads to adhesion and to closer approximation of the blastocyst to the uterine lining. Cytoplasmic processes of the syncytiotrophoblast push between the epithelial cells, probably aided by trophoblast-derived enzymes which metabolise extracellular materials. As the defect in the endometrial epithelium is enlarged the blastocyst sinks into it and the advancing trophoblast erodes the connective tissue stroma of the endometrium. Finally the blastocyst sinks entirely beneath the epithelial surface; the only evidence of implantation detectable from the uterine lumen is a small elevation of the epithelium with a central defect plugged by a fibrin clot.

Shortly afterwards the epithelium regenerates to repair the gap.

As erosion of the endometrial stroma proceeds blood vessels are penetrated and blood flows into the space surrounding the blastocyst. The surface area of the syncytiotrophoblast is greatly amplified by the development of spaces within it, the *lacunae*, which are open to the trophoblastic surface and so fill with maternal blood. Thus the surface of the conceptus is brought into contact with an abundant supply of nutrients and oxygen. Even before contact with the mother's blood is established, the blastocyst lies in a pool of extracellular fluid containing nutrients produced by hydrolysis of maternal tissue by trophoblastic enzymes; it is very probable that the blastocyst makes extensive use of this source of nutrients between the onset of implantation and the establishment of a functional contact with maternal blood.

The main phases of implantation are illustrated in figure 5.2. The subsequent development of the interface between embryonic and maternal tissues is considered in the context of the placenta in chapter 7.

5.7 Maternal responses to implantation

Trophoblastic invasion induces a local response in the endometrial stroma which, although well documented, is very poorly understood. This so-called *decidual reaction* is characterised by changes in the cells of the endometrial stroma. Initially these cells appear to be perfectly normal fibroblasts or fibrocytes, but when stimulated by implantation those nearest to the trophoblast enlarge and become polygonal rather than spindle-shaped. Their nuclei become large, round and pale-staining and the cytoplasm becomes more basophilic and acquires substantial quantities of stored glycogen. Apart from the glycogen, these changes are typical of increased protein synthesis. Stromal transformation by the decidual reaction is initially localised but spreads to affect the entire subplacental zone of the decidua as the placenta grows. The permeability of the stromal capillaries also increases.

Little is known about the function of the decidual reaction, although it is apparently obligatory for further placental and embryonic development. It may be significant that the highly invasive human trophoblast gives rise to a strong decidual reaction, whereas less invasive placentae in other species produce a much weaker response. In consequence it has been suggested that the decidual reaction may serve in some way to limit the invasive properties of the trophoblast.

Establishment of pregnancy is dependent upon the suppression of the menstrual cycle. In the absence of any such mechanism menstruation would occur about a week after implantation and would terminate the pregnancy. Since menstruation occurs as a result of withdrawal of progesterone and oestradiol when the corpus luteum involutes, implantation must somehow suppress luteolysis so that the corpus luteum may continue to secrete steroids. This is accomplished by secretion of human chorionic gonadotropin (hCG) from the trophoblast into the uterine vessels; this hormone maintains luteotropic support of the corpus luteum thus maintaining progesterone and oestradiol secretion. Failure of hCG secretion at the correct time results in loss of the pregnancy at the next menstruation. Normally hCG appears in maternal blood within a few days of implantation and can be detected in urine by immunoassay methods shortly after the first missed menstrual period. The properties of hCG are discussed more thoroughly in chapter 7.

5.8 Maintenance of an established pregnancy

The 40 weeks or approximately 9 calendar months of human pregnancy are often divided for descriptive purposes into three *trimesters* or periods of three months. This may seem arbitrary but in fact forms a useful basis for subdivision of the developmental phases of the embryo and of the pregnancy itself.

In the latter part of the first trimester the role of the corpus luteum in the maintenance of pregnancy is supplanted by synthesis of steroids

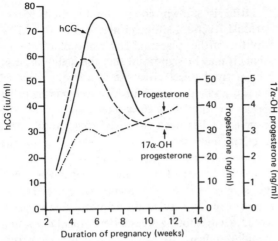

Figure 5.3   Hormone secretion in early pregnancy as determined by measurement of plasma levels

by the trophoblast. There is usually a slight fall in maternal plasma progesterone levels at the time of this changeover, and the relationship between maternal plasma progesterone and hCG levels in early pregnancy is shown in figure 5.3. Failure of the placental steroid secretion results in breakdown of the endometrium and termination of pregnancy, and it is thought that a proportion of early spontaneous abortions may arise in this way. It is interesting that the pre-changeover decline in maternal plasma progesterone levels occurs while hCG levels are still high because it suggests that the steroid synthesising activity of the corpus luteum cannot be maintained indefinitely even in the presence of the continuing luteotropic stimulus. However, the assumption of the main progesterone-secreting role by the placenta does not result in atrophy of the corpus luteum, because it persists as a *corpus luteum of pregnancy* and only undergoes regression to form a fibrous scar in the ovary (the *corpus albicans*) after parturition. However during the second and third trimesters the release of steroids from the corpus luteum is insignificant compared to placental output.

5.9   Abnormal implantation sites

The preceding discussion on the mechanism of implantation implies that a blastocyst finding

itself in the wrong region of the female reproductive tract when syncytiotrophoblast formation occurs might attempt to implant in an unsuitable site. This is a fairly common occurrence; a significant proportion of implantations occur in the lower segment of the uterus rather than the normal fundic region, and these may cause obstetric problems such as placental haemorrhage during labour. Less commonly implantation takes place at a site outside the uterus; situations of this type are called *ectopic pregnancies* and occur with a frequency of about 1 in 300. These relatively rare events are of importance because they may lead to death of both mother and fetus if unrecognised and untreated. The most serious form is tubal pregnancy, in which implantation occurs in the lumen of the uterine tube. This usually results in extensive invasion of local vessels and release of high pressure blood into the space surrounding the conceptus. Tubal rupture may then occur producing disastrous haemorrhage. Termination is the only possible course to take if such a pregnancy is detected. Very rarely the zygote implants in the peritoneal cavity; such pregnancies are not likely to go far unless they occur in tissues such as mesentery which have a good blood supply. If this occurs the pregnancy may occasionally go to term, although this would not be recommended if detected. Such a fetus must obviously be delivered by caesarean section.

Possibly the most curious feature of ectopic pregnancies is the fact that implantation and a decidual reaction can occur in such physiologically unsuitable sites. It demonstrates that loose connective tissues in general can undergo a decidual reaction, and makes one wonder why the conditions for uterine implantation are so stringent.

5.10   The foreign fetus

The fetus inherits half of its nuclear genes from its father, and this includes genes coding for histocompatibility antigens. This means that the antigenic differences between the fetus and mother are likely to be so great that a tissue graft from fetus to mother would be rapidly rejected. As the fetal trophoblast is in direct contact with maternal blood rich in lymphocytes, conditions for sensitisation and rejection appear to be ideal. The fact that the fetus is not rejected makes it clear that there are powerful mechanisms protecting the fetus from immune attack. In fact there are examples of some bizarre crosses between species such as lion/ tiger or horse/donkey which result in liveborn offspring in which the antigenic differences between mother and fetus must be enormous.

It can also be demonstrated that the maternal immune system is sensitised against fetal antigens but the trophoblast is somehow not attacked. The means by which this is achieved are still unknown, but it is possible to suggest a few feasible mechanisms as well as some which are known not to operate. The hypothesis that the uterus is an immunologically privileged site, like the brain or testis, is attractive but unfortunately untenable because ectopic pregnancies are not rejected either. The most plausible alternative is that antigenic sites on the trophoblast are somehow masked so that sensitised lymphocytes cannot interact with them to produce cellular injury. The placental hormones human chorionic gonadotropin and human placental lactogen are both capable of suppressing cell-mediated immune responses *in vitro*; both are present in high concentration in the placenta and hCG can be adsorbed on to the trophoblast surface and may possibly have a shielding action. This cannot, however, provide a universal explanation for protection of the fetus because chorionic gonadotropins only occur in primates and equidae, whilst all mammalian species obviously tolerate their own fetuses.

In general the potential for immunological damage to the fetus is restricted to the cell-mediated, T lymphocyte-based system. Maternal immunoglobulin G is transported into the fetus in large quantities (see chapter 7) but does no damage. One very significant exception to this generalisation is *rhesus isoimmunisation* (or rhesus haemolytic disease of the newborn), see section 10.6, which results from the leakage of rhesus positive fetal red cells into the blood of a rhesus negative mother. This usually occurs at parturition so the first rhesus positive fetus is not affected. However, the mother may produce anti-rhesus antibodies which in subsequent pregnancies cross the placenta to produce lysis of fetal red cells. The damage is severe and requires exchange transfusion of the fetus *in utero* or, failing that, of the newborn infant.

Further reading

Brachet, J. (1974). *Introduction to Molecular Embryology*, English Universities Press/Springer-Verlag, New York

Greep, R. O. (ed.) (1973). 'Female reproductive system', in *American Handbook of Physiology*, sec. 7, Endocrinology, vol. II, pt 2, American Physiological Society, Washington

Johnson, M. H. (ed.) (1977). *Development in Mammals*, North-Holland, Amsterdam

Odell, W. D. and Moyer, D. L. (1971). *Physiology of Reproduction*, C. V. Mosby Co., St Louis

6

Contraception

6.1 Population growth, family planning and contraception

There is little doubt that world population is increasing at an alarming rate, and that urgent action in the form of provision and use of contraceptives is required to limit population growth. Many would argue that the control of human fertility is the most important biosocial and medical problem that we face today.

Figure 6.1 shows world population growth, and the contributions to the numbers made by the affluent 'developed' regions, such as Europe, North America, Australasia, Japan and the USSR, and by the 'developing' regions of Africa, Asia and Latin America. The subdivision of nations in this way is to some extent arbitrary, although conventional, and there are obvious exceptions to the rule. The graph shows that world population is growing at an exponential rate, and emphasises that the enormous increase is dominated by numbers in the developing nations, that is in those countries which are in general poorer and less capable of supporting their rapidly increasing numbers.

The dramatic meaning of exponential population growth is well illustrated by considering the doubling time of the human population. It is calculated that the population at the time of Christ took 1500 years to double and that a century ago the doubling time had reduced to about 100 years. It is likely that the present world population of 4000 million will have doubled within 30–50 years. Few people believe that the earth possesses sufficient resources to support this population. Indeed, such growth might instead be forcibly restrained by catastrophes like famine, pestilence or war as Malthus predicted. It is estimated that malnutrition already affects half the world's population and the situation is unlikely to improve greatly even in spite of advances in the technology of food production and distribution.

The most important factors determining overall population growth are the birth and death rates, but other variables, such as migration, may also be significant. There are considerable differences between the developing and developed nations in birth and death rates, and these largely account for the differing rates of population growth referred to above.

The birth rates of different nations vary between about 14 and 50 live births per thousand population. However, if a rate of 25 per thousand is taken as an arbitrary dividing line, then the worldwide statistics show that the affluent developed countries all have birth rates lower than this, whereas nearly all the developing nations have higher rates. Death rates also vary considerably and are highest in the poorest nations, at 20–25 per thousand, and lowest in the developed nations (8–10 per thousand). The effect of these differences in death rates may be summarised in terms of life expectancy: at birth, life expectancy is still only about 40 years in parts of Africa, India and other tropical regions, whereas it is over 70 years in most of Europe and North America.

The high rate of population growth in the

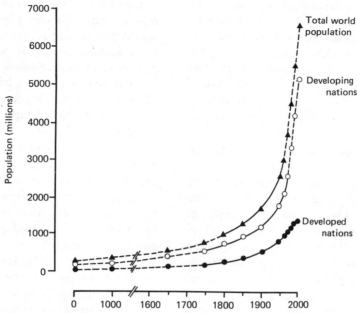

Figure 6.1 World population. Graph of past and estimated future growth of the world population, showing the contributions to total made by the developing and developed nations. Dashed portions of the curves are estimates or predictions

developing countries results from the large excess of live births over deaths. In rough terms, this excess varies between about 20 and 30 per thousand, compared with values of about 8–14 in the developed nations. Furthermore, it is likely that this excess may increase even further as health and hygiene standards improve, because this reduces the death rate, particularly in infancy.

These data give a clear general impression of the worldwide situation but are insufficient to enable satisfactory prediction of future population growth trends as they are influenced by other variables. For example, it is important to know such things as the age and sex composition of the population, particularly the number of women who are in the reproductive age group, age at marriage, infant mortality rate, rate of abortion, and so on. Such information, together with an adequate assessment of the conception rate, would enable a demographer to predict future population growth. One important consideration concerns the age distribution of a population. The growth potential of a predominantly young

population, as found today in many developing nations, is clearly much greater than that of an equal population of older people, since the young people will themselves mature to swell the ranks of the fertile.

It has been argued that population growth in developing countries might diminish if there is substantial economic and material progress. Such an association has been offered as an explanation for the *demographic transition* from high to low birth and death rates and consequent reduction in rate of population growth which has occurred in the post-industrialisation societies of the West. Such economic and social change would probably be far too slow to have much effect on the population crisis in the developing nations.

The preceding comments strongly imply that voluntary limitation of fertility by one means or another is an absolute prerequisite, at least for many nations if not necessarily for individuals. This could be achieved by introducing widespread and vigorous family planning campaigns which advocate the use of contraceptives. Contraception is already practised voluntarily on a wide scale by a large number of couples, particularly in the West and China. The means for achieving effective contraception on a worldwide scale already exist, since there is a sufficient variety of efficient contraceptives available, as discussed below. Strenuous efforts are also being made to develop alternative methods of efficient contraception, some of which are described briefly in this chapter, so as to increase the range and acceptability of available methods.

In most developed and several developing countries, family planning facilities and contraceptives are provided by the government as part of health care or population programmes. In many other countries fertility control has not advanced very far, due to political or economic inertia or because social, religious or cultural practices preclude change. Education is as important a part of an effective population planning programme as the provision of the contraceptives themselves. It should also be noted that the governments of certain countries currently pursue a philosophy of population expansion.

Although many contraceptive methods, often involving bizarre folk remedies, have been known or attempted for a very long time, widespread advocacy of contraception as a means for a couple to regulate their family to the desired size, or as part of a national policy for population planning, is comparatively recent. Thus, condoms have been used quite widely in Britain since the mid-Victorian era, but only since the Second World War has their sale and family planning become respectable, and governmental participation in the form of provision of other birth control facilities extends back for only some 15 years. In part, the slow progress resulted from apathy or even opposition by legal, religious and medical groups as well as reluctance to discuss sexual matters in public. The history of human fertility control offers examples of reformers or champions of the poor, who attempted to make contraception available to the masses in the face of considerable hostility and resistance.

It is interesting that until about 10 000 years ago the human population was almost constant, with an estimated annual population growth rate

of the order of 0.001 per cent over a period of a million years or more, compared to the present annual growth rate of 2.0 per cent. The evidence available from studies of primitive societies that have survived to the present day suggests that this was not due to a balance between high birth and death rates or to natural physiological fertility-limiting mechanisms which apply to some animal populations, but resulted from certain consciously applied ritual or cultural practices. The three methods of importance are infanticide, abortion and abstention from intercourse.

Abstention from intercourse is obviously a legitimate and effective 'contraceptive method', but would hardly be adopted today by many couples as first choice in competition with other less restrictive methods. Abortion is still used as a means of last resort by many women when contraception has not been used or has failed, but in many societies abortion is forbidden for cultural or religious reasons. However, it is generally acknowledged that facilities for safe and effective abortion must be available if the concept that a woman should herself be the final arbiter of whether or not she has a child is to have real meaning. In certain societies, for example Japan, abortion is widely used to limit fertility. The ethical beliefs of most societies prohibit infanticide, but the practice of allowing weaker, ill or handicapped babies to die because of lack of care or attention persists in some cultures even today. This practice could be regarded as infanticide and might perhaps be justified in eugenic and evolutionary terms as a means of preserving the fitness of the species.

The different contraceptive techniques used today are listed below in table 6.1, and are separated into groups according to whether they are practised by the male or female partner. The table only includes methods of acknowledged importance. Some data are also given for their relative effectiveness and for the prevalence of their usage as determined from large-scale retrospective surveys. The table includes sterilisation as a contraceptive method, but this obviously differs from the others because it is irreversible.

Of the reversible methods, all but oral contra-

Table 6.1   Effectiveness and use of different contraceptive methods*

Method	Failure rate (pregnancies per 100 women per year)	Usage (percentage of all couples using contraception)	
		Denmark (1970)	England & Wales (1970)
Male methods:			
condoms	10	10	46
coitus interruptus	33	0	7
vasectomy (irreversible sterilisation)	0.05	–	–
Female methods:			
oral contraceptives	0.1	66	31
intrauterine device	1.5	10	5
diaphragms	15	10	6
rhythm method	20	0	2
spermicidal substances	30	0	3
tubectomy (irreversible sterilisation)	0.05	–	–

* The table shows average figures taken from a number of representative surveys of contraceptive use. The effectiveness of a given type of contraceptive often varies widely from study to study, depending on variables such as motivation of user, age and social status, etc. The variation is greatest for the least effective methods, such as coitus interruptus, rhythm method and spermicidal substances. There is also wide social and geographical variation in the choice of different contraceptive method as well as in the overall use of contraceptives.

ceptives and the intrauterine device can be used without any special medical or paramedical supervision or facilities. However, they are less reliable methods in terms of contraceptive protection, even though they have the virtue of simplicity, and they will therefore be discussed below in less detail. Oral contraceptives and the intrauterine device provide a greater measure of contraceptive protection if used correctly, and owe their effectiveness to the way in which they interfere with specific physiological processes in the female. Their use is increasing at the expense of the less reliable methods, and they will be considered in some depth.

6.2   Male contraceptive methods

In many societies the man has most responsibility for decisions concerning the family and it is desirable that effective contraceptives for male use should be developed. Unfortunately, male reproductive physiology does not lend itself so readily to successful intervention as does that of the female. Millions of sperms are formed continuously rather than a single egg being shed at a specific monthly interval, and interference with the hormonal functions of the testis has far-reaching effects outside the male reproductive tract. Some future possibilities for male contraception are mentioned at the end of this section.

Condoms

A condom is a sheath of latex rubber which is unrolled over the erect penis so as to collect the ejaculate, thus preventing its access to the female reproductive tract. Condoms are cheap, easy to use and reliable, since they are electronically tested for perforations. Their manufacture was revolutionised by the invention of rubber vulcanisation in the mid-nineteenth century, and of latex moulding in the 1930s. Condoms may provide some protection against the transmission of venereal disease, and allow the male to retain full responsibility for contraception.

There are no side effects associated with their use but some couples find them distasteful or messy, and they can be put on only when erection has been achieved. In Western countries the use of condoms is declining in the face of increased acceptance of other methods of contraception, but they are still used more than any other single method. The correct use of condoms by sufficiently motivated couples allows a considerable degree of protection against unwanted pregnancy, but their efficacy falls far short of that of oral contraceptives or the intrauterine device. Additional protection may be gained by applying spermicidal creams or jellies to the vagina.

The cheapness, simplicity of use and freedom from required medical supervision make condoms an ideal method of contraception for family planning programmes in rural areas.

Coitus interruptus

Consistently successful contraception by coitus interruptus (withdrawal of the penis just before ejaculation) is difficult to achieve as it requires considerable skill and self-control, but the method is not associated with any side effects. The failure rate of coitus interruptus is thus very high compared to other methods, but fortunately its popularity as sole method of contraception is waning.

Vasectomy

Vasectomy is performed by sectioning the paired ducti deferentes. This prevents the passage of spermatozoa from the testis to the accessory sex glands and the urethra, and thus produces effective sterility. It is not equivalent to castration since the endocrine function of the testis proceeds unim-

paired; testosterone secretion from the interstitial cells continues and libido, secondary sexual characteristics and normal sexual performance are retained. Spermatozoa are still formed in the testis, but cannot escape and are digested by macrophages. Sterility is not immediate since viable sperm are sequestered in the accessory reproductive organs, and fertility may persist for as many as 15 ejaculations. Additional contraceptive precautions should be maintained until analysis of seminal fluid confirms that no active spermatozoa are present.

Vasectomy is irreversible, although occasional successful re-anastomoses have been achieved, and is therefore suitable only for men who do not wish to have any more children. The operation is simple and quick, requiring local anaesthesia of the scrotum, and can be performed on an outpatient basis, or under field conditions. No serious side effects have been noted. Although vasectomy is still relatively uncommon as a contraceptive method of choice in Europe, several hundred thousand men in India have been so treated as part of a vigorous family planning campaign. Vasectomy is likely to increase in popularity as an alternative to female sterilisation by tubectomy (see section 6.3) because most men find the results acceptable and it is absolutely reliable.

Future developments in male contraception

Small-scale trials of a male pill containing the oestrogen ethinyloestradiol and methyltestosterone taken orally showed that sterility occurred after several weeks of treatment. This was probably due to inhibition by the oestrogen of gonadotropin secretion from the pituitary as occurs in women taking a combined oral contraceptive (see section 6.4). As FSH and LH levels decrease, testicular spermatogenesis and testosterone secretion both decline gradually and sterility results. Testosterone must be added as a supplement to avoid regression of secondary sexual characteristics and breast development and to retain libido. Some androgens themselves, for example the synthetic weak androgen analogue danazol, also inhibit pituitary gonadotropin release. The future potential of this type of male pill appears to be very limited by comparison with the female oral contraceptive, because interruption of the male pituitary—gonad axis has several drastic consequences.

Although numerous chemicals which interfere with spermatogenesis have been identified in tests on animals, they are all too toxic to be of any clinical value. Most of them interfere with cell division, but a degree of selectivity has been achieved by developing compounds such as the α-chlorohydrins which interfere with sperm maturation in the epididymis. Another possible site for selective attack of spermatozoa would be to develop acrosin inhibitors. Acrosin is an enzyme found in the acrosome and is involved in the fertilising ability of sperms (see chapter 4); certain polypeptides secreted by the male accessory glands inhibit acrosin activity before sperm capacitation takes place. These substances may yield useful clues for a new type of male contraceptive.

Inhibin is a small protein first found in bovine testis and seminal fluid, but now also identified in smaller amounts in ovarian extracts, which selectively inhibits release of FSH. An inhibin analogue with a similar action would be of great promise as a male contraceptive since it might block spermatogenesis without diminishing testosterone secretion, known to be principally dependent upon LH. This would be a considerable advance over the male pill mentioned above.

6.3 Female contraceptive methods

Apart from the contraceptive pill and intrauterine device, which are considered in later sections, the most important female contraceptive methods are the diaphragm, rhythm method, sterilisation by tubectomy, the local application of spermicidal substances and lactational amenorrhoea.

Rhythm method

The teaching of Thomas Aquinas forbade any practice which impedes the generation of offspring, that is any form of artificial contraception, and is still followed by strict adherents to the Roman Catholic Church. The only method of birth control open to Catholics is the rhythm method, which is based on abstinence from intercourse during periods when the female is potentially fertile. For this purpose it is considered that the egg remains viable for up to 2 days after ovulation and that sperm can survive for 3 days inside the female tract. In practice it is recommended that sexual intercourse should be avoided for 7—12 days during the cycle, depending on the duration of and variation between cycles. The major defect of the method, apart from the considerable restriction of connubial bliss, is that it is often not certain when ovulation occurs since it is difficult to detect and often varies in timing, even in the same woman. A common way of trying to pinpoint ovulation is to measure body temperature on awakening; there is often a small rise of up to 0.5°C after ovulation at the onset of the luteal phase of the cycle. It is necessary to keep accurate calendar records of menstrual behaviour for this method of contraception, and it is generally very unreliable in comparison with other techniques. Fortunately it is not the method of choice for many couples (see table 6.1).

Spermicidal substances

A large number of astringent or antiseptic substances are known to be harmful to spermatozoa. Many ancient folk remedies for contraception, such as the introduction of vinegar or potions into the vagina, depend on this sort of direct spermicidal action. A number of more effective chemicals are now available and can be introduced into the vagina in the form of foams, sprays, pessaries or creams. Their use is recommended in conjunction with condoms or diaphragms, but they do not provide sufficient contraceptive protection if used on their own (see table 6.1).

Lactational amenorrhoea

The mechanisms whereby lactation and breast feeding inhibit the return to fertility are discussed in chapter 14. It is relevant to mention here that this is a natural method for the spacing of births, and that breast feeding is therefore indirectly very important for population control. The reliability of lactational amenorrhoea as a contraceptive 'method' is low, however, so on its own it could hardly be recommended.

Diaphragms

The diaphragm or cap is a hemispherical dome of soft rubber attached to a circular sprung rim, and is inserted into the vagina so as to block the passage of sperms to the cervical canal. Diaphragms are fitted over the cervix itself, or high in the vagina, so as to occlude the cervix. The sizes of the appliances vary to suit individual women, and initial instruction for learning how to insert the device requires skilled help and advice.

The diaphragm is inserted before intercourse and, unlike the condom, is designed to be re-used many times. Its contraceptive efficacy depends upon the skill and motivation with which it is used, and may be enhanced by concurrent application of spermicides. The diaphragm is considerably less effective than the IUD or contraceptive pill (see table 6.1). As a method of contraception it is not very widely used and until recently was declining in importance in the face of more efficient methods, but has the advantages of simplicity, low cost and freedom from side effects. Like the condom, its value for family planning programmes might have been underestimated in the past.

Sterilisation

There is now increasing demand for voluntary sterilisation, either male or female, and it is estimated that almost one-sixth of couples in the USA will adopt sterilisation as a means of permanent fertility control. Vasectomy was discussed in the previous section.

Female sterilisation is nowadays performed principally by *tubectomy*, that is, by severance of the uterine tubes. The practice of *hysterectomy*,

removal of the uterus, has been largely superseded except when medically indicated, as it is a much more traumatic and extensive procedure. After the uterine tubes are severed or cauterised, eggs can no longer pass from the ovary to the uterus, and so fertilisation and implantation are impossible. The surgical methods used for female sterilisation involve manipulation of the tubes after approach via either the vaginal, transcervical or transabdominal route, and are comparatively minor procedures with rapid patient recovery and few side effects. As a contraceptive method, tubectomy is virtually 100 per cent certain. The ease and cheapness of the different procedures now available for tubectomy have also contributed to the adoption of these methods in preference to hysterectomy. However, female sterilisation cannot be applied on a mass basis, as can vasectomy, because the technique is not of comparable simplicity.

6.4   Oral contraceptives

The oral contraceptive for women has revolutionised family planning and the control of a woman over her fertility. No other pharmaceutical product has been awarded the definite article so emphatically as 'the pill'. Oral contraceptives have gained widespread international acceptance since they were first used in large-scale trials in Puerto Rico in the mid-1950s, and it is estimated that more than 50 million women worldwide are taking the pill as a daily basis for contraception.

Oral contraceptives are simple, safe and socially acceptable and, if taken correctly, provide contraceptive protection that is virtually 100 per cent certain. They contain mixtures of steroid sex hormones which as might be expected have widespread actions on the body. Thus many side effects have been attributed to the pill and the most important ones will be discussed below. Fortunately many of the minor side effects disappear after regular use of the pill has been established. More rarely, the pill has been considered to be responsible for serious adverse effects, and the identification of long-term but rare hazards due to prolonged medication with oral contraceptives is of major concern. That a number of serious but occasional reactions to the pill have been identified is not surprising in view of the potency of its ingredients and the very large number of women using it. Another matter for concern is the effect of long-term pill-taking on subsequent fertility of women who wish to start families after a prolonged period of pregnancy avoidance.

Despite these reservations about the possible harmful effects of oral contraceptives, the pill has established itself as the contraceptive method of choice in the West. Its use is increasing at the expense of less reliable methods of contraception. This has been fostered by the efforts of governments and of the medical profession to provide low cost professional family planning services offering a choice of the most effective contraceptive methods.

Historical background and types of contraceptive pill

The development of oral contraceptives is based upon a detailed knowledge of the hormonal basis of control of ovarian function and a source of cheap orally active analogues of the female steroid sex hormones. Thus their development is relatively recent. It has been known for a long time that ovulation is inhibited during pregnancy, and the presence of a blood-borne factor was postulated from ovary transplant experiments. Oestrogens and progesterone were identified and purified by the mid-1930s and their inhibitory effects on pituitary control of reproductive function were clarified at this time by animal experiments. Although the possibility of using these hormones to suppress ovulation in women was suggested, it could not be attempted because the purified hormones were very scarce and expensive and could be used only by injection because they are inactivated if taken orally. Further advances came in the 1940s when semi-synthetic analogues of oestrogens and progesterone were made by synthesis from plant steroid precursors. These

derivatives contain substituents which prevent their metabolism, but full oestrogenic or progestational potency is retained.

Development of oral contraceptives using these synthetic steroids proceeded rapidly, especially once it was realised that an ideal combination resulted from the daily administration of milligram quantities of a progestogen combined with microgram quantities of an oestrogen. Preparations containing either type of steroid alone can also be used as contraceptives but are either less effective or cause more side effects.

Three types of contraceptive pill are in use today, although other ways of using female steroid hormones as contraceptives have been devised and will be discussed later. The *combined pill* is the most important and widely used type of preparation; it comprises a course of 21 tablets containing a mixture of 0.5—5.0 mg of a synthetic progestogen and 30—80 μg of a synthetic oestrogen. These tablets are presented in specially designed tear-off foil packs or dated push-out plastic mounts or dials and are taken every day for 21 days, starting on day 4 or 5 after the first day of menstrual bleeding. There is a week when no tablets are taken, during which bleeding occurs due to the withdrawal of progestogen in a manner similar to that occurring in the normal menstrual cycle. Very regular cycles are established after a few months of this treatment. There are almost 30 combined pill formulations currently available in Britain, made up of different combinations of the various synthetic steroids, and this allows some scope for finding a suitable preparation for each woman. It also reflects the keen competition between rival pharmaceutical houses for a lucrative market.

The *sequential pill* also comprises a course of 21 tablets, but oestrogen is taken alone for the first two weeks and is then supplemented with a progestogen for a further week. These pills attempt to mimic the normal pattern of changes in ovarian steroids during the menstrual cycle, and the removal of progestogen at the end of the treatment period precipitates regular withdrawal bleeding. The popularity of sequential pills has now declined, and only a handful of different brands are available. In some formulations dummy tablets or iron or

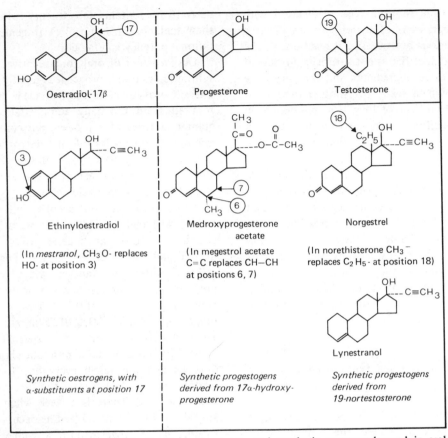

Figure 6.2 Structures of steroid sex hormones and synthetic compounds used in oral contraceptives, showing the two different types of progestogen based on the 17α-hydroxyprogesterone and 19-nortestosterone structures. Note that dashed lines represent α-substituents that are oriented below the plane of the steroid nucleus, i.e. away from the reader, and that the 3- and 17-substituents of the natural hormones have the β-configuration

vitamin supplemented placebos are added for the fourth week so that pills are taken continuously, thus simplifying pill-taking.

The development of the *progestogen mini-pill* is more recent. A low dose of progestogen, 0.2–0.5 mg, is taken without a break. This dosage of progestogen, lower than that for the same compound used in the combined pill, is sufficient to have a contraceptive effect, although its mode of action at this dose may be different. The mini-pill does not promote the same degree of cycle regularity as the other types of pill because progestogen is not withdrawn, and bleeding may be irregular or sometimes occur during the middle of the 'cycle'.

Some of the most important synthetic steroids used in contraceptive pills are depicted in figure 6.2, and the structures can be compared to those of progesterone and oestradiol-17β themselves. These compounds all have alpha substituents at carbon-17, and it is this which confers oral activity by providing resistance to enzymatic breakdown. Some of these substances are more potent in biological tests of oestrogenic or progestational activity than the parent compounds, although this may be due to differences in absorption or metabolism.

Two synthetic oestrogens are commonly utilised in contraceptive pills — ethinyloestradiol and mestranol. Mestranol owes its biological action exclusively to conversion *in vivo* to ethinyloestradiol. Oestrogens have many important and widespread actions in the body which are discussed in chapters 2, 14 and elsewhere, such as promoting and maintaining the female secondary sexual characteristics, and on the reproductive organs and breasts. They also cause salt and water retention, affect protein, fat, and carbohydrate metabolism, and have vital positive and negative feedback effects on the hypothalamo—pituitary control of gonadotropin release.

It is surprising that many non-steroid compounds containing substituted phenols have oestrogenic activity because, as a rule, it is not possible to alter the structure of a hormone very much without losing its specific biological properties. Diethylstilboestrol is the best known of these compounds and is a very potent oestrogen which was used until recently for oestrogen replacement therapy in the menopause, for control of painful menstruation and as a post-coital contraceptive. It is not recommended nowadays for this latter use as there is evidence that it may increase the susceptibility to vaginal cancer of the daughters of women who used the drug. Another interesting example of oestrogenic substances concerns the isoflavones which occur in certain clovers. They can be converted by animals to equols which have weak oestrogenic actions, and this explains 'clover disease' which once resulted in infertility in sheep in Australia. The equol acted as a contraceptive and inhibited ovulation.

The three important synthetic progestogens illustrated in figure 6.2 belong to two general classes of compounds. Most synthetic progestogens are 19-nortestosterone derivatives, and as expected some of these compounds may have weak androgenic actions because they are similar in structure to testosterone as well as to progesterone. The other progestogens, such as medroxyprogesterone acetate, are derivatives of 17α-hydroxyprogesterone and contain a substituent at carbon-6 to prevent breakdown by the enzyme which metabolises 17α-hydroxyprogesterone during steroid biosynthesis. All these steroids have the properties expected of progestogens: they modify or amplify the effects of oestrogens on steroid-sensitive

tissues, cause the endometrium to become oedematous and secretory, promote fluid retention and have effects on the hypothalamo—pituitary gonadal axis. Some of the synthetic progestogens also have other unexpected effects. For example, norgestrel has some anti-oestrogenic properties, whereas some of the other 19-nortestosterone steroids may be converted in small amounts to oestrogenic compounds by aromatisation. These various additional effects make it difficult to predict or interpret all the effects seen when using these substances therapeutically, and they may also help to explain some of the variations in side effects between individuals and between different types of pill.

Mode of action and metabolic effects of oral contraceptives

The very high efficiency of the combined and sequential oral contraceptives is due to the fact that they inhibit ovulation by negative feedback action at the hypothalamus and anterior pituitary. Negative feedback by oestrogens and progestogens also occurs naturally during the luteal phase of the menstrual cycle (see chapter 2) and during pregnancy. The consequences are that FSH and LH release are much reduced, follicles are not selected for maturation, ovulation does not occur and steroid hormone synthesis by the ovary is not stimulated. Radioimmunoassay of plasma FSH, LH, oestrogens and progesterone during the menstrual cycle of women taking combined or sequential pills shows that levels are low throughout the cycle and do not fluctuate cyclically in the normal manner. Before the advent of radioimmunoassay, limited evidence for this mechanism of action was obtained by bioassay for the steroid hormones of plasma samples and by analysis of urinary pregnanediol excretion, which is much reduced in the luteal phase of women taking oral contraceptives. When the ovary is examined at laparotomy, developing follicles can be recognised in normal fertile women but not in those on the pill. The progestogen mini-pill may also inhibit ovulation, but less reliably so than the other types of oral contraceptives as determined by plasma hormone measurements. This explains why it is not quite such an effective contraceptive.

There is no evidence that the pill can induce the LH surge by positive feedback. This can be achieved artificially by administering oestrogens at a critical time before the mid-point of the menstrual cycle, but hormonal interference by oral contraceptives does not do this.

The pill also modifies the endometrium so as to make it unsuitable for implantation of the embryo. There is a very short phase of proliferation, rapidly followed within a few days by secretory changes which differ qualitatively from those seen in the normal luteal phase. The histological appearance of the endometrium is also much altered, with evidence of glandular exhaustion towards the end of the cycle. Nourishment of the blastocyst is probably impeded. The progestogen mini-pill causes similar endometrial changes and this is probably important for its contraceptive action.

Progesterone promotes the secretion of a thick tenacious cervical mucus in which spermatozoa find movement difficult compared with the abundant watery secretion normally found at ovulation. This probably reduces the penetration of sperm into the uterine cavity and adds to the contraceptive effect, particularly of the combined pill and mini-pills.

It is also possible that the pill has direct actions on the ovary and on uterine motility which enhance its contraceptive effectiveness, but these effects are likely to be secondary to those mentioned above.

The administration of oral contraceptives leads to numerous biochemical changes, many of which are also observed during pregnancy as a result of high steroid hormone levels. In general, these changes are of small consequence, unless the responses are exaggerated. High doses of oestrogens sometimes cause the release of enzymes from the liver and may even lead to biochemical manifestations of hepatocellular damage such as elevated plasma levels of bilirubin and lactate dehydrogenase. At worst, jaundice may occur. Women with histories of liver failure or jaundice are obviously vulnerable and probably should not use an oestrogen-containing contraceptive pill.

Glucose tolerance is reduced in women taking oral contraceptives, perhaps due to complex synergistic effects of both oestrogen and progestogen components. This is usually not serious except in diabetics, who may have to increase their daily insulin dose, but this alteration in carbohydrate metabolism could contribute to some of the other side effects of the pill. Levels of plasma triglyceride, cholesterol and very low density lipoprotein are often elevated in women taking combined oral contraceptives and this reflects oestrogen and progestogen-dependent alterations in fat metabolism by the liver.

Blood clotting factors are usually slightly raised in pregnancy, and may also change during medication with the pill. Taken overall, there appears to be an increase in blood coagulability, particularly in women taking pills containing high doses of oestrogens. This may explain the increased incidence of venous thromboembolism associated with the pill.

Many of the potentially serious biochemical consequences of the combined pill noted above are probably due to the oestrogenic component. Recognition of this fact within the past 10 years has prompted the recommendation that the daily oestrogen dose should be minimised as much as possible; in most preparations it is now limited to 30–80 μg daily. This fact also lends impetus to the search for effective contraceptives based solely on progestogens.

Side effects and adverse reactions to oral contraceptives

Although a large number of side effects to oral contraceptives have been noted and widely discussed, most do not represent a hazard to life and are not of sufficient seriousness to influence the high acceptability of oral contraceptives as the preferred means of contraception for many women in the developed nations. Many of the more commonly reported side effects may be subjective in nature and difficult to measure, and similar effects are often experienced by women not taking the pill or during pregnancy. Thus it is difficult to assess the extent to which oral contraceptives should be biamed. Anticipation of side effects may also bias both patients and doctors. In many cases minor side effects are more frequent when starting the pill, and disappear after two or three cycles.

Minor side effects include initial menstrual irregularity, increased premenstrual tension with depression and irritability, increased or decreased libido, increased appetite and weight, breast tenderness, nausea and vomiting, and increased frequency of headaches. Facial hyperpigmentation sometimes results, particularly in tropical countries. Acne may be improved by taking oral contraceptives, as oestrogen opposes the actions of androgens on sebaceous gland secretion. Menstrual bleeding and discomfort is usually reduced and this is generally appreciated, and may be beneficial if the nutritional state of the woman is poor. Irregular bleeding may occur with the low dose preparations, particularly the mini-pill, especially for the first few months.

More seriously, the pill may occasionally precipitate migraine, jaundice, hypertension, gall bladder disease with gallstone formation, and cervical erosion, and it is sometimes diabetogenic. It should not be used by women who suffer from these complaints. The reasons for some of these effects have been discussed above in the context of the biochemical changes produced by oestrogens and progestogens. Although certain neoplasms are known to be steroid-dependent, there is no sound evidence that prolonged use of the contraceptive pill leads to any increase in susceptibility to the common types of cancer seen in women, despite extensive research to check for any such association. One progestogen used in pills, megestrol acetate, was withdrawn recently in Britain because it was shown to cause mammary gland tumours in beagles when administered for long periods at very high doses. However, the relevance of such animal experiments to the human is questionable.

There is more certainty about the association between oral contraceptives and deep vein thrombosis, pulmonary embolism and acute myocardial infarction. It has been established beyond reasonable doubt that the susceptibility of women to these potentially fatal episodes increases with age

and smoking and also with pill-taking. Fortunately, the chances of suffering such an attack remain very low: for every 100 000 women in the age groups 20–34 and 35–44 years, the number of deaths per year are about 1.5 and 3.9 for users of oral contraceptives, compared to 0.2 and 0.5 for non-users in the two age groups. These effects on the cardiovascular system probably depend on the oestrogenic component of the pill as noted earlier. It should be borne in mind that it is very difficult to prove beyond all doubt that extremely rare side effects are due specifically to oral contraceptives (or to any other cause, for that matter) because of the many variables that could be considered, and because the small numbers of events demand huge groups of women.

There is natural anxiety about the long-term hazards of the contraceptive pill since many women take it continuously for years on end. Considering the potency of steroids used, there appear to be relatively few serious adverse effects compared to the benefits it offers in terms of freedom from anxiety about pregnancy or from the dangers of pregnancy itself. A comparison of the risks and benefits of the pill compared to the intrauterine device and diaphragm is made in section 6.7.

Many women are concerned that prolonged use of the contraceptive pill might impair subsequent fertility. There is evidence that there may be a temporary impairment, but it seems most unlikely that any women become permanently sterile through taking the pill. In a recent study of 1200 women who stopped taking the pill, 30 per cent became pregnant within 3 months, 70 per cent within 9 months and 85 per cent within 2 years. About 10 per cent of these women would be expected to be sterile in any case, and the figures for pregnancy after 2 years were the same for women stopping the pill as for those stopping using the diaphragm or who had not previously used any type of contraceptive.

New formulations of steroid contraceptives designed for long duration of action

Several methods for administering contraceptive progestogens in long-acting forms which require only infrequent administration have been developed. The most useful are the injectable steroids, such as norethindrone oenanthrate or depomedroxyprogesterone acetate, which are administered by intramuscular injection once every 3 or 6 months respectively. The steroids are very slowly released from these insoluble salts. Long-acting injectable contraceptives seem to be particularly well suited to developing countries and there is high demand for them, perhaps because many people are accustomed to receiving injections for disease control. The method places much less emphasis on continuing self-motivation than the conventional oral contraceptive taken daily. Disadvantages are that there is considerable menstrual irregularity and amenorrhoea during treatment, the medication is essentially irreversible over the period in question and that fertility after discontinuing the treatment is impaired for a year or more.

Another promising method of administering slowly released progestogens is to incorporate them into silastic capsules which are implanted subdermally. In all cases, the objective is to produce a depot source of steroid from which the active molecule is slowly released or leached out at a constant and dependable rate.

6.5   The intrauterine contraceptive device

Although intrauterine devices (IUDs) such as the small pliable silver ring of Gräfenburg were used successfully in the 1920s, this method of contraception went out of fashion, mainly because of the risks of uterine infection and because it was thought to be too unphysiological. Interest was revived in the 1960s and intrauterine devices are now widely used for contraception. They are promoted by family planners and the medical profession because of their reliability and acceptability. An advantage of the IUD is that once inserted further motivation is not required for its use, in distinction to all other contraceptive methods.

Present-day IUDs (illustrated in figure 6.3) are made of flexible plastic which can be sterilised before insertion by irradiation or soaking in

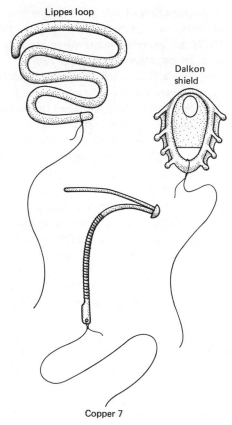

Figure 6.3   **Three commonly used intrauterine contraceptive devices, drawn to actual size**

antiseptic. They are introduced into the uterus through the cervical canal by means of a tubular applicator, inside which the device is collapsed, and regain their original shape inside the uterine cavity. This new method of insertion represents an advance, because the older inflexible IUDs could be introduced into the uterus only after considerable dilation of the cervix, and this was often a disagreeable and traumatic experience. Insertion must be done by trained and experienced medical or paramedical personnel, and sterile precautions are obviously most important, as the uterus is highly vulnerable to infection.

It seems as though the contraceptive efficacy of the IUD is dependent upon its size and area of contact with the uterus. However, this also increases the tendency of the device to increase menstrual bleeding, and cause other harmful effects such as uterine perforation, so a balance must be struck between efficacy and acceptability. An important advance was the discovery that additions of small amounts of copper increase contraceptive efficiency, but not side effects. This is exploited in the 'copper 7' or 'copper T' which contain a spiral of thin copper wire wound around the vertical arm. The copper slowly leaches away, and the device must be renewed after several years. Medicated IUDs containing a slowly released progestogen have been tested experimentally and they seem to be effective contraceptives which reduce the extent of excessive menstrual bleeding.

The IUD prevents implantation, perhaps by increasing local motility of the myometrium, but the detailed mechanism of its action is not known. It is possible that the presence of an IUD stimulates macrophage activity in the uterus and this may prevent implantation by encouraging a local sterile inflammatory focus. Prostaglandins have been implicated, and they may also affect uterine motility, thus contributing to the effects of the IUD. The effects of copper on the uterus and fertilised ovum are not known.

Many women find that they cannot tolerate IUDs and the acceptability of this type of contraception is lower than for oral contraceptives. Increased and painful menstrual bleeding and abdominal cramps are the commonest causes of discontinuance. IUDs may be expelled spontaneously, for example within the first year of insertion in up to 10 per cent of women, and the presence of the nylon thread protruding through the cervix is helpful for checking that the device is still in place. More rarely, an IUD may perforate the uterus and even move into the peritoneal cavity. The failure rate of the IUD is higher than that of the pill (see table 6.1) and it has been noted that the frequency of ectopic pregnancy and spontaneous abortion is higher in women who become pregnant while using an IUD than in normal pregnancies. The frequency of pelvic inflammatory disease (which can result in permanent infertility) has been much reduced with advances in IUD technique. Most of the side effects mentioned above are more frequent or intense with the larger devices.

6.6 Possible new methods of female contraception

It is realistic to suppose that most major advances in contraception will come from the development of female-oriented methods because the single monthly event determining fertility, ovulation, is much more susceptible to attack than the continuous process of spermatogenesis in the male. Moreover, it is the female who actually becomes pregnant and is therefore more strongly motivated. There are several very promising possibilities for new female contraceptives.

The recent synthesis of the decapeptide gonadotropin releasing hormone (GnRH) has prompted searches for orally active analogues which might be capable of blocking rather than stimulating LH and FSH release. These would prevent ovulation if administered at suitable times during the menstrual cycle. No such compounds have yet been identified, but the prospects are good. An alternative approach would be to develop an antibody to GnRH.

Another exciting possibility concerns the development of an immunisation against pregnancy, and work on this is well advanced. Antibodies to the β-subunits of hCG have been prepared in monkeys by injection of β-subunits coupled to a protein carrier such as tetanus toxoid. The beta chain complex thus becomes 'foreign' and antigenic to the species into which it is injected, and stimulates antibody formation. These antibodies are capable of neutralising hCG, thus preventing its action, and in the monkey such immunisation has been shown to prevent pregnancy. This is because hCG secreted from the trophoblast is required in the early stages of pregnancy for correct blastocyst implantation and early development. Trials of this method in the human are awaited with great interest, since pregnancy is disrupted in the animal experiments for up to two years before another immunisation is required.

Nevertheless, the desire for progress must be tempered with caution since it is possible that the anti-hCG antibodies may cross-react with LH, and thereby neutralise it and disrupt physiological function, since the beta chains of hCG and LH contain homologous sequences. This possibility might be minimised by utilising the terminal 30 amino acid fragment of hCG which has no counterpart in LH, rather than the whole beta chain.

There is much impetus for the development of a postcoital pill (or 'morning-after pill') which could be used to prevent fertilisation after unprotected intercourse, and for the development of a pill capable of inducing menstruation which has been delayed, perhaps because of pregnancy. There is an evident need for such methods of 'contraception with hindsight', as many women do not plan ahead and use reliable contraceptives.

A substance capable of stimulating menstrual bleeding would be suitable, and both oestrogens and prostaglandins have been suggested for this purpose. Large doses of oestrogens stimulate myometrial contractions and cause 'menstrual' bleeding if administered for several days. They may also have a contraceptive action by accelerating the transport of the ovum down the uterine tube, thus reducing the chances of a successful fertilisation. However, there are a number of unpleasant side effects. Diethylstilboestrol was used until recently, but has now been abandoned

because of doubts concerning its safety (see section 6.4). Prostaglandin analogues prepared in gel pessaries for vaginal administration appear to be much more promising and effective; menstrual induction occurs in a high proportion of women. It is suggested that this method might be suitable for self-administration since the side effects of treatment are slight. Of course, it must be remembered that in the minds of many people 'menstrual induction' may be synonymous with 'early abortion', so it is probable that this issue will be controversial.

6.7 Assessment of risks and benefits of different types of contraceptive

All human activities carry risks and it is important in the field of contraception to bear this in mind. The *ideal* contraceptive would be 100 per cent effective and would have no side effects and no risks. Unfortunately, the most effective contraceptives, the pill and the IUD, both have some serious side effects or adverse reactions as des-

Table 6.2   Cost—benefit analysis of risks from contraception*

Contraceptive method	*Mortality due to*	*Age of women in years*	
		(20—34)	(35—44)
Pill	Method	2.4	11.5
	Accidental pregnancies	0	0.1
Diaphragm	Method	0	0
	Accidental pregnancies	0.5	2.4
Intrauterine device	Method	0.2	0.2
	Accidental pregnancies	0.7	1.5
Mortality due to pregnancy (per 100 000)		22.8	57.6
Mortality from other causes:			
cancer		13.7	70.1
traffic accidents		5.9	4.6
murder and manslaughter		1.2	1.0
suicide		4.4	7.7
Deaths from all causes		52.8	155.2

(Based on Vessey, M. P. & Doll, R. (1976). *Proc. Roy. Soc. B,* **195,** 69 and other sources.)
* Mortality rates per 100 000 women using differing methods of contraception, allowing for the dangers of the methods and for the dangers of the pregnancies which result from contraceptive failure, and for some other selected causes.

cribed, although their incidence is reassuringly low. By contrast, those methods which are safe in terms of absence of side effects are relatively inefficient contraceptives. Individuals must obviously reach a decision if they are faced with choosing a method, and it should be based on proper information.

Table 6.2 gives a cost—benefit analysis of three female-oriented contraceptive methods — the pill, IUD and diaphragm — in terms of associated mortality, together with some other information about risks to life. It should be borne in mind that not only is unwanted pregnancy highly undesirable and unfortunate for all parties, but also carries its own substantial risk to life.

Further reading

Frisch, R. E. (1978). 'Population, food intake and fertility', *Science*, **199**, 22

Llewellyn-Jones, D. (1974). *Human Reproduction and Society*, Faber, London

May, R. H. (1978). 'Human reproduction reconsidered', *Nature*, **272**, 491

Peel, J. and Potts, M. (1971). *Textbook of Contraceptive Practice*, Cambridge University Press

Short, R. V. and Baird, D. T. (eds.) (1976). 'Contraceptives of the future', *Proc. Roy. Soc. B.*, **195**, 1—224

7

The Placenta

7.1 Nutrition of developing organisms

During embryonic development animals require a substantial and constantly available source of nourishment, and in addition must be able to respire and excrete. This is accomplished in vertebrates in one of three principal ways.

(1) *Simple eggs* contain nutrients in the form of yolk, and are found in fish and amphibians. Respiratory and excretory exchange occurs by diffusion between the shell-less egg and its watery environment. While suitable for fish and for the aquatic larval stage of amphibians, such a stratagem is useless for a fully terrestrial animal as dehydration of the egg cannot be prevented.

(2) The *amniote egg* of the bird or reptile (figure 7.1) represents an important evolutionary advance since it permits a fully terrestrial life cycle. The egg is surrounded by a shell which retains water but allows gaseous exchange. The embryo develops in a fluid-filled sac, the amnion, and its non-gaseous metabolic wastes, such as uric acid, are stored in another sac, the allantois. The membranes of both these sacs are vascular and are involved in gas exchange. The food source is yolk contained within a yolk sac as in the lower vertebrates. In reptiles the eggs are most often incubated by absorption of heat from the environment, thus limiting reproduction to certain habitats or seasons. In birds, incubation of the eggs requires parental care and thus demands more elaborate behaviour such as pairing and nesting.

(3) *Placentation*. The most primitive mammals are the prototherians, such as the platypus, which lay reptile-like amniote eggs. A major reproductive achievement of all other mammals was the evolution of *placentation*, the association between certain tissues of the female reproductive tract and embryonic membranes. This association permits the exchange of substances between embryo and mother, and allows much better and more prolonged embryonic nutrition, thus supporting intrauterine development of a much more complex fetus. The membranes which form the placenta are homologous with those of the amniote egg of reptiles; maternal tissues make contact with the external surface or chorion of the embryo, which in turn is closely applied to the vessels of the allantois or of the yolk sac. Thus placentae may be either of the *chorioallantoic* or *yolk sac* type (figure 7.2). In the marsupials the association is transient and this placenta can only support the embryo in the early stages of its development; gestation in such species is short and the newborn is very immature. In contrast, the true placental mammals have greatly elaborated the transport capacity of the chorioallantoic placenta so that a well-developed fetus may be delivered.

The development of placentation means that the offspring can be fed, protected and transported within the mother's body. Furthermore the needs of mother and fetus can be satisfied jointly rather than in competition, and fetal homeostasis is improved by indirect access to the fully developed maternal systems. However, these advantages are obtained at a price: the metabolic demands of the

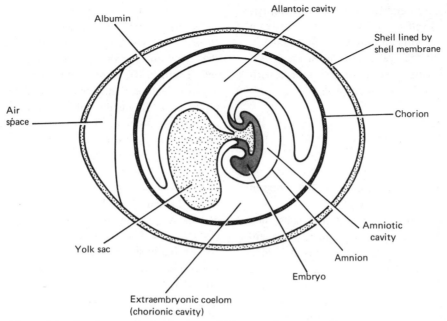

Figure 7.1   Amniote egg in development. This type of egg occurs in reptiles and birds, but the same membranes are present in mammalian development

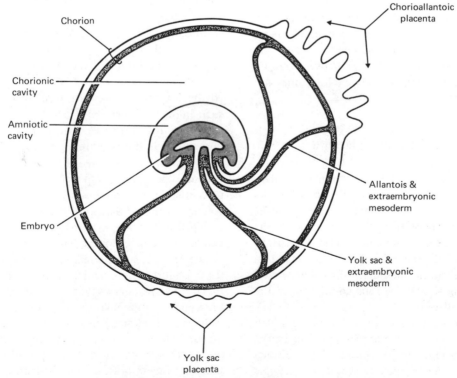

Figure 7.2   Yolk sac and chorioallantoic placentae

fetus impose a considerable burden on the mother, and parturition itself carries significant risks from hazards such as trauma and infection. In summary, the development of placentation substantially improves the survival chances of the embryo with a slight increase in risk to the mother.

7.2 The yolk sac placenta

A placenta may develop where the vascular connective tissue of an embryonic membrane comes in contact with the inside of the trophoblastic covering of the conceptus. In many mammals such contact forms between the yolk sac and trophoblast, giving rise to a yolk sac or choriovitelline placenta (see figure 7.2). This is often a transient structure which regresses when a chorioallantoic placenta is established. In some groups, notably rodents, the ventral parts of the chorion and yolk sac disappear so that the yolk sac cavity opens into the uterine lumen. This 'inverted' yolk sac placenta persists throughout gestation and is important as a route for antibody transfer from mother to fetus. In the human embryo the very early development of the extraembryonic coelom prevents the establishment of any vascular link between chorion and yolk sac, so yolk sac placentation does not occur.

7.3 The chorioallantoic placenta

The allantois is a ventral outgrowth of the hindgut endoderm into the presumptive body stalk. Its duct plays an important role in the development of the lower urinary tract (chapter 9), whilst its covering of extraembryonic mesoderm is crucial to development of the chorioallantoic placenta. Within this allantoic mesoderm the blood vessels develop giving rise to the fetal component of the placental circulation.

In chapter 5 we described the manner in which the blastocyst invades the uterine wall. The extent of this invasion varies considerably between species; it may be completely absent, for example in ruminants and horses, or at the other extreme

can cause extensive erosion of maternal vessel walls, as in man and rodents. This invasion is carried out by the epithelial layer of the chorion, the trophoblast. During the implantation phase cell fusion in the outer trophoblast gives rise to a multinucleate surface layer called the syncytiotrophoblast, while deeper cells retain their individuality forming a cellular layer known as the cytotrophoblast; in man these two placental components can be recognised throughout gestation.

Invasion of maternal tissue occurs by the penetration of syncytial processes, the primary villi, through the endometrial epithelium and connective tissue into the endometrial vessels (figure 7.3). The maternal tissue is broken down but probably serves as a source of nutrients for the conceptus prior to the establishment of a placental circulation. When the maternal capillaries have been penetrated the villi are bathed in maternal blood which now flows sluggishly through the intervillous spaces. Initially the villi consist of trophoblast alone, but soon acquire a core of allantoic mesoderm which subsequently becomes vascularised.

Initially the entire trophoblastic surface is covered with villi, but as growth continues they become concentrated over the embryonic pole, and those on the rest of the surface atrophy (figure 7.4). The composite layer of trophoblast, extraembryonic mesoderm and vessels is termed the *chorion*, and may be divided into the smooth, unspecialised chorion covering most of the surface (chorion laeve), and the villous area which will become the fetal component of the definitive placenta (chorion frondosum). The human placenta belongs to the *haemochorial* group of chorioallantoic placentae since maternal blood is directly in contact with the chorion. The early development of the chorion and its relationship with maternal tissue is illustrated in figures 7.3 and 7.4.

The invasive and cytodestructive behaviour of the syncytiotrophoblast is very reminiscent of a malignant neoplasm. This resemblance goes further than merely invasiveness, as fragments of syncytium often become detached from the placenta and sometimes metastasise to maternal sites, especially the lungs. Such 'secondaries' regress after parturi-

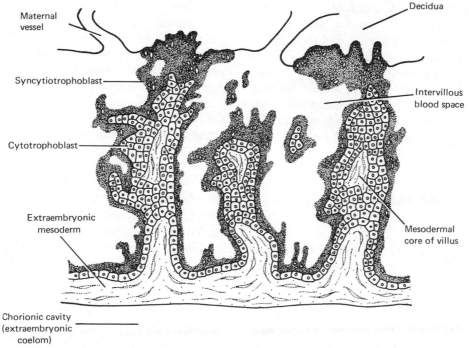

Figure 7.3   Placenta at the stem villus stage. Chorionic villi have eroded away the maternal tissue so that maternal blood now flows between the villi. The cyotrophoblast still forms a continuous layer and the villi are not yet vascularised

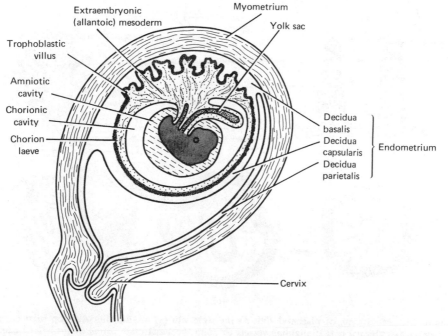

Figure 7.4   Placenta in relation to adjacent structures. With further development the embryo and amniotic cavity enlarge more rapidly than the other intrauterine structures

tion, presumably due to lack of hormonal support. Occasionally trophoblast invasion gets out of control; the embryo is destroyed and the trophoblast forms a malignant, life-threatening neoplasm called a *choriocarcinoma*. Apart from its clinical importance this neoplasm is of interest for two reasons: its growth often remains dependent on the hormones of pregnancy, and it is of immunological interest as it has fetal rather than maternal genotype.

7.4 Development of the 'definitive' placenta

It is not entirely logical to attempt to describe the 'definitive' placental form, as is common practice, because the structure of this organ changes throughout its life. Indeed, at term it is probably senescent rather than mature or 'definitive'. However, by the end of the first trimester the placenta has become a stable structure which persists until term with only minor morphological changes apart from growth. During the phase of invasion and villus formation in the first month the essential interface between maternal and fetal circulations is established. Further cellular changes at this interface lead to an increase in the vessel surface area available for exchange, reduction in thickness of the barriers between maternal and fetal blood and establishment of an efficient pattern of blood flow.

The villi described so far are completely covered in syncytiotrophoblast. This soon disappears from the tips of the villi and cytotrophoblast grows out through the gaps. Outgrowths from adjacent villi fuse so as to form a plate of cytotrophoblast separating the maternal blood spaces from the underlying endometrial tissue (figure 7.5). This layer is perforated only by the maternal vessels carrying blood to and from the intervillous spaces, and is known as the *basal plate* to distinguish it from the *chorionic plate* from which the villi originally developed. The villi .are therefore no longer free, but extend like pillars from the

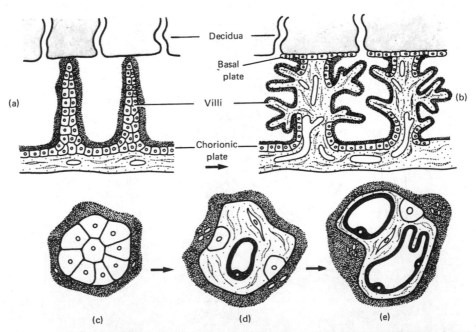

Figure 7.5   Maturation of placental villi. As the stem villi (a) mature they develop branches and acquire a mesodermal core containing vessels (b), and the basal plate forms by growth of trophoblast over the decidual surface. The transverse sections (c)–(e) show enlargement of fetal vessels and thinning of the trophoblast as the villi mature

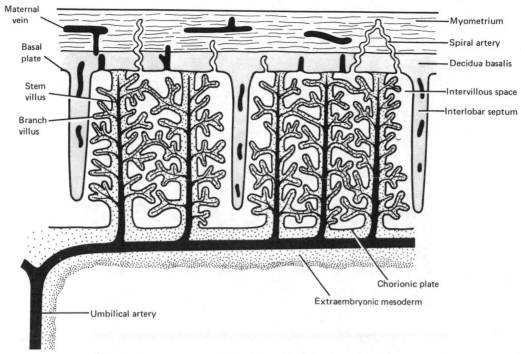

Figure 7.6   Organisation of the term placenta. The maternal blood space is incompletely divided into lobes by the septa

chorionic plate on the fetal side to the basal plate on the maternal side. Around them flows the maternal blood, while within their cores of mesoderm lie the fetal capillaries (figure 7.5). The maternal blood space becomes incompletely divided into lobar regions by septa growing out from the basal plate, but as these do not reach the chorionic plate, blood can in principle flow from one lobe to the next (figures 7.6 and 7.7). Placental blood flow is discussed in relation to placental exchange in section 7.6.

During the phase of rapid placental development in the first and second trimesters abundant lateral branches sprout from the stem villi. These also acquire mesodermal cores and vascularisation from fetal capillaries, becoming the most important sites of exchange between mother and fetus. The outgrowth of these lateral villi requires the formation of large amounts of new syncytiotrophoblast by incorporation of cytotrophoblast cells; this raised rate of recruitment exceeds the capacity of the cytotrophoblast to proliferate. Thus the new

branch villi lack a complete layer of cytotrophoblast under the syncytium, and only contain occasional scattered clusters of cytotrophoblast cells. This may be advantageous as it reduces the thickness of the barrier separating the two circulations. As the branch villi mature the syncytium itself thins until it becomes attenuated, organelle-poor *alpha-syncytium*. This contrasts with the thicker, organelle-rich regions, found primarily on the stem villi, which are concerned with synthetic rather than exchange functions and are known as *beta-syncytium*. During the thinning phase the amount of connective tissue in the villi is reduced and the diameter of the fetal capillaries increases. All of these changes potentially increase the efficiency of the villi as an exchange interface. This is vital because the rate of fetal growth outstrips that of the placenta from the 14th week onwards (figure 7.8).

The area of membrane exposed to blood in the placenta is very large. Reliable figures based on electron microscopy are not available for man, but

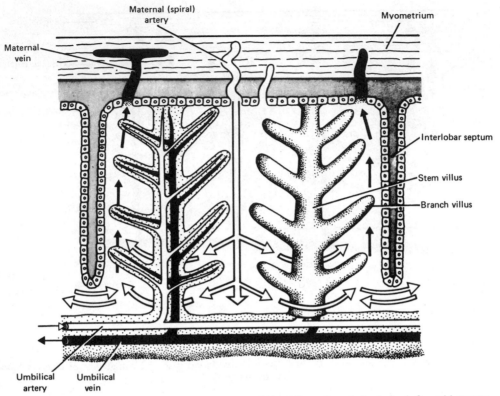

Figure 7.7   Blood flows in mature placenta. Maternal blood from the spiral arteries is forced between the villi, exchanging materials with the fetal blood perfusing them

in the guinea-pig the total area of blood-contacting membrane is as much as 750 mm² per cubic millimetre of placental tissue at term.

7.5   Factors affecting placental exchange

Normal growth and development of the fetus is only possible if there is adequate placental exchange of nutrients, oxygen and metabolic wastes. These transport processes appear to be fulfilled almost exclusively by the chorioallantoic placenta. The rate of exchange of any particular substance depends on a number of factors, the most important of which are:

(1)   Area available for exchange.
(2)   Thickness of the barrier between circulations.
(3)   Permeability of the barrier.

(4)   Concentration gradient.
(5)   The rate of blood flow on each side.
(6)   Relative flow geometry of the two blood streams.
(7)   Removal or production of substance by the placenta itself.
(8)   Special transport or binding systems.

This is not an exhaustive catalogue, nor are all these factors necessarily important for every substance. Penetration of substances such as salts, nutrients and macromolecules which are exchanged or accumulated relatively slowly by the fetus is limited by the barrier characteristics of the placenta. By contrast the rate of placental blood flow is the most important limiting factor for highly diffusible substances such as the blood gases. It must be emphasised that this subject is still poorly understood because the techniques for measuring blood concentrations of substances in both fetal

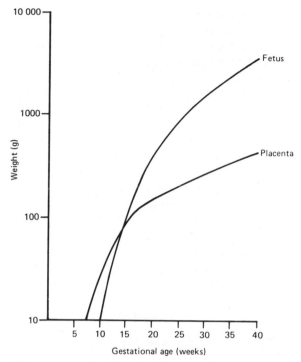

Figure 7.8 Fetal and placental growth. Fetal and placental weights as a function of gestational age. Weights are plotted on a logarithmic scale

and maternal placental circulations are difficult and of uncertain reliability. Furthermore it is not safe to extrapolate animal results to man due to the great variation in structure and function found in the placentae of different species.

7.6 Placental blood flow

It is evident that the magnitude and direction of the concentration gradient of a substance across the placental barrier will be a major determinant of its transfer rate. This gradient is in turn dependent on the rate and pattern of blood flow, provided that the solute transfer rate is fast enough to cause significant depletion from one stream and accumulation in the other. This is certainly so in the cases of blood gases and nutrients, and indeed inadequate maternal perfusion may sometimes limit fetal growth.

The relationships between maternal and fetal blood have already been indicated in section 7.4

and are summarised in figure 7.7. Measurement of the perfusion rate of the maternal vessels is fraught with difficulty because the uterine arteries supply the rest of the uterus as well as the inter-villous spaces of the placenta. Total uterine flow can be measured by a method based on the Fick principle, using nitrous oxide as the indicator substance, and gives values of about 13 ml blood per 100 g per minute for the human uterus at term (figure 7.9). Comparison of such results for the pregnant and the non-pregnant uterus permits an indirect estimate of maternal placental flow. There are other more accurate methods which are unfortunately invasive, but the several methods used to date all give values near term of about 100 ml/100 g placental tissue per minute, equivalent to a total placental blood perfusion rate of 650 ml/min for an average-sized placenta. Uterine and fetal placental flow is of course much lower earlier in gestation and increases about tenfold between the tenth week and term (figure 7.10), although the rate of blood flow per unit uterine weight remains fairly constant throughout gestation (figure 7.9). Thus maternal perfusion of the placenta is very high in relation to the tissue mass and has a flow rate similar to that of brain in the adult and some 50

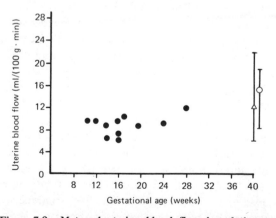

Figure 7.9 Maternal uterine blood flow in relation to uterine weight. The total uterine weight has been used to calculate blood flow which was determined by the Fick principle with nitrous oxide as the indicator. Solid points are flow rates obtained at hysterotomy and the open triangle and circle the mean flow rates obtained at caesarean section in two different investigations (Redrawn from Carter, A. M. (1975). *Comparative Placentation* (Ed. Steven, D. H.), Academic Press, London)

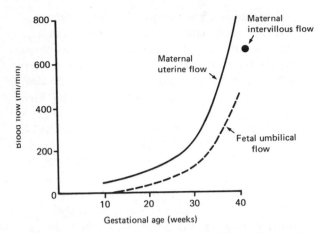

Figure 7.10 Total maternal uterine blood flow and umbilical blood flow during pregnancy. Note the rapid increase in perfusion of both sides of the placenta during the final few weeks of pregnancy. A single point for maternal intervillous flow is plotted for comparison (Modified from Rhodes, P. (1969). *Reproductive Physiology for Medical Students.* **J. & A. Churchill, London)**

times larger than that of adult resting skeletal muscle. It represents about 10 per cent of cardiac output at term (see chapter 11).

Since the volume of the intervillous blood space at term is about 250 ml, the measured flow rate implies that the blood is totally replaced 2.5 times every minute. This sounds extremely sluggish, but in fact the blood is very well mixed and reaches the steady-state values found in the venous outflow very rapidly. Blood enters the intervillous spaces at the high pressure of 100 mmHg, and injection of radio-opaque dyes into the spiral arteries of the uterus shows that it penetrates through the mass of chorionic villi, reaching the chorionic plate as a mushrooming jet. Blood then flows back along the interlobar septa to drain from the intervillous space through the decidual veins (see figure 7.7). The mean transit time for an erythrocyte is about 15 s. The dye technique also reveals that the interlobar septa effectively isolate blood flow within an individual lobe even though they are not fused to the chorionic plate, although the gaps in these septa may allow the pressures in adjacent lobes to equalise. The blood pressure in the intervillous spaces is about 10–15 mmHg, falling to a typical venous pressure of 5 mmHg in

the decidual veins. Therefore with such a high arteriovenous pressure gradient, any breakdown in the attachment of the trophoblast to the decidua would lead to haemorrhage and thus endanger the pregnancy.

There is little evidence for active autoregulation of maternal blood flow through the placenta; it appears to be a relatively constant fraction of the mother's cardiac output, and falls during maternal sleep. The uterus has a sympathetic innervation but there is conflicting evidence regarding its importance in regulating maternal placental perfusion. The uterine circulation is certainly sensitive to circulating hormones and drugs: adrenaline and noradrenaline reduce uterine perfusion whereas acetylcholine and histamine increase flow. Oestrogens also increase uterine blood flow in the long term, but are unlikely to be involved in active regulation of the vascular bed. Maternal hypertension arising from generalised vasoconstriction may also reduce uterine blood flow significantly and impair fetal growth.

In principle it is easier to measure fetal blood flow as the umbilical arteries supply the entire fetal aspect of the placenta and nothing else; therefore the flow in the umbilical arteries should equal that in the umbilical veins. The main practical problem is that the techniques required are invasive and cause the extremely irritable umbilical vessels to contract, thus reducing flow.

Most observations have been made at hysterotomy or immediately after delivery; in both cases the umbilical circulation is still intact but changing and the measurements may not be truly representative. In 10–28-week-old fetuses umbilical flows of about 11.0 ml/100 g fetus per minute have been obtained. Extrapolation of this value to the average term fetus yields a total fetal–placental blood flow of 360 ml/min, that is over one-half of the entire fetal cardiac output. Although umbilical blood flow remains relatively constant per unit weight of fetus, as does maternal placental perfusion, total flow increases during gestation (see figure 7.10).

The fetal capillary volume of the term placenta is about 45 ml, and thus blood is replaced 8 times per minute as compared with 2.5 times per minute on the maternal side. The fetal blood spaces of the placenta may therefore be regarded as a low volume—high turnover compartment, whereas the maternal side has large volume—slow turnover characteristics, an arrangement which may favour dialysis of materials from maternal blood. An advantage of this is that if the uterine circulation is temporarily obstructed, the fetus may be able to continue to extract materials from the intervillous blood pool for a limited period.

It is hard to determine whether the fetus actively controls placental perfusion. Although the umbilical arteries and veins are only innervated in their short intra-abdominal segments, it is possible that the substantial smooth muscle coats of these vessels may regulate flow during gestation and at birth if exposed to suitable concentrations of vasoactive agents. Local hormones such as bradykinin and the prostaglandins and thromboxanes, as well as adrenaline and noradrenaline, produce powerful constriction of umbilical vessels *in vitro*, and such agents may be involved in the autoregulation of the umbilical circulation. In addition these vessels are very sensitive to oxygen tension: hypoxia causes vasodilation, whereas a rise in oxygen tension produces vasoconstriction.

Reflex control of fetal cardiac output is established during the final trimester of pregnancy, and this permits some measure of regulation of fetal placental perfusion. Mild fetal hypoxia, hypercapnia or both cause a rise in fetal heart rate and mean blood pressure, thereby increasing placental perfusion so as to restore homeostasis.

7.7 Barrier characteristics of the placenta

As stated in section 7.5, the thickness and permeability of the tissue layer separating maternal and fetal circulations may be important determinants of the transfer rates of many substances. It has already been pointed out that the syncytiotrophoblast undergoes differentiation into thin (alpha) and thicker (beta) regions, and that the former are the main transport areas. Some data comparing oxygen transport in the placenta with neonatal lung are collected in table 7.1 and demonstrate that the diffusion capacity for oxygen of the placenta is similar to that of the neonatal lung even though its thickness is considerably greater, However, evidence from animal experiments suggests that barrier characteristics may be much more important determinants of the transfer of less freely diffusible substances.

The structure of the human placental barrier in a typical alpha-syncytial region is illustrated in figure 7.11. The scattered nature of the cytotrophoblast means that only two continuous cellular

Table 7.1 Oxygen transport across the placenta and neonatal lung

	Fetus	*Neonate*
Body weight (kg)	3.3	3.3
Thickness of barrier (μm)	2.0—5.5	0.3—2.5†
Exchange surface area (m^2)	11	3
Oxygen diffusion capacity (ml/mmHg min))	1.2‡	2.5
Oxygen diffusion gradient across barrier (mmHg)	19—24	11†
Nominal transfer capacity* (ml/kg body wt)	6.9—8.7	8.3
Oxygen consumption (ml/kg)	5—7	6—8

* Calculated as (diffusion capacity × diffusion gradient)/(body weight).
† Based on adult values.
‡ This value may be too low because of oxygen consumption by the placenta itself.

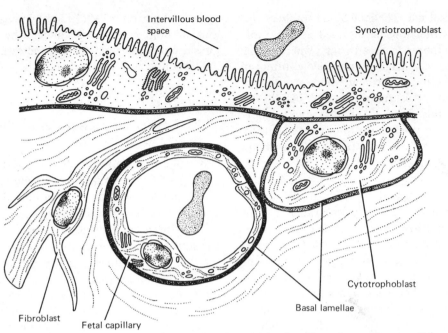

Figure 7.11   Ultrastructure of the human placental barrier. The only continuous cellular layers between the two circulations are the syncytiotrophoblast and the fetal endothelium, each attached to its own basal lamella. The intervening connective tissue is thin and is unlikely to form an important barrier

layers are interposed between the circulations: the syncytiotrophoblast and the fetal endothelium. The syncytiotrophoblast forms a continuous sheet without intercellular channels, while the endothelium lacks fenestrations and has well-developed tight junctions spanning the intercellular spaces. The features of both cellular layers in the human therefore favour the idea that the transfer of substances across the barrier must be transcellular rather than intercellular and must involve passage across four plasma membranes. However, experimental evidence from rodents and other animals with haemochorial placentae implies the existence of paracellular hydrophilic channels across the barrier, although admittedly these species generally have a fenestrated endothelial layer. The mechanism for transport across the syncytiotrophoblast is still obscure, but an endocytosis–exocytosis mechanism involving the numerous membrane-bounded vesicles is a possibility. It is unfortunate that there is no convenient experimental animal with the same placental barrier structure as man.

7.8   Placental transport functions

Gas transport

Transport of gases across the placenta is believed to be dependent on simple diffusion alone, with transfer rate proportional to the difference in partial pressures across the barrier. The rate at which any particular gas crosses the interface is determined by its diffusion coefficient, which falls with increasing molecular size. In practice the diffusion coefficients of the respiratory gases are so large that blood perfusion rates limit their transfer and small variations of the barrier characteristics do not affect the rate of gas exchange. Values for respiratory gas partial pressures and for pH in the uterine and umbilical blood vessels are given in figure 7.12.

Oxygen

The diffusion capacity of the placenta for a gas can only be calculated accurately if the partial

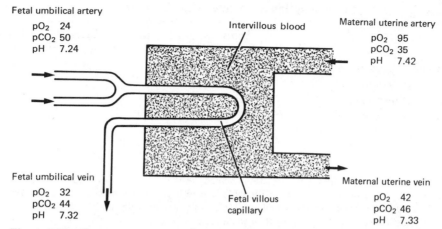

Fetal umbilical artery
pO$_2$ 24
pCO$_2$ 50
pH   7.24

Intervillous blood

Maternal uterine artery
pO$_2$ 95
pCO$_2$ 35
pH   7.42

Fetal umbilical vein
pO$_2$ 32
pCO$_2$ 44
pH   7.32

Fetal villous
capillary

Maternal uterine vein
pO$_2$ 42
pCO$_2$ 46
pH   7.33

Figure 7.12 Gross arrangements of the placental circulations and typical blood gas concentrations (in mmHg) and pH values in inflow and outflow blood. Note that shunts occur on the maternal and probably also the fetal side so that not all of the blood in the venous outflows has been in contact with the exchange surfaces

pressure gradient between the two circulations is known. It is difficult to obtain values for the gradient within specified placental areas because of the problem of identifying the exact source of the samples. The gradient is usually estimated by measuring oxygen tension in both the uterine and umbilical veins; the mean pressure gradient of oxygen between maternal and fetal blood is 19–24 mmHg, which is relatively large compared with that in the adult lung in which complete equilibration of oxygen tension occurs between alveolar gas and blood. This finding implies that the placenta has a rather low diffusion capacity for oxygen, which might thus be a limiting factor for the supply of oxygen to the fetus. However this is probably not so, because the presence of shunts on the maternal and perhaps fetal sides causes venous oxygen tensions to deviate from the equilibrium values achieved at the exchange interface.

Another difficulty in measuring oxygen transport is that the placenta is metabolically active and itself utilises up to 20 per cent of the extracted oxygen. Therefore there is always an oxygen concentration gradient between maternal and fetal blood irrespective of any diversion of blood through shunts. Furthermore, this means that oxygen transfer across the placenta cannot be measured by the

Fick principle using oxygen as a marker. In the sheep this problem has been overcome by determining the permeability of the placenta to carbon monoxide which is not metabolised. The relative diffusibilities of oxygen and carbon monoxide in the lung are known accurately, and so values for the placental diffusibility of oxygen can be estimated from those measured for carbon monoxide. These experiments suggest that oxygen is about four times more diffusible than is implied by measurements of the venous partial pressures. Diffusional resistance is therefore unlikely to limit the supply of oxygen to the fetus.

The oxygen consumption of the uterus and its contents at term are shown in table 7.2. Although the placenta has the highest oxygen consumption per unit mass, its relatively small mass compared with the other components means that its share of the total oxygen extraction from the uterine flow is fairly small. The entire fetoplacental unit at term extracts between 19 and 27 ml of oxygen per minute from the blood perfusing the intervillous space.

Release of oxygen from the maternal blood to the placental tissue is determined by the same factors that operate in other tissues; oxygen dissolved in the plasma determines the diffusion

Table 7.2   Oxygen consumption by the uterus and its contents*

	Fetus	Placenta	Uterus	Total
Estimated oxygen consumption at term (ml/kg min))	5–7	7–10	3.5	15.5–20.5
Weight at term (kg)	3.3	0.42	0.98	4.7
Calculated oxygen consumption (ml/min)	17–23	2.9–4.2	3.4	23.3–30.6

* The cord and membranes have not been included in these calculations because their oxygen consumption is not accurately known. Although the cord is greatest in mass, it has a low oxygen consumption per unit mass and the membranes, although metabolically active, contribute little to the total oxygen consumption because of their small mass.

gradient and therefore the direction and rate of transfer, but itself only forms a small proportion of the total oxygen content of the blood.

The haemoglobin content of fetal blood is about 18 g/100 ml and the haematocrit is 60 per cent, both significantly higher than the maternal values. The red cell count is within the normal adult range but the cells are larger, increasing the oxygen-carrying capacity of fetal blood by as much as 50 per cent.

Transfer of oxygen to the fetus is also facilitated by the high affinity of fetal haemoglobin for oxygen. A structural difference in the globin chains of fetal haemoglobin (see chapter 11) causes it to have a lower binding affinity for 2,3-diphosphoglycerate, a product of the glycolytic pathway which reduces the affinity of haemoglobin for oxygen. Maternal and fetal erythrocytes contain similar concentrations of this metabolite, but the lower affinity of fetal haemoglobin for it effectively shifts its oxygen dissociation curve to the left of the maternal curve (figure 7.13). Thus at normal oxygen tensions fetal haemoglobin operates within a more steeply rising portion of the dissociation curve than that of the mother; this means that a small change in oxygen partial pressure causes a much larger change in oxygen saturation in the blood of the fetus (figure 7.13).

Efficiency of oxygen transfer is also influenced by carbon dioxide movement in the opposite direction, which causes the pH of maternal blood

to fall from 7.42 to 7.33, while fetal blood pH rises from 7.24 to 7.32. These changes in hydrogen ion concentration also alter the oxygen affinity of haemoglobin (*the Bohr shift*). A rise in pH increases oxygen affinity in the fetal blood (shifting the curve to the left in figure 7.13) whilst a fall shifts the maternal affinity curve to the right. This increases the separation of the two curves and so enhances oxygen transfer to fetal blood.

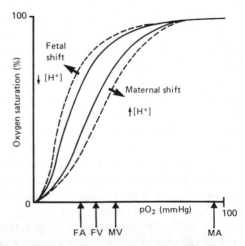

Figure 7.13   Dissociation curves of maternal and fetal haemoglobin (FA, fetal umbilical arterial pO_2; FV, fetal umbilical venous pO_2; MV, maternal uterine venous pO_2; MA, maternal uterine arterial pO_2). Maternal blood becomes more acidic and fetal blood less acidic as they pass through the placenta. This produces the unique 'double Bohr effect' which greatly facilitates oxygen transference from maternal to fetal blood

Carbon dioxide

Blood flow and diffusion gradients affect carbon dioxide transport in much the same way as oxygen. Since carbon dioxide is far more soluble and permeant than oxygen, conditions which are adequate for transplacental oxygen transport have a large reserve capacity in respect of carbon dioxide. None the less, shunting prevents complete equilibration of carbon dioxide between the two circulations (figure 7.12). In both fetal and maternal plasma about 60 per cent of carbon dioxide is carried as bicarbonate, about 30 per cent as carbamino complexes with proteins and only about 8 per cent in physical solution.

Diffusion of dissolved carbon dioxide down the concentration gradient from the fetal to the maternal blood shifts the maternal and fetal equilibria between bicarbonate and carbon dioxide so that bicarbonate is formed in the mother and lost in the fetus (figure 7.14). Attainment of the new equilibrium is accelerated by erythrocyte carbonic anhydrase activity, but this activity is much lower in the fetus than in the mother. In addition, oxygenation of fetal blood causes release of hydrogen ions which associate with bicarbonate and shift the equilibrium in favour of carbon dioxide.

The placenta has a very low permeability to bicarbonate ions; indeed a significant net flux of any anion would require either a concurrent loss of cations or a counterflow of another anion species such as chloride, and either of these mechanisms would lead to an ionic imbalance in the fetus.

Water transport

A large bidirectional water flux across the placenta can be demonstrated using isotopically labelled water. This flux increases during pregnancy and by the 35th week there is an exchange of about 35 l/h. A net flux of water from mother to fetus or vice versa occurs in the presence of an osmotic gradient. If the osmolarity of maternal plasma is raised by intravenous injection of sucrose, fetal dehydration occurs due to rapid passage of water across the placenta into maternal plasma until osmotic equilibrium is restored.

Although the fetus accumulates water in step with its growth, there is no demonstrable osmotic gradient across the placenta; the osmolarities of the maternal and fetal circulations are always found to be equal, as are the osmolarities of umbilical arterial and venous blood. The best explanation for the net gain of water by the fetus is that fetal accumulation of osmotically active material generates a potential osmotic gradient which is immediately cancelled by the entry of water from the mother.

The placenta may not be the only site at which the fetus can exchange water. Exchange with amniotic fluid coupled with a possible water flux across the amnion may also occur (see chapter 11).

Cation transport

The exchange of sodium across the placenta (figure 7.15) is remarkably similar to that of water. The decline in placental exchange after 35 weeks may be attributable to ageing processes in the placenta such as fibrinoid deposition or infarction of portions of the fetal vascular bed, and probably applies to most substances towards term. Sodium transfer is membrane-limited and depends on the characteristics of the tissue layer

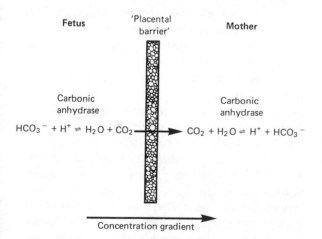

$$HCO_3^- + H^+ \rightleftharpoons H_2O + CO_2 \longrightarrow CO_2 + H_2O \rightleftharpoons H^+ + HCO_3^-$$

Concentration gradient

Figure 7.14   Carbon dioxide transfer from fetal to maternal blood

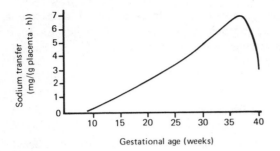

Figure 7.15 Sodium exchange across the placenta in relation to gestational age (Redrawn from Dancis, J. and Schneider, H. (1975). *The Placenta* **(ed. Gruenwald, P.), MTP, Lancaster)**

separating the two circulations. The direction of net sodium exchange appears to be determined by the concentration gradient which favours movement into the fetus as its extracellular fluid volume increases during growth, but there is a very large margin of safety since the bidirectional exchange rate for sodium is about 1000 times the net rate of accumulation of sodium by the fetus.

There is experimental evidence in animals for the existence of a placental sodium–potassium pump which probably contributes significantly to transplacental potassium balance. Any effect on sodium concentrations is overwhelmed by the very large passive fluxes. Fetal and maternal plasma potassium levels are both normally between 3.6 and 4.6 mmol/l. However, experiments on rodents show that the fetal plasma potassium level can be protected by the potassium pump which is probably located in the syncytiotrophoblast.

Fetal blood levels of both free and protein-bound calcium are higher than the corresponding maternal values, implying that this ion is actively transported. By contrast magnesium ions equilibrate freely across the placenta.

Iron transport across the placenta is of particular importance during the last trimester for the maintenance of fetal erythropoiesis. In the rabbit it has been shown that iron is actively removed from maternal transferrin by the placenta and transported against its concentration gradient into the fetal circulation.

Anion transport

Chloride concentrations on both sides of the placenta are very similar and its transfer probably closely follows that of sodium, thereby preserving electrochemical equilibrium.

In many species the fetal plasma levels of free iodide are higher than in the mother due to active transplacental transport which can be inhibited by thiocyanate. However, maternal and fetal plasma levels of protein-bound iodine are equal.

Metabolite transport

Glucose is by far the most important metabolic substrate for the fetoplacental unit. It is a relatively polar molecule and so its transfer across the placenta would be slow if limited by diffusion alone. In fact the rate of glucose transport is much higher than expected because it is carried by facilitated diffusion; fructose has exactly the same molecular weight and diffusion coefficient as glucose but is transported only one-tenth as fast. Maternal and fetal fasting plasma glucose concentrations are fairly similar, the maternal level usually being higher by some 0.4 mmol/l. One consequence of this rapid transport is that mothers with uncontrolled diabetes mellitus and high plasma glucose levels tend to have heavy babies because the rate of glucose entry into the fetus is increased. Such babies have a thick layer of subcutaneous fat and also hyperplastic pancreatic islet tissue due to the active secretion of insulin which lowers fetal blood glucose and favours fat synthesis.

The levels of free amino acids in fetal umbilical venous blood are higher than the levels for the same amino acids in maternal arterial blood. Amino acid transport is active, can be slowed by metabolic inhibitors, and predictably is stereospecific for the L isomers. Transport can occur against a concentration gradient and some amino acids show competition with one another for transport sites. Figure 7.16 shows the results of an experiment in which an isolated living cotyledon from a human placenta was perfused with Ringer solution containing equal amounts of L- and

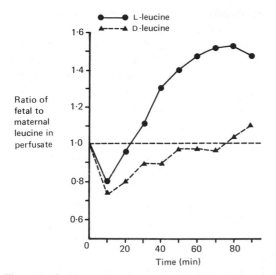

Figure 7.16   Transport of L- and D-leucine in an isolated perfused human placental lobule. Fetal concentrations of leucine appear to fall at the beginning of the experiment. This is due to dilution by buffer containing no amino acid which has been retained in the fetal circulation during tissue preparation (Redrawn from Dancis, J. and Schneider, H. (1975). *The Placenta* (ed. Gruenwald, P.), MTP, Lancaster)

D-leucine on both maternal and fetal sides. The L isomer was readily transported into the fetal compartment but the D form was not.

In general, proteins and polypeptides cannot cross the placenta in significant amounts. An important exception to this is immunoglobulin G antibody which is actively transported from mother to fetus. The transport system involves specific pinocytosis and can produce fetal plasma immunoglobulin G titres well in excess of maternal levels at a time when the fetus is synthesising little immunoglobulin of its own. This antibody transport provides the newborn with passive immunity to some antigens previously encountered by its mother and thus gives it some measure of protection against infection during the first few weeks of postnatal life.

Human fetal and maternal plasma levels of free fatty acids are similar. Lipoproteins are not transported intact across the placenta; instead the phospholipid is hydrolysed and the resulting free fatty acids enter the fetus to be resynthesised into phospholipids in the fetal liver. Cholesterol is able to cross the placenta freely.

Hormone transport

The ability of hormones to cross the placenta depends on their physicochemical properties. The placenta is impermeable to polypeptide, protein and glycoprotein hormones, and their levels in fetal and maternal circulations may fluctuate independently. By contrast, unconjugated steroids such as oestrogens, progesterone, cortisol, cortisone and testosterone can cross the placenta as readily as cholesterol by virtue of their high solubility in membrane lipids. Conjugated steroids such as sulphates and glucuronates are polar and cannot be transported without prior hydrolysis; the placenta contains sulphatases but not glucuronidases.

Thyroid hormones cross the placenta relatively easily and some of the fetal circulating thyroid hormone, essential for its normal development, is of maternal origin. On the other hand, the catecholamines adrenaline and noradrenaline do not easily cross the placenta because they are polar and also because they are inactivated in the syncytium which contains abundant monoamine oxidase.

Urea transport

Although the fetus has a positive nitrogen balance overall, protein catabolism is significant and excess fetal nitrogen returns to the mother as urea. The placenta is freely permeable to urea which diffuses into the maternal circulation down a concentration gradient, since fetal plasma levels are usually higher. About 40 per cent of the nitrogen that enters the fetus as amino acids returns to the mother as urea.

Drug transfer

Many drugs administered therapeutically to pregnant women cross the placenta. Sometimes they produce undesirable effects in the fetus. In addition environmental chemicals, including pollutants, absorbed inadvertently by the mother may have adverse effects on the fetus (see chapter 10).

The general considerations applicable to the placental transport of other substances also apply to drugs. Thus smaller, less polar substances penetrate at the fastest rates. Placental transfer of almost all drugs is diffusion limited, although rarely a substance may be stereochemically acceptable to a transport mechanism and be actively accumulated by the fetus. The placenta contains large amounts of enzymes capable of metabolising acetylcholine, histamine and oxytocin and other naturally occurring vasoactive substances, and until recently it was believed that it could also inactivate foreign chemicals and drugs by the same enzymatic routes as in the adult liver. Recent studies have disproved this, so it seems that the placenta does not protect the fetus from such foreign substances; however, the human fetus, unlike all other species so far studied, possesses its own drug metabolising enzymes in the liver and adrenals which are capable of inactivating many foreign substances by oxidation and conjugation reactions. Interestingly it has been observed that the placentae of mothers who smoke heavily contain detectable amounts of enzymes which hydroxylate polycyclic aromatic hydrocarbons and steroids. Their presence probably reflects enzyme induction in response to the polycyclic hydrocarbons in cigarette smoke. Similar enzyme induction occurs in liver and represents an adaptive response to an external chemical insult. After birth the liver of all species including man rapidly acquires the drug metabolising enzymes, often within a few days.

The powerful local anaesthetics used for spinal nerve or pudendal block are lipid-soluble and are not hydrolysed by cholinesterases present in plasma and placenta. Thus they pass readily across the placenta. Fetal bradycardia and neonatal depression sometimes occur when these drugs are used in labour if they reach significant concentrations in maternal plasma. General anaesthetics and the lipid-soluble short-acting barbiturates cross the placenta very rapidly and at the doses used for light anaes-

thesia of the mother often cause fetal depression.

Opiate analgesics are routinely used to relieve pain during labour. That they can cross the placenta is evident from the fact that they cause respiratory depression and characteristic pinpoint pupils in the newborn. Thus these analgesics are normally given only in early labour rather than close to the expected time of delivery.

It is also significant that the newborn babies of habitual users of barbiturates and opiates show dangerous withdrawal symptoms when they are removed from the maternal source of the drug at birth. This shows that these drugs can cross the placenta into the fetus in amounts sufficient to stimulate the biochemical changes of drug dependence and cellular tolerance.

Ethanol is occasionally used to inhibit threatened labour; it crosses the placenta freely but is only metabolised slowly by the fetal liver and has a depressant action on the fetus:

Infections during pregnancy are often treated with antibacterial drugs. Many of them cross the placenta relatively rapidly and attain effective antibacterial concentrations in the fetus. Placental transfer may be retarded by high plasma binding, for example of certain penicillins, or by low lipid solubility, as with some sulphonamides. Some antibiotics have harmful effects on the fetus and their use in pregnancy should obviously be avoided. For example, tetracyclines are avidly taken up by growing hard tissues and may cause permanent discoloration of a child's teeth and retard normal skeletal growth. It is thought that this may also predispose to arthritis. Streptomycin can damage the auditory nerve in the developing fetus and cause congenital deafness. Sulphonamides should not be used near term since they enter the fetus and may displace bilirubin from its plasma globulin carrier protein. In some cases the free bilirubin may produce kernicterus and cause permanent brain damage.

Many other commonly used drugs, such as the thiazide diuretics, cardiac glycosides, beta-adrenergic blockers, tranquillisers and antidepressants all enter the fetal circulation but as yet there is fortunately little evidence to suggest that these drugs may have a harmful effect.

7.9   Hormone production by the placenta

In addition to its transport and barrier functions the placenta is also an endocrine organ of crucial importance during pregnancy. It synthesises steroid hormones (oestrogens and progestogens) and also two polypeptide hormones, human chorionic gonadotropin (hCG) and human placental lactogen (hPL). All of these hormones are synthesised in the trophoblast which at term has a mass of about 60 g, which means that it is a very large endocrine organ indeed. The placenta helps to provide a correct hormonal environment in both the mother and the fetus for the maintenance of pregnancy (see chapter 5).

Steroid hormones

The maternal plasma concentrations of the steroid hormones of pregnancy are illustrated in figure 7.17. It can be seen that although the plasma levels of all of these hormones rise during pregnancy, that of progesterone is dominant. There are three major oestrogens of pregnancy: oestriol, oestrone

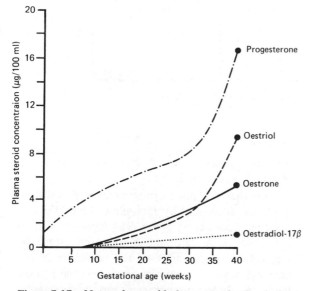

Figure 7.17   Maternal steroid hormone levels during pregnancy (Redrawn from Odell, W. D. and Moyer, D. L. (1971). *Physiology of Reproduction*, C. V. Mosby, St Louis, USA)

and oestradiol. In the menstrual cycle oestradiol is the dominant oestrogen, but in pregnancy its concentration is lower than that of oestriol or oestrone.

The placenta shares a common general pattern for the biosynthesis of steroid hormones with the adrenal cortex and gonad, although some important differences exist. Figure 7.18 is a simplified diagram of placental pathways of steroid biosynthesis. The placenta is unable to synthesise steroids from acetate and is therefore dependent on fetal and maternal cholesterol as a precursor. Progesterone can be synthesised directly from cholesterol and after the 12th week of pregnancy the placenta is the major source of this hormone; after this time the corpus luteum of pregnancy contributes little. The fetus is unable to synthesise progesterone but can modify it in its own adrenal cortex to produce glucocorticoids. At term the placenta synthesises about 350 mg progesterone per day, 90 per cent of which becomes bound to protein in maternal plasma. It is rapidly metabolised by the maternal liver and excreted in maternal urine as pregnanediol. The rate of excretion is lower than the rate of production so the plasma progesterone level rises throughout pregnancy.

Oestrogens are not directly synthesised by the placenta because it lacks the enzyme necessary to convert pregnenolone to dehydroepiandrosterone. This step is effected by the fetal adrenal cortex and the sulphated dehydroepiandrosterone which is produced is then hydroxylated in the fetal liver to produce 16α-OH dehydroepiandrosterone. This is then utilised by the placenta to produce the oestrogens of pregnancy. A smaller part of the placenta's supply of dehydroepiandrosterone is synthesised in the maternal adrenal cortex (figure 7.18). About 60 per cent of the oestrone and oestradiol and 90 per cent of the oestriol are synthesised from fetal precursors. Near term about 12 mg of oestrone, 15 mg of oestradiol and 19 mg of oestriol are secreted daily by the placenta. Figure 7.17 shows that these secretion rates are not reflected in the maternal plasma concentrations of these oestrogens since they and their conjugates are metabolised at differing rates.

The differing patterns of synthesis of the placental steroids make their levels in plasma

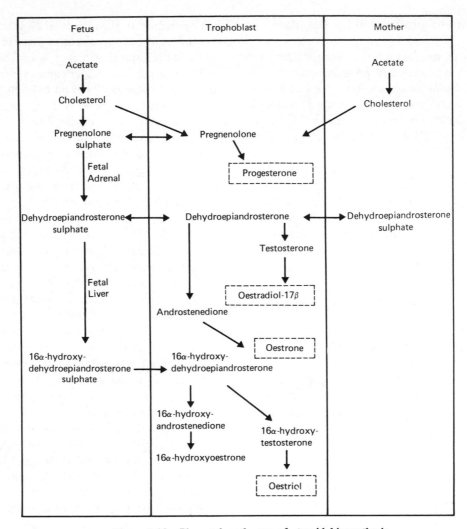

Figure 7.18   Placental pathways of steroid biosynthesis

particularly useful as indicators of fetoplacental function. Progesterone is produced by the placenta alone, so its levels in maternal plasma reflect placental function; by contrast oestrogens, particularly oestriol, are largely dependent on fetal precursors and are therefore a useful indicator of fetal well-being. For example, if the maternal oestriol level declines but the progesterone level remains constant, fetal death with a continuance of placental function is indicated. Useful information can therefore be obtained by comparing the maternal plasma steroid hormone levels with standard curves similar to figure 7.17.

Both maternal plasma progestogen and oestrogen levels are influenced by intervillous blood flow by a simple mass action effect. The higher the blood flow the more hormone is removed from the intervillous space and thus the equilibria in the placenta move in favour of greater synthesis. Low levels of both progestogen and oestrogen in maternal plasma may indicate inadequate maternal placental perfusion.

Polypeptide hormones

Human chorionic gonadotropin (hCG)

Human chorionic gonadotropin is secreted from the trophoblast extremely early in pregnancy, possibly even before implantation. The presence of hCG is thus one of the earliest diagnostic signs of pregnancy. Its function is to provide a continuous luteotropic stimulus to the corpus luteum so that luteal function extends beyond the duration of the normal menstrual cycle. In this way, continued secretion of progesterone and oestrogens is maintained so that the endometrium remains in a state favourable for implantation and embryonic nutrition (see chapter 5).

In the human, steroid secretion from the corpus luteum is only necessary until the placenta can take over this endocrine function. The very earliest that this 'independence' of the fetoplacental unit can be achieved is about 30 days. Thereafter, ovariectomy of a pregnant woman does not necessarily terminate the pregnancy. In many other mammals the corpus luteum is required for the whole duration of pregnancy as the placenta cannot itself supply all the hormones required.

Human chorionic gonadotropin can be detected in urine within a few days of conception by various highly sensitive and specific immunological assays and this forms the basis of the most reliable simple pregnancy tests available at the present time. Diagnosis of pregnancy can be made two weeks after the first missed period with 97 per cent certainty.

Levels of hCG reach a peak in early pregnancy and decline from the seventh or eighth week onwards (figure 7.19) but the hormone remains detectable until term. The levels vary widely between women. Little is known about the factors which control hCG synthesis and secretion by the placenta, but there is speculation that it may be repressed by increasing levels of progesterone of placental origin in a manner analogous to the feedback inhibition of luteinising hormone secretion from the pituitary by circulating progesterone secreted in the luteal phase of the menstrual cycle.

Human chorionic gonadotropin is one of four closely similar glycoprotein hormones. FSH, LH, TSH and hCG all share a common subunit structure

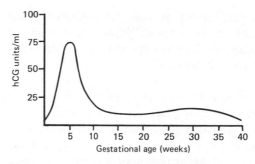

Figure 7.19 Maternal plasma hCG during pregnancy (Redrawn from Allen, W. R. (1975). *Comparative Placentation* (ed. Steven, D. H.), Academic Press, London)

of alpha and beta peptide chains linked together non-covalently. The alpha subunits of all four hormones are virtually identical, and the individual biological properties typical of each hormone are conferred by the differing beta chains. The beta chains also confer immunological specificity on each of the four hormones and this is of great practical use in the development of specific radioimmunoassays. The carbohydrate moiety of the hormones varies, but is necessary for their hormonal activity and also increases their survival in the circulation by conferring some protection against metabolism in the liver. Human chorionic gonadotropin most resembles LH and shares many of its properties, with alpha and beta chains of 90 and 145 amino acids, respectively. The beta chain of hCG has 30 more amino acid residues than LH at the carboxy-terminal end, and this is believed to enhance its luteotropic action by reducing its vulnerability to metabolism. The placenta also secretes free alpha and beta subunits of hCG but the physiological significance of this is unknown.

The measurement of maternal plasma levels of hCG is of use for the diagnosis or management of certain disorders of pregnancy such as choriocarcinoma or hydatidiform mole, both of which secrete hCG. It has also been shown that some spontaneous abortions in the first two months of pregnancy are associated with abnormally low levels of hCG production and therefore inadequate luteal function.

Purified preparations of hCG obtained from pregnant women's urine are used in conjunction with FSH for the treatment of disorders of female fertility characterised by gonadotropin deficiency. Its relatively long plasma half-life and similarities to LH are advantageous.

Human placental lactogen (hPL)

Human placental lactogen is first detectable in maternal plasma at 6–8 weeks of gestation and is secreted by the placenta in increasing amounts throughout pregnancy until the last 4–5 weeks (figure 7.20). It is produced in enormous quantities by the placenta, as much as 1 g per day in the third trimester, accounting for up to 10 per cent of the total protein output of the placenta. It has a half-life in plasma of 10–20 min and is secreted unidirectionally into maternal plasma in contrast to hCG, some of which appears in the fetal as well as in the maternal circulation. Human placental lactogen has lactogenic, luteotropic and growth hormone-like actions, and is structurally very

closely related to prolactin and growth hormone. All three hormones contain 190 amino acids; in GH and hPL 160 or more are identical. A more detailed comparison of these hormones is made in chapter 14.

Broadly defined, the functions of hPL are twofold. It stimulates mammary gland development in concert with the placental steroid hormones and pituitary prolactin. However, it is questionable whether hPL is of vital importance for the preparation of the breast for lactation as its lactogenic potency is only very slight, comparable to that of GH, and much less than that of prolactin. In any case, prolactin secretion from the pituitary increases towards the end of pregnancy, and its effects on the breast far outweigh those of hPL.

A second function assigned to hPL concerns its growth hormone-like actions, and suggests that the hormone serves to regulate metabolic turnover to meet the demands of pregnancy. Human placental lactogen promotes lipolysis and produces a rise in the levels of plasma free fatty acids and triglycerides, antagonises the peripheral glycolytic but not lipogenic or glycogenic actions of insulin and enhances amino acid incorporation into protein, probably in association with insulin. These actions of hPL on carbohydrate metabolism probably explain why glucose tolerance is moderately depressed during pregnancy and why the pregnant diabetic mother often requires to increase her insulin dosage for adequate control of plasma glucose levels. There is evidence that hPL secretion and glucose and insulin levels are related: hPL causes insulin release from pancreatic tissue *in vitro*, and elevated blood glucose levels depress hPL secretion from the placenta. However, hPL has low potency in this respect and it is doubtful whether it is essential for successful gestation in the adequately nourished mother, although it may be of prime importance for the survival of both mother and fetus in times of nutritional deficiency.

Human placental lactogen is a specific product of the placenta and so is a useful indicator of placental function; low maternal plasma levels usually indicate poor placental function. Levels of

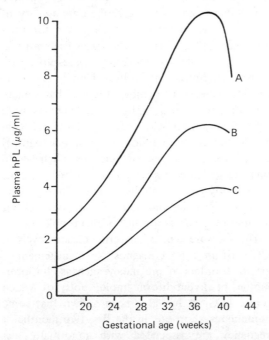

Figure 7.20 Maternal plasma hPL during pregnancy. Curve B shows mean values for all women in the sample, while curves A and C lie two standard deviations above and below the mean respectively (Redrawn from Chard, T. (1974). *Clinics in Obstetrics and Gynaecology*, 1(1), pages 85–101)

hPL also decline after fetal death. Maternal hPL levels are correlated with placental mass and are therefore high in multiple pregnancies.

Other polypeptides
The trophoblast also secretes a number of polypeptides, called 'specific proteins of pregnancy', which may be of use for early pregnancy diagnosis. They are produced in huge quantities throughout pregnancy, one of them even in excess of hPL, but their function if any is unknown.

Further reading

Boyd, J. D. and Hamilton, W. J. (1970). *The Human Placenta*, Heffer, Cambridge

Brosens, I. A., Dixon, G. and Robertson, W. B. (eds.) (1975). *Human Placentation*, Excerpta Medica, Amsterdam

Gruenwald, P. (1975). *The Placenta*, MTP, Lancaster

Steven, D. H. (1975). *Comparative Placentation*, Academic Press, London

8

Embryogenesis and its Mechanisms

8.1 Approaches to development

The first three months of human intrauterine development are conventionally referred to as the *embryonic period*, and the last six months as the *fetal* period. This apparently arbitrary distinction is of some value since the embryonic period is the phase of establishment of external and internal body form whereas the fetal period involves mainly the growth and maturation of origins already present.

Human embryology has traditionally been a descriptive discipline offering little insight into the underlying mechanisms of development. This is not to imply that it lacks value, since descriptive embryology helps in the understanding of both normal anatomy and of congenital malformation. The emphasis in this book is on developmental mechanisms, much of our understanding of which is derived from non-mammalian systems. Details of descriptive human embryology are given a very brief treatment in this and the following chapter, so students requiring more detailed information on aspects of structural development in man should refer to one of the more comprehensive texts listed at the end of chapter 9.

8.2 The mechanics of development

The central question of developmental biology is how the descendant cells of the zygote come to show characteristic structure and behaviour appropriate to their positions in space and time. Currently available information suggests that, with few exceptions, all somatic cells of a given individual vertebrate have identical genetic information in their nuclear DNA. Thus differentiation, defined as the development of structural and functional differences between the cells in a single organism, must be a consequence of differential control of gene expression in cells in various parts of the embryo. The nature of such control is the main issue to be discussed in the next few sections.

The character of the problem is well demonstrated by the first cleavage division of the zygote, which yields a two-celled embryo. If left without interference, each cell at this stage gives rise to about half the body of the new individual. However, if the two daughter cells resulting from the first division are separated and allowed to develop independently, each can produce a complete viable individual. A mechanism of this sort is well recognised as the basis for identical twinning, but from the point of view of the developmental biologist it illustrates an important principle. This is that a cell in a developing system has a *presumptive fate* that can be altered if its relationships with other cells are changed; in other words, developing systems show regulative capacity.

However, a cell isolated from an embryo at about the 50-cell stage cannot regulate so as to give rise to a complete embryo; at best if isolated it can generate an incomplete, malformed and nonviable part of an embryo. Regulation can therefore only occur within certain limits, and increasing developmental age tends to result in a decrease in the growth potential and options open to any particular cell.

Two sets of factors appear to determine an embryonic cell's behaviour: the information reaching it regarding its spatial relationships with other cells, and its own capacity to make a response to such positional information. Although a cell from a two-celled embryo is provisionally destined to form about half an embryo, this fate is dependent on its relationship with the other cell. It must therefore be able both to sense the presence of the other cell and to make a response to this presence. This contrasts with the 50-celled embryo, in which the recognition—response mechanism no longer allows the regeneration of an entire embryo from a single cell. This commitment or restriction of potential is known as *determination*; it may be accompanied by structural differentiation, although in most cases determination occurs before any signs of differentiation are apparent. Once a cell or group of cells is determined, it can only show regulation within a limited repertoire; such limiting of the number of roles a cell can play generally increases with time, and is a key factor in the unfolding of development. Cells in development can thus be viewed as running through a genetic programme which includes a number of choices. At each fork in the programme the choice is made according to the presence of certain signals to which the cell can respond at that time.

8.3   Early choices

The suggestion that developing cells make a series of choices in a branching programme implies that the same choice-determining signal could be used at a number of different branch points, acting merely as a trigger to activate a mechanism established as a result of choices already made. We thus have a picture of a system with a complex programme, common to all cells and contained in the DNA, controlled by perhaps a very limited repertoire of simple signals. It is logical to look at very early development if we wish to see the decision-making process in its simplest forms.

We shall consider the consequences of repeated mitotic division of a cell with essentially homogenous cytoplasm. Since mitosis is considered to produce genetically identical daughter cells, we anticipate that the only differences that can arise are in the positional relationships of the cells to one another. Division of this type is likely to give rise to a spherical mass of cells, such as a mammalian morula. Within this mass we can recognise two major categories of cells differing from each other in terms of their positions: some cells are entirely surrounded by other cells, while some lie at the surface of the sphere and thus have a surface not in contact with other cells (figure 8.1). If a sensing system capable of detecting this positional difference is present, this could cause the two categories of cells to respond differently,

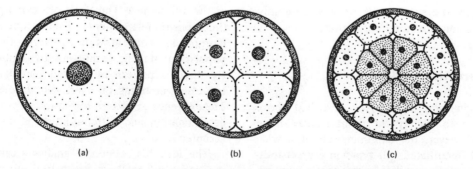

(a)	(b)	(c)

Figure 8.1   Inside—outside positional information: (a) single cell; (b) early cleavage, no positional information; (c) later cleavage, positional information of inside—outside type

and thus produce divergence of their differentiation. Such a system could readily account for the divergence of trophoblast (outer) and inner cell mass during blastocyst formation, and transplantation experiments on early mammalian embryos have indeed shown that this early differentiation choice is based on cell position.

This type of autonomous differentiation is obviously very limited in its potential; at best it could only give rise to an organism consisting of concentrically arranged layers of cells. It cannot account for the bilateral symmetry characteristic of vertebrates and many other animals. In fact there is no conceptual difficulty in modifying our scheme to allow for the establishment of body axes, as a number of plausible mechanisms can be suggested. The main problem lies in determining which ones are actually used in a particular situation.

In our discussion of a dividing cell it was assumed that the cytoplasm was effectively homogenous. It is obvious that in many vertebrate zygotes this assumption is totally unjustified. In yolk-rich non-mammalian eggs the yolk is concentrated to one pole of the egg, and this unequal distribution of yolk determines the orientation and rate of cleavage divisions, resulting in the yolk mass lying at the ventral aspect of the embryo. The fact that mammalian eggs lack yolk and look cytoplasmically homogenous does not exclude the possibility that polarity is present but is so subtle as to have escaped detection. Apart from intrinsic asymmetry of this kind, the egg may develop polarity in response to a stimulus such as sperm penetration, or even as a result of the amplification during cleavage of any randomly arising deviation from a spherical form.

8.4   Instructions and cues

Crude mechanisms of the type described above may suffice to specify the primary axes of an embryo. However, the determination of a wide range of differentiated cell types in correct locations presumably requires more subtle control. We have already indicated that choices in the programme are made on the basis of the signals received acting on cells with a particular previous developmental history. It is now useful to consider signals on the basis of their information content. At one extreme is an *instructional signal*, with a high information content; a molecule of messenger RNA is a good example. At the other end of the spectrum is an *elicitive signal* or *cue*, which only provides information in that it can be recognised by its target, thus activating a programmed set of responses in the genome of the target. Hormonal and neurotransmitter signals are clearly of this type. Our knowledge of both types of signal predisposes us to expect that signalling from one cell to another will usually be by elicitive signals. Such a view fits our hypothesis that development proceeds through local signals acting on the branch points of the complex developmental programme in the genes.

8.5   Pattern and differentiation

In principle the number of signals required for the control of development could be reduced if cells could discriminate between different concentrations of a signal substance. The establishment of a simple diffusion gradient of such a substance, known as a *morphogen*, would allow cells to differentiate along several different lines according to the point on the gradient at which they lie. This concept therefore implies that the cell's interpretation of the presence of a morphogen depends on the concentration present, which in turn depends on the position of the cell in relation to the source of the morphogen. The effect of the morphogen is thus position-dependent. Establishment of a morphogen concentration pattern through a population of cells competent to respond could lay down a pattern of commitment, later to be expressed in terms of overt cell differentiation. The existence of pattern formation steps preceding determination and differentiation is now widely accepted.

The idea that chemical gradients can provide *positional information* for pattern formation is well illustrated by Wolpert's 'French flag' model

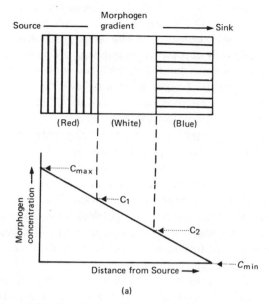

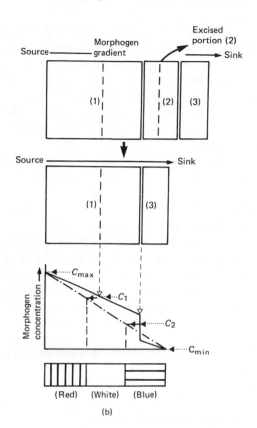

Figure 8.2 The French flag model: (a) shows how a morphogen gradient between fixed limits can generate a pattern; (b) shows how re-establishment of the gradient after partial excision of the field yields a proportionally correct pattern. In (b) the solid line represents the morphogen gradient immediately after surgery, and the broken line that after equilibration

(figure 8.2). Suppose that cells in a rectangular field have the capacity to differentiate into red, white or blue types, and that the choice is determined by the concentration of a particular morphogen to which they are exposed. It is postulated that the morphogen is produced at one end of the field and destroyed at the other, so that across the field lies a concentration gradient between fixed limits. Coded in the genome of all the cells are interpretation rules reading as follows:

(1)   If morphogen concentration is between C_{max} and C_1, turn red.
(2)   If morphogen concentration is between C_1 and C_2, turn white.
(3)   If morphogen concentration is between C_2 and C_{min}, turn blue.

By following these rules the cells in the field will differentiate into a French flag, as shown in

figure 8.2(a). It is clear that exchange of cells within the field prior to pattern formation will be without effect, as each cell derives its *positional value* from the positional information provided when pattern formation occurs. Exchange after pattern formation is completed will result in field distortion as the cells are committed to their old positional values and cannot adopt new ones. This simple model gives an elegant explanation of the capacity of fields to *regulate* or make compensatory adjustments after excision of large areas. As figure 8.2(b) shows, excision of a large slice of the field prior to pattern formation results in the establishment of a shorter, steeper gradient *between the same limits*. Regulation gives a French flag which is smaller than the original but has the correct proportions of red, white and blue.

A single linear gradient of this type can only specify position along a single axis. In order to specify the position of a cell in a solid mass of tissue three gradients would be needed. Although the French flag illustration only considers three differentiated states, it is obvious that each cell has a unique positional value in the gradient. Three gradients therefore suffice to define the position of a single cell uniquely in its field, provided that the cell's capacity to discriminate between concentration differences is sufficiently acute.

We must now consider what relevance such simple and elegant models have to real embryos. The first point is that these models imply certain predictions about the effects of experimental interference on developing systems. Some of these predictions have been tested in a variety of vertebrate and invertebrate systems, in general producing results remarkably consistent with the view contained in the models. Naturally the investigation of complex real systems has led to considerable elaboration of models, but the idea of morphogen gradients specifying positional values is conserved and is a concept of great predictive value.

8.6   Developmental fields

Any mechanism of pattern formation based on gradients would not be likely to operate effectively over a very great distance; the gradient would not be steep enough to be maintained in the face of disruptive influences, and in any case would take too long to be established. Estimates based on the time required to set up a gradient imply that a field of about 50–100 cells in length would probably be the limit. In practice the length of tissue areas responding to a single set of pattern forming signals seem to be of this order of size. The term *developmental field* is generally defined as a volume of tissue responsive to a single coordinate system. This is good as a theoretical definition, but until it is known how the coordinates are generated it is rather hypothetical. A much more practical definition is to call any volume of tissue within which regulation can occur a developmental field.

As the embryo grows the number of developmental fields increases owing to subdivision of existing fields. At first sight this might seem to imply a parallel proliferation of morphogens, but this is not necessarily the case. Developing cells are usually only capable of responding to a particular influence for a limited period, and soon become refractory to further patterning by that factor. Thus the same morphogen could affect the same cell or its descendants at a later time as part of a new field system, probably producing quite different effects. To summarise, it is proposed that the response of a cell to a particular morphogen is a function of its age and previous experience as well as of the morphogen concentration. This implies that there is a developmental 'clock' as well as the 'map' provided by morphogen gradients. This idea is examined further in the context of limb development in chapter 9.

It is important to realise that morphogens are purely a theoretical concept invented to explain the existence and observed properties of developmental fields; at the time of writing, not a single morphogen has been identified in an embryological system. This is hardly surprising in view of the minute quantities likely to be involved, but is less than satisfactory. None the less some clues as to the general nature of morphogens may be obtained by examining the possible structural sites for gradient formation in tissues.

In principle a chemical gradient could be created either in the extracellular or intracellular compartments. Although the extracellular region seems the more obvious choice, it would have certain disadvantages. The extensiveness of the space beyond the limits of any single field creates problems both of limiting a gradient and of avoiding disruption of it by bulk movements of extracellular fluid. In addition, the effects of an extracellular morphogen would have to be communicated across the plasma membranes to the interior of the target cells, presumably by means of a specific receptor system. By contrast, an intracellular gradient is confined and protected, and permits direct action of a morphogen on metabolic or genetic systems of the target cell.

The feasibility of an intracellular system depends on the availability of a suitable coupling system for propagation of the gradient from one

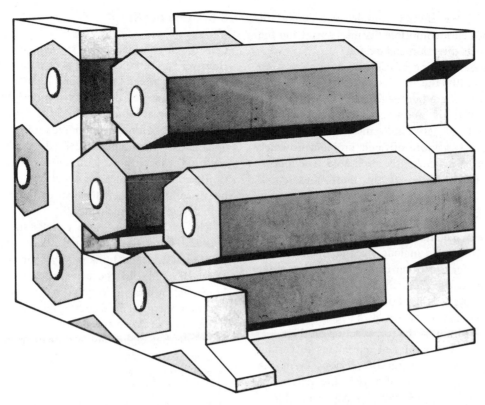

Figure 8.3   Cutaway diagram of a gap junction. The hollow hexagonal rods span both membranes, passing from one cell interior to another. Molecules small enough to pass through the central channels of the rods can pass from one cell to another

cell to the next within the field. Currently the most likely site for such coupling is thought to be the *gap junction*, shown diagrammatically in figure 8.3. Gap junctions consist of areas of close approximation of the plasma membranes of adjacent cells, with hollow channels spanning the gap and penetrating both membranes so as to couple the two cytoplasmic spaces. In many tissues these junctions have been shown to mediate cell coupling effects demonstrable by intracellular recording and by tracer methods. Recent studies suggest that the structure of these junctions does not permit the transfer of molecules with molecular weights larger than about 1000; large, information-rich molecules such as proteins and nucleic acids are certainly unable to cross them. This observation is consistent with our earlier speculation that developmental regulators such as morphogens might be

simple molecules with little information content. In addition, this limit is consistent with the size range of known mediators of cellular regulation in single cells, such as cyclic nucleotides and calcium ions.

8.7   Cell migration

Pattern formation and subsequent differentiation of cells cannot provide a complete basis for animal development since in the genesis of most body structures active migration of cells plays a prominent part. Migrations may be long-range movements of individual cells (as in the colonisation of the gonads by germ cells) or they may be coordinated movements of entire sheets or masses of cells (as in the formation of intraembryonic mesoderm or notochord). We should consider two important aspects of cell locomotion: its mechanism and the control of its direction and extent.

Our understanding of cell locomotion has been advanced with the realisation that the actin—myosin type of contractile filament system is not a special feature of muscle cells but is found in all cells capable of active movement. Control of cell locomotion is a more difficult problem in which many factors are currently implicated. The following are merely three of the most conspicuous headings:

(1) Chemotactic migration of cells along extracellular gradients of morphogens. This could include fixed gradients on the surface of other cell aggregates, or masses of extracellular material. One possibility is a gradient of adhesiveness along which moving cells could be guided by the resultant of the forces acting on them.

(2) Restriction of cell movement to certain paths as a result of previous events. A good example of this is the pattern of migration of invaginating cells during intraembryonic mesoderm formation (see section 8.11).

(3) Passive dragging and distortion of cells by nearby active growth or movements.

It is evident that a detailed insight into the control of developmental cell movement depends largely on understanding how the plasma membrane interacts with the intracellular contractile system and with extracellular contact surfaces. One intriguing aspect of the problem is the apparent relationship between cell polarisation and microtubules. Cells undergoing elongation during development show arrays of microtubules which form along the axis of elongation; inhibition of microtubule formation results in failure of organised elongation. Similarly axial movements of organelles and directed cell locomotion seem to depend on the integrity of microtubule assembly mechanisms. The system is evidently vital to many polarised cellular processes, but its interactions with both membranes and filament systems are still obscure.

8.8   Cell death

Cells die in all organs at all stages of development. However, in certain sites synchronised cell death occurs as an integral part of development; it can be regarded as a special form of terminal differentiation forming a definite part of the developmental programme. Although hundreds of instances of apparently programmed cell death have been reported, the purpose is unknown in most cases. Conspicuous examples for which some reason may be discernible are mentioned in the context of limb development in chapter 9.

The mechanism of such cellular suicide is also in doubt. Early views favoured lysosomal autolysis, but this now seems unlikely. Lysosomal activity is often elevated, but the evidence suggest that the lysosomal system is usually engaged in recycling the components of dead cells or damaged organelles rather than in doing the original damage. It is not clear whether embryonic cell death is in any way related to the general problem of cellular ageing (see chapter 15).

8.9   Explaining development

The main intention of this chapter so far has been to suggest that the trend of current work supports the view that development can be understood by reference to familiar physical and chemical principles. We may still be impressed by the complexity of developmental events, but can at least begin to see how these events could be regulated by the delivery of a modest number of simple chemical signals distributed in space and time according to a genetic programme. This does not reduce the complexity or subtlety of the events in even the simplest developing system, but at least there is a conceptual framework within which to begin analysis.

In the rest of this chapter and the whole of chapter 9, the early development of the human embryo and the origins of several of its major systems will be briefly described. As most of these systems have so far not contributed much to ideas about developmental mechanisms, the account is largely descriptive. Comments on mechanisms will only be made where experimental evidence is available.

8.10 The bilaminar embryo

At the point at which the embryo was left in chapter 5, it had developed into a blastocyst consisting of two parts: the outer hollow sphere of the trophoblast and the inner cell mass (figure 8.4). We have already examined the fate of the trophoblast in chapter 7, and must now follow the further development of the inner cell mass which gives rise to the embryo.

Initially the inner cell mass is a solid cluster of cells, attached to the inner surface of the trophoblast and projecting into the blastocyst cavity or *primary yolk sac*. At the end of the first week after ovulation the cells facing the primary yolk sac become cuboidal. The resulting layer of cells is known as the *primary embryonic endoderm*. The cells lying between this and the trophoblast differentiate into a single columnar layer, the *primary embryonic ectoderm*. Accumulation of fluid in intercellular spaces leads to the formation of a cavity between the ectoderm and the trophoblast known as the *amniotic cavity*. These changes are illustrated in figure 8.5 in which it is seen that the inner cell mass has been transformed into a double layer of epithelioid cells attached to the trophoblast

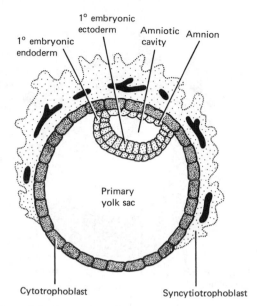

Figure 8.5 **Formation of embryonic ectoderm and endoderm and of the amniotic cavity**

at the margin and suspended between the amniotic cavity and the primary yolk sac. This *bilaminar disc*, and in particular the ectodermal component of it, appears to give rise to the entire embryo.

8.11 The trilaminar embryo

In chapter 7 the origin of the extraembryonic mesoderm and endoderm was discussed in the context of the further development of the trophoblast. It will be appreciated that the extraembryonic endoderm is continuous at its edges with the primary embryonic endoderm, the two together bounding the yolk sac (figure 8.6). As yet the extraembryonic mesoderm has no counterpart within the embryonic disc. This extraembryonic mesoderm becomes extensive and loosely packed as many fluid-filled cavities develop within it (figure 8.7). The cavities coalesce to form a single space splitting the extraembryonic mesoderm into two layers in all regions except that of the body stalk; this new space is known as the *extraembryonic coelom of chorionic cavity* (figure 8.8). The very early development of this space in the human

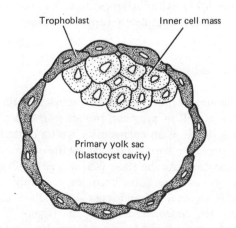

Figure 8.4 **Blastocyst showing separation into external trophoblast and an inner cell mass**

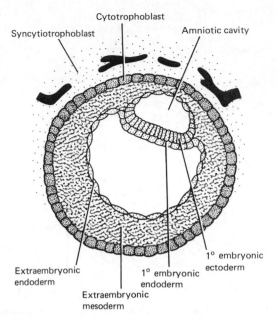

Figure 8.6 **Differentiation of extraembryonic mesoderm and yolk sac mesoderm**

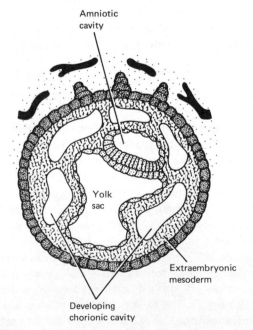

Figure 8.7 **Splitting of extraembryonic mesoderm. Fluid-filled cavities become confluent to form the extraembryonic coelom or chorionic cavity. Formation of the cavity pinches off the ventral part of the yolk sac and the isolated segment undergoes atrophy**

embryo cuts off the yolk sac from the trophoblast and thus prevents the development of a yolk sac placenta (see chapter 7).

After the establishment of the bilaminar disc a small patch of ectodermal cells increases in height. This *prochordal plate* lies at the presumptive cranial end of the disc, and is thus the first outward expression of anteroposterior polarity. This process of polarisation is carried further after the second week of development by the changes associated with the formation of the intraembryonic mesoderm. Initially ectodermal cells near the posterior end heap up along the midline to form a ridge, the *primitive streak*, in which rapid cell proliferation takes place (figure 8.9). Cells in the streak lose their epithelioid features, migrating downward and then laterally so as to form a layer between the primary ectoderm and endoderm. This new layer of *intraembryonic mesoderm* becomes continuous with the extraembryonic mesoderm at the disc margins (figure 8.10). At the prochordal plate region the mesoderm cells fail to penetrate between ectoderm and endoderm, presumably due to the resistance offered by unusually strong cell adhesion at this site.

A similar effect occurs caudally where another midline patch of tight adhesion is present. These two tightly adherent ectoderm–endoderm associations are known as the *buccopharyngeal* and *cloacal membranes* respectively, and mark the presumptive cranial and caudal ends of the gut (figure 8.11). Although mesoderm does not invade these plates it completely surrounds them.

8.12 The notochord

While mesoderm invagination through the primitive streak is still in progress, the anterior end of the streak develops an enlargement with a central pit. This *primitive knot* is a specialised site of mesoderm invagination. As the (now pear-shaped) embryonic disc grows the knot becomes relatively more caudal, laying down an invaginated midline tube of cells, the *notochordal process* (figure 8.11). Initially the process becomes intercalated into the endoderm as a midline strip, but later moves

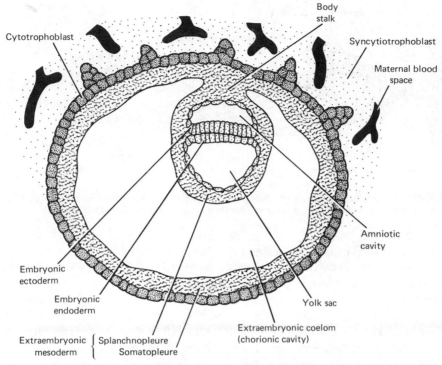

Figure 8.8   Completion of the chorionic cavity. The cavity isolates the embryo, amniotic cavity and yolk sac from the trophoblast except at a narrow body stalk

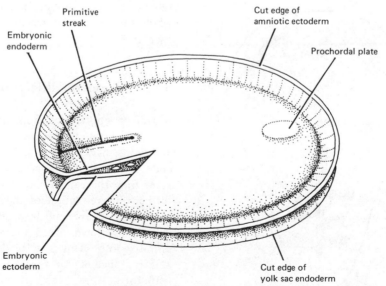

Figure 8.9   Bilaminar embryo at the primitive streak stage. The embryonic disc has been cut free from its marginal attachments. The upper ectodermal surface faces the amniotic cavity while the lower endodermal aspect faces the yolk sac. The marginal groove is the zone of contact with the extraembryonic mesoderm and chorionic cavity

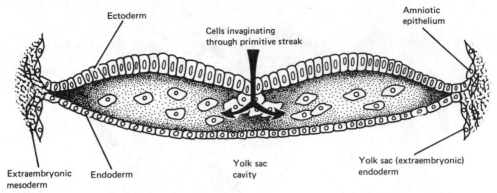

Figure 8.10   Invagination of mesoderm through the primitive streak. This drawing corresponds to a transverse section through the posterior third of the embryo shown in figure 8.9

dorsally again to form a solid midline rod between ectoderm and endoderm, the definitive *notochord* (figure 8.12). As the figure shows, the hollow notochordal process forms a transient communication channel between the amniotic cavity and the yolk sac. The midline parts of these cavities become trapped within the embryo as the neural canal and the gut lumen respectively, so the temporary link

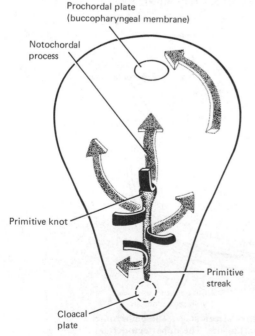

Figure 8.11   Migration of prospective mesoderm through the primitive streak. The unlabelled arrows represent typical paths of mesodermal invagination

between them is known as the *neurenteric canal*; very rarely this persists as a congenital malformation.

The notochord forms a midline structure around which the axial skeleton develops; during this phase the notochord itself becomes less prominent, being ultimately reduced to the nucleus pulposus of the intervertebral discs. Nevertheless it has one other important role in development, by acting as the inducer triggering development of the neural tube from the overlying midline ectoderm. The whole of neural tube development is discussed in chapter 9.

8.13   Mesoderm differentiation

It will be appreciated from the previous section that formation of the notochord starts cranially and works backward. Thus the cranial end of the embryo appears to be more advanced in development than the caudal end at any given time; the further differentiation of mesoderm around the notochord occurs cranially while the caudal end is still laying down chord mesoderm through the primitive knot. This time-lag along the embryonic axis is apparent for the rest of the embryonic period.

Once the notochord is established cranially further mesodermal changes occur. The mesoderm adjacent to the notochord proliferates to form a longitudinal column on each side, the *paraxial*

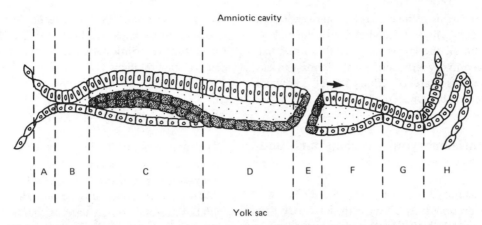

Figure 8.12   Sagittal section of a primitive streak embryo showing notochord formation. The rearward movement of the primitive streak makes it possible to see all the stages of notochord formation in one section. Working forwards from the primitive pit: E shows notochordal process invagination, D shows intercalation into the roof of the yolk sac, and C shows reinstatement of the definitive notochord to its final position. Zone F has not yet taken part in notochord formation, which cannot in any case proceed beyond the prochordal plate B or the cloacal plate G. Note the allantois growing out from the yolk sac in zone H

mesoderm. This later undergoes transverse segmentation to form about 44 pairs of blocks, the *somites.* Later these differentiate to give rise to skeletal, muscular and connective tissues. Lateral to the somites lies an unsegmented zone, the *intermediate mesoderm,* which gives rise to many of the components of the urinary and genital tracts. Most laterally lies the *lateral plate meso-*

derm, which develops into the serous linings of the pleural, pericardial and peritoneal cavities and also forms the mesenchyme of the limb buds. At its periphery the lateral plate becomes continuous with the extraembryonic mesoderm (figure 8.13).

Recent evidence suggests that, in rodents at least, the definitive endoderm which comes to line the gut tube and its derivatives originates from the

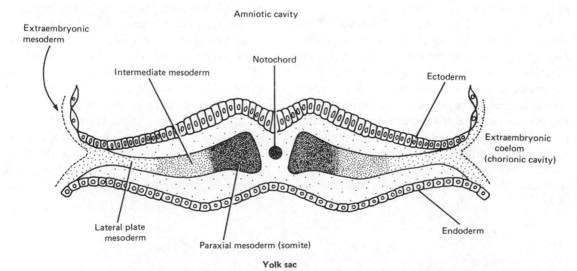

Figure 8.13   Mesoderm differentiation at the third week. Transverse section

mesoderm. If this is the case the primary endoderm contributes to the yolk sac but not to the embryo proper, and all the layers of the embryo originate from the primary ectoderm. This is not too surprising as this state of affairs is well known to occur in the avian embryo.

8.14   Intraembryonic coelom and body folds

The extraembryonic coelom or chorionic cavity has been present from a very early stage. After the establishment of the lateral plate mesoderm a corresponding mesodermal cavity appears within the embryo (figure 8.14). It begins as a series of fluid-filled enlargements of the intercellular space of the lateral plate mesoderm, which soon coalesce to form a horseshoe-shaped channel passing anterior to the buccopharyngeal membrane and opening into the extraembryonic coelom on each side. This cavity later becomes segmented to form the pleural, pericardial and peritoneal cavities. Its existence means that the lateral plate mesoderm is split into the *somatopleure*, associated with the ectoderm and hence the future body wall, and the *splanchnopleure* adherent to the endoderm and thus the prospective viscera. These two layers eventually give rise respectively to the somatic and visceral linings of the body cavities.

Until the fourth week of development the embryo remains essentially flat, apart from a slight dorsal bulge into the amniotic cavity. After this time the marginal parts of the now very elongated embryonic disc tuck in ventrally so as to enclose the dorsal part of the yolk sac. which now becomes the gut lumen. Thus the marginal parts of the disc form the ventral parts of the later embryo (figure 8.15). The originally extensive body stalk attaching the embryo to the trophoblast is now more circumscribed and is attached to the posterior end

of the embryonic disc; as a result of its marginal position it participates in body folding and assumes its definitive position on the ventral surface at the site of the umbilicus.

8.15   Endodermal derivatives

The main embryonic derivative of the endoderm is the gut and its glands, which are described in chapter 9. Apart from the gut itself there are two diverticula requiring discussion. The first is the vitellointestinal duct, a narrow channel formed by the pinching off of the yolk sac from the gut at body folding. This decreases in size and significance as development proceeds and in most cases is eliminated completely before birth, although the sac itself may persist until term as a vestigial structure attached to the placental end of the umbilical cord. Of greater interest is the *allantois*, an outgrowth of the hindgut endoderm already discussed in chapter 7. Apart from the involvement of the allantoic mesoderm in placental development, the endodermal allantoic duct persists in part after birth, giving rise to the major part of the bladder. This association between the development of the bladder and the placenta explains why the umbilical and superior vesical arteries arise in common from the internal iliac artery. The positions of the yolk sac and allantois during and after folding are shown in figures 8.16 and 8.17.

In this chapter we have not discussed two systems which are already prominent by the body fold stage. These are the nervous system, derived from midline ectoderm, and the blood vascular system, arising in the mesoderm. These have been omitted partly in the interests of clarity, to avoid simultaneous description of too many systems, and partly so that the description of the development of both systems can be covered in a unified way in chapter 9.

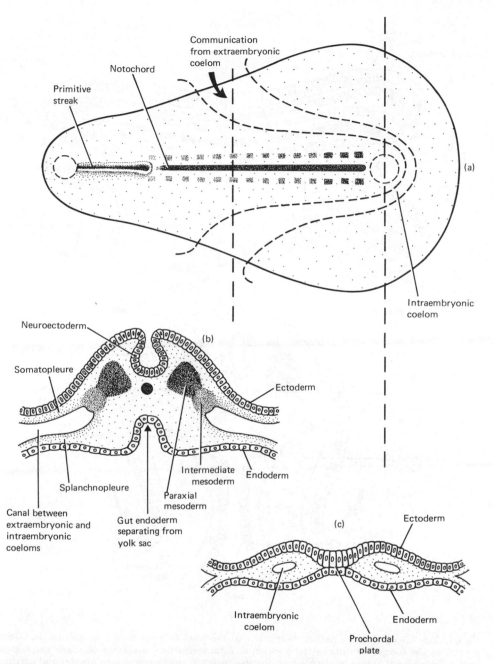

Figure 8.14   Position of the intraembryonic coelom: (a)   shows the position of the horseshoe-shaped channel in top view – note that it passes in front of the prochordal plate and opens into the extraembryonic coelom on both sides; (b)   shows that the cavity develops in the lateral plate mesoderm – at the level of the prochordal plate the relationships are as seen in (c)

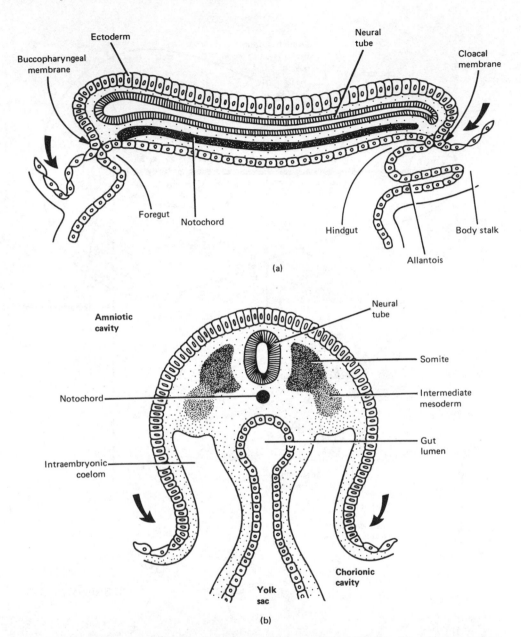

Figure 8.15   Body fold formation. Formation of the head fold (a) brings the preoral mesoderm ventral to the foregut into the correct position to form mediastinal structures. Similarly the tailfold brings the allantois ventral to the hindgut, foreshadowing its development into bladder and urachus. Lateral folding (b) isolates the gut within the mesodermal partition separating the two sides of the intraembryonic coelom; the partition will form the dorsal and ventral mesenteries

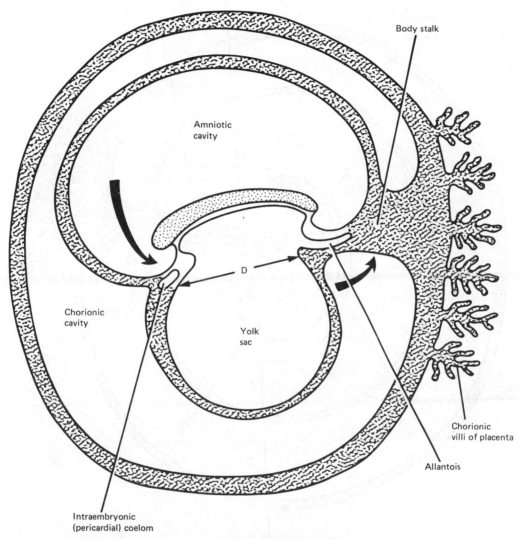

Figure 8.16   Embryo and membranes during folding. As the margins of the embryonic disc become tucked underneath, the amniotic sac enlarges to surround the embryo. The anterior membrane attachments are swept towards the body stalk as the gap D narrows, constricting the neck of the yolk sac to form the vitello-intestinal duct, which becomes incorporated into the definitive body stalk, the umbilical cord

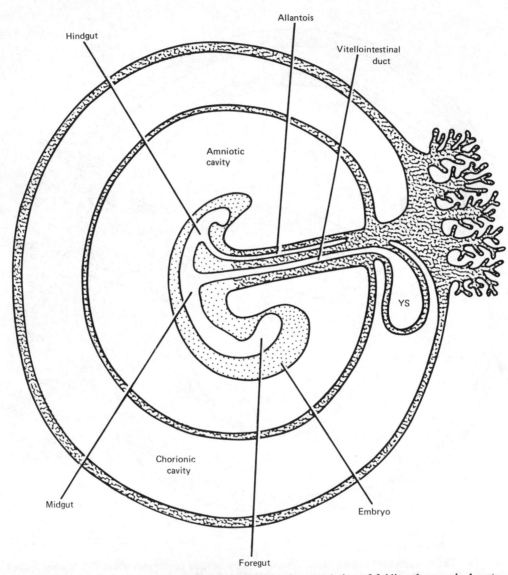

Figure 8.17   Embryo and membranes after folding. At the completion of folding the marginal parts of the embryonic disc have all been tucked on to the ventral surface. The embryonic margins have been drawn into the new stalk, the umbilical cord, while the old body stalk is incorporated into the inner face of the placenta. The allantois terminates blindly in the cord, while the yolk sac just projects into the chorionic cavity

Further reading

Ashworth, J. M. (1973). *Cell Differentiation*, Chapman and Hall, London

Ede, D. A. (1978). *An Introduction to Developmental Biology*, Blackie, Glasgow

Garrod, D. R. (1973). *Cellular Development*, Chapman and Hall, London

Greaves, M. F. (1975). *Cellular Recognition*, Chapman and Hall, London

Gurdon, J. B. (1974). *The Control of Gene Expression in Animal Development*, Oxford University Press

Harris, H. (1970). *Nucleus and Cytoplasm*, Oxford University Press

Wolpert, L. (1971). 'Positional information and pattern formation', *Current Topics in Developmental Biology*, **6**, 183

9

The Development of Organ Systems

9.1 Embryogenesis and organogenesis

In chapter 8 we examined the origins of the cell communities which give rise to the definitive organ systems. We must now consider some features of the processes by which these organ rudiments acquire the characteristics of the definitive organs. This process of *organogenesis* continues throughout development both before and after birth. However, many of its most striking features are seen in the third and fourth months of intrauterine development. The changes occurring in this period are complex and poorly understoood; with few exceptions our knowledge is largely descriptive and there is little insight into the mechanisms responsible. None the less the importance of this phase is enormous because during organogenesis the embryo is most vulnerable to infective and chemical agents capable of producing malformations (*teratogens*) as described in chapter 10. It is evident that any detailed understanding of teratogen action must await insights into the mechanisms of normal organogenesis.

In this chapter we shall consider briefly the pattern of organogenesis in selected major body systems and regions. In no sense is this either comprehensive or detailed; the main purpose is to illustrate the types of process involved by reference to a small number of important examples. Readers requiring a more complete account of human organogenesis should consult one of the excellent embryology texts listed at the end of this chapter.

9.2 The musculoskeletal system

Most of the structures in the musculoskeletal system are regarded traditionally as being of mesodermal origin. However, it is probably not very helpful to overstress this point as the mesoderm and probably also the definitive endoderm are derived from the ectoderm; it is likely that further cells are recruited into the musculoskeletal apparatus after the formation of the primary germ layers. Thus although most musculoskeletal structures are derived from the somites, the branchial arches arise from neural crest ectoderm (see section 9.3).

The differentiation of intraembryonic mesoderm into somitic, intermediate and lateral plate types was illustrated in figure 8.13 and described in the accompanying text. After about four weeks of development the somites undergo differentiation as illustrated in figure 9.1. Each somite, starting with the most anterior pair, develops a central cavity and becomes somewhat flattened to give a dorsolateral and a ventromedial wall. The dorsolateral portion is destined to become the dermis of the skin and is therefore known as *dermatome*. The lower part of the ventromedial wall is called the *sclerotome*; this disperses to form mesenchyme-like cells which largely become arranged around the notochord and neural tube, giving rise to the cartilaginous precursors of the vertebrae and their derivatives. Sclerotome not used for axial skeleton formation probably contributes to the paraxial mesenchyme generally.

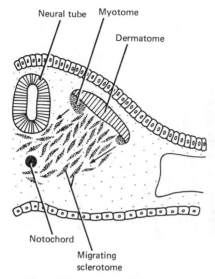

Figure 9.1 Somite differentiation

any particular muscle can often only be inferred from its nerve supply. The myoblasts present in a muscle field undergo end-to-end fusion thus forming the large multinucleate skeletal muscle fibres. Once the fibres are fully established further growth and hypertrophy occur by increase in size rather than by formation of new fibres or recruitment of myoblasts.

Segmentation is also modified in the development of the axial skeleton, although in a less drastic manner. Each vertebra is formed not from a single pair of somites but from fusion of the posterior half of the sclerotome derived from one pair of somites with the anterior half of that derived from the succeeding pair (figure 9.2). The splitting of the segmental sclerotome is thought to be dependent upon the presence of the spinal ganglia which develop at the same time (see figure 9.2 and section 9.3).

One specialised axial area deserves some further comment. This is the so-called *branchial arch region* which lies on either side of the presumptive pharynx. In fishes the body wall is pierced in this region by a series of vertically arranged gill slits, each with its own skeletal supports, muscles, and vascular and nerve supplies. In mammals the gill slits do not develop, but their skeletal, muscular, vascular and nervous elements appear during embryogenesis and are then subverted for other purposes. The main structures derived from each skeletal arch are indicated in figure 9.3. The majority of the skeletal elements are probably

The more dorsal part of the ventromedial somite wall is termed the *myotome* and gives rise to most of the somatic muscles. Although small at first, this portion of the somite rapidly enlarges and grows ventrally to meet its opposite number. These proliferating cells, known as myoblasts, regroup and migrate as required to form the characteristic muscle groups of the body axis and probably also of the limbs. In this process much of the somitic segmentation is lost due to longitudinal fusion or more complex rearrangement of originally segmented elements and the segmental origin of

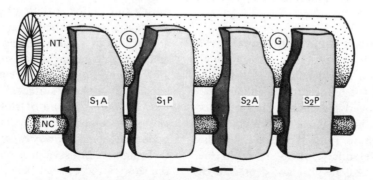

Figure 9.2 Formation of vertebrae from segmental sclerotomes (NT, neural tube; NC, notochord; S_1A and S_2A, anterior parts of first and second segmental sclerotomes; S_1P and S_2P, posterior parts of the first and second segmental sclerotomes; G, spinal ganglion)

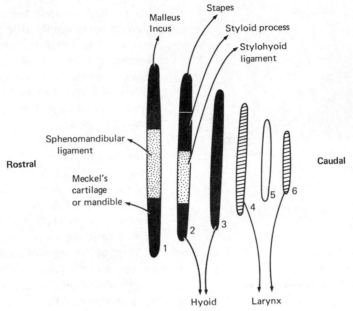

Figure 9.3   Branchial arch cartilages. Their fates are indicated by the arrows

derived from neural crest cells (see section 9.3). The origin of the muscles is not very certain; they are definitely not of somitic origin, but probably arise from local mesenchyme cells. The fate of the vessels of each arch is discussed in section 9.4, whilst the special derivatives of the endodermal lining of the gut in this region are briefly considered in section 9.5.

The musculoskeletal development of the limbs shows some special features and is dealt with in the context of limb development in section 9.7.

9.3   The nervous system and neural crest

After the mesoderm has invaginated to form the trilaminar embryo the notochord has an inductive influence on the overlying midline strip of ecto-derm. Starting at the anterior end, this ectoderm becomes thickened to form a plaque called the *neural plate*. Differential growth results in the raising of the edges of the plate and depression of the centre, producing a pronounced neural groove. Continuation of this process causes the raised edges to meet one another in the midline forming

a *neural tube* buried under the ectoderm (figure 9.4). Neural tube formation (*neurulation*) occurs during the somite phase of development. Initially both anterior and posterior ends of the tube remain open to the amniotic cavity, but closure of these *neuropores* usually occurs by the fifth week of development.

However, neural tube and neuropore closure are very susceptible to disturbance, and several teratogens are known which cause neural tube defects in animals if administered experimentally during this period. Failure of posterior closure of the neural tube is relatively common in the human and results in varying degrees of *spina bifida*, in which the neural arches of some lower vertebrae are incomplete so that neural tissue may be exposed at the body surface. Even more severe but less common is failure of closure of the anterior neuropore which results in almost total failure of brain development (*anencephaly*).

From an early stage it is possible to distinguish the shorter and broader part of the tube, destined to form the brain, from the longer, more slender spinal cord precursor. The cerebral portion becomes segmented into fore-, mid- and hindbrain

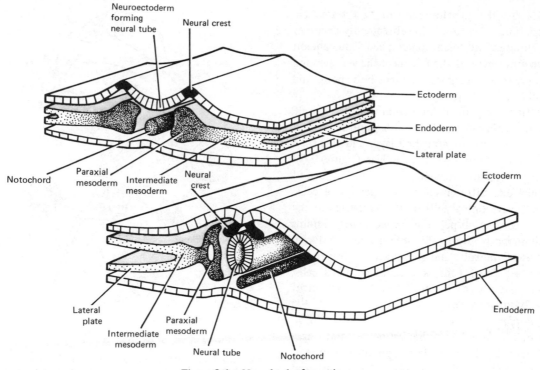

Figure 9.4   Neural tube formation

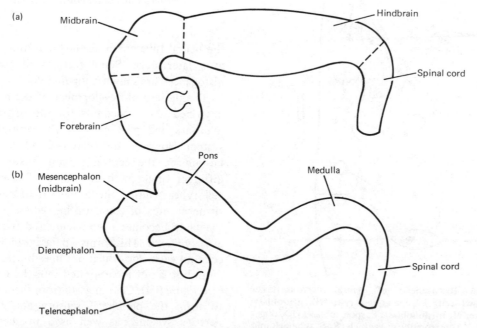

Figure 9.5   Development of brain form at formation of primary (a) and secondary (b) flexures

vesicles by the development of two transverse constrictions. The forebrain subsequently becomes differentiated into telencephalon and diencephalon by the outgrowth of the telencephalic vesicles, and the hindbrain becomes divided into pons and medulla (figure 9.5).

At first the wall of the neural tube is a simple columnar epithelium. Cell proliferation leads to a thicker, more pseudostratified layer and this then differentiates into several cell lines (figure 9.6). One type remains attached to the inner surface of the tube and differentiates into ependymal cells, the definitive lining cells of the ventricles of the brain. Another type, the *spongioblast*, retains attachments to both the internal and external surfaces of the tube and subsequently gives rise to astrocytes. Some cells, known as germinal cells, remain initially as a proliferative compartment but subsequently give rise to two cell lines, the *medulloblasts* and *neuroblasts*. The former differentiate into late-developing astrocytes and oligo-dendrocytes, while the latter produce neurones. The microglial phagocytes do not develop from

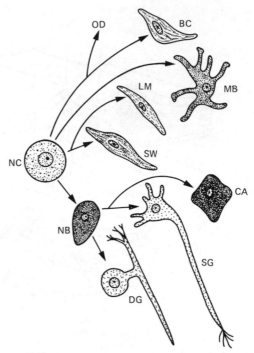

Figure 9.7   Neural crest derivatives (NC, neural crest cell; NB, neuroblast; DG, neurone of dorsal root (sensory) ganglion; SG, neurone of sympathetic ganglion; CA, chromaffin tissue, mainly adrenal medulla; SW, Schwann cell; LM, leptomeninges; MB, melanoblast; BC, branchial cartilage; OD, other possible derivatives)

the neural tube but enter the brain from the blood at a later stage. Some features of neural tube histogenesis are shown in figure 9.6.

The pattern of development of the neural tube described above accounts for the origins of the neurones and glial cells of the central nervous system. However, the nerve cells whose perikarya lie outside the central nervous system share a different origin with a number of non-neuronal cell types. During the induction of neural plate tissue an area of ectoderm immediately lateral to the plate becomes a semi-neuralised tissue known as *neural crest*. This forms a parasagittal column of cells on each side which becomes buried in meso-derm but is not incorporated into the neural tube (see figure 9.4). Cells migrate from the neural crest to form the peripheral sensory and autonomic nervous systems, as well as a number of non-neuronal tissues as indicated in figure 9.7.

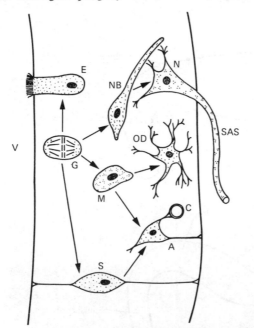

Figure 9.6   Histogenesis of central nervous tissue (G, germinal cell; E, ependymal cell; NB, neuroblast; N, neurone; M, medulloblast; S, spongioblast; OD, oligo-dendrocyte; A, astrocyte; V, ventricle; SAS, subarachnoid space; C, capillary)

Further development of both spinal cord and brainstem starts with the formation of a longitudinal groove on each side of the neural tube separating the dorsal and ventral parts. This divides the neuronal components of the tube into the *alar lamina*, concerned with sensory functions, and the *basal lamina*, concerned with motor functions, out of which develop the cranial and spinal nerve nuclei, both somatic and visceral (figure 9.8). Further details of the development of the central nervous system may be found in the specialised embryological and neuroanatomical textbooks recommended at the end of the chapter.

One important feature of early brain differentiation is the downgrowth of a part of the diencephalic floor to form the neural part of the pituitary gland, the *neurohypophysis*. This is considered with the development of the pituitary as a whole in section 9.5.

9.4   The cardiovascular system

With increasing embryonic size the need arises for a circulatory system to supplement diffusional processes in nutrition, respiration and excretion. The first elements of a circulatory system appear during the third week of development in the mesoderm of the yolk sac, body stalk and chorionic villi and of the embryo itself. Clusters of mesenchyme cells assemble and differentiate into endothelial and blood-forming cells. This generates a number of isolated endothelium-bounded spaces containing blood cells, usually described as *blood islands*. These enlarge and sprout, linking up with one another to form a vascular network which progressively becomes organised so that a few channels take the bulk of the blood flow; among the earliest to appear are the *vitelline* and *umbilical* vessels in the extraembryonic area and the *heart*

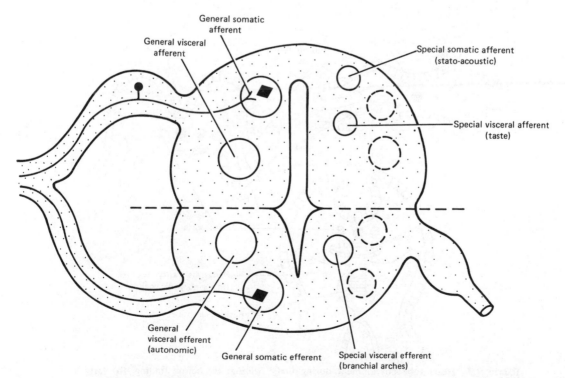

Figure 9.8   Pattern of origin of nerve nuclei of spinal cord and brainstem

tubes and *dorsal aortae* within the embryo. The heart tubes originate from a horseshoe-shaped plexus lying ventral to the intraembryonic coelom prior to body folding – figure 9.9(a). As folding progresses the limbs of the horseshoe are swept towards each other below the foregut and eventually fuse to form a single heart tube – figure 9.9(b) – which bulges into the pericardial cavity formed around it by the folding of the intraembryonic coelom. The dorsal aortae develop above the gut on either side of the notochord and are relatively unaffected by body folding – figure 9.9(c). This phase of development is reached during the fourth week, i.e. when the embryo is at an early somite stage. At this time the preoral mesoderm surrounding the heart tubes differentiates into cardiac muscle and a coordinated heartbeat is established.

The early embryonic heart is therefore a single tube which receives blood from the vitelline, umbilical and intraembryonic veins at its posterior end and expels it at its anterior end. Blood leaving this anterior or arterial end flows dorsally on either side of the foregut in a series of paired arteries which develop within the newly acquired branchial arches. These empty into the dorsal aortae through which arterial blood is distributed (figure 9.10). Continued growth of the heart tube means that it can only be accommodated by folding within the pericardial cavity so that a ventrally directed loop is formed which becomes folded caudally to give an S-shaped heart (figure 9.10). Thus the anterior parts of the tube, the *bulbus* and the *ventricle*, now lie ventrally, whilst the posterior *atrium* and *sinus venosus* are more dorsally placed. The ventricle enlarges and bulges leftward, displacing the bulbus to the right. In its turn the atrium enlarges to bulge downward on each side of the bulbus (figure 9.11).

The heart now outwardly resembles the adult condition, since it appears to have two chambers which are dorsal (the two lobes of the atrium)

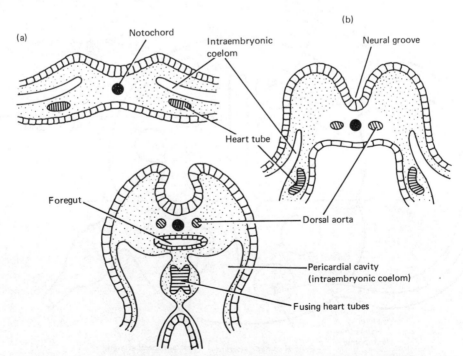

Figure 9.9   Heart tube development during body folding: (a) before folding; (b) early folding; (c) late folding

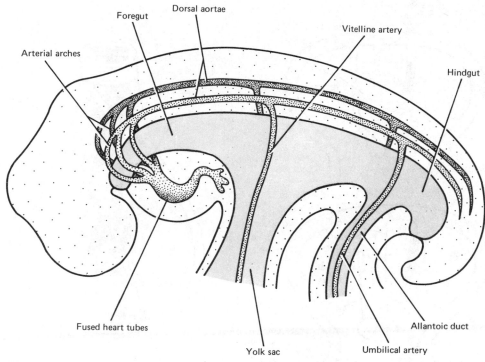

Figure 9.10   Heart tube, arches and dorsal aortae after body folding

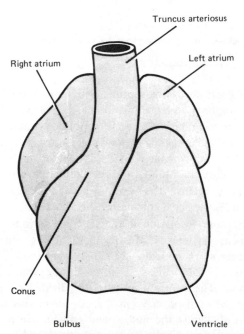

Figure 9.11   Ventral view of the folded heart tube before septum formation

and two ventral (the ventricle and the bulbus). However, functionally it is still a single tube and is only capable of driving a single circulation. The establishment of a double circulation starts with remodelling of the sinus venosus at the venous end of the heart, which has remained a paired structure because heart tube fusion was never completed. Additionally, the left umbilical and vitelline veins are obliterated early so that most venous drainage comes to the right side of the heart. Both horns of the sinus drain into the right side of the primitive atrium, thus preparing the way for the definitive pattern in which all venous return from the systemic circuit drains to the right atrium. Division of the heart chambers into right and left sides then proceeds during the fifth week with the development of septa in the atrium, ventricle and arterial trunk (figure 9.12).

Development of the atrial septum — figure 9.12(a) — starts with the formation of a crescent-shaped ingrowth, the *septum primum*, to the left of the entry of the sinus venosus into the atrium.

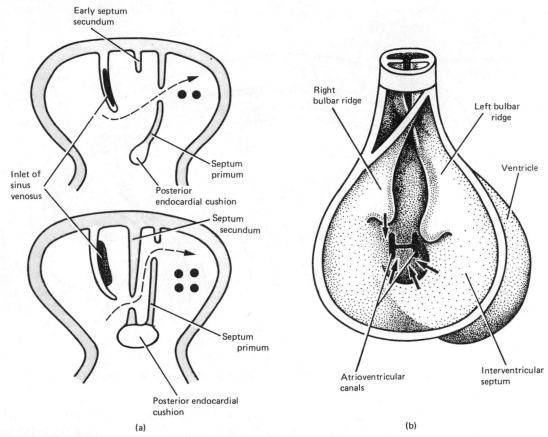

Figure 9.12   Septal development: (a) development of interatrial septum – ventral view; (b) development of interventricular and truncoconal septa

Enlargement of the right and left wings of the atrium increases the size of the septum primum, which grows down towards the atrioventricular canal. At the same time a pair of swellings called *endocardial cushions* grows on the anterior and posterior walls of the atrioventricular canal; these meet and fuse so as to divide the canal into right and left channels. Further downgrowth of the septum primum leads to its fusion with the endocardial cushions, thus completely dividing the atrium. Before this occurs, however, a secondary perforation of the septum primum develops (the ostium secundum), allowing continued flow of blood from right atrium to left atrium. Backflow is prevented by the growth of another crescentic partition, the *septum secundum*, between the entry of the sinus venosus and the septum primum.

The aperture of the septum secundum, known as the *foramen ovale*, does not lie in line with the ostium secundum. Since the septum secundum is thicker and more rigid than the septum primum, flow of blood from right to left is not impeded, but reflux of blood presses the mobile septum primum against the septum secundum and so occludes the canal connecting the two atria.

Septum formation in the ventricle, bulbus and truncus arteriosus – figure 9.12(b) – is rather simpler as there is no need to retain blood flow between right and left sides during the fetal period. The ventricle is partially divided by the upgrowth of a crescent-shaped *interventricular septum*, whilst the bulbus and truncus are partitioned longitudinally by the outgrowth and fusion of a pair of *bulbar ridges*. One of the channels so formed leads from the right ventricle to the sixth (the pulmonary) arch, while the other connects the left ventricle with the fourth (the aortic) arch. Division of right and left sides is completed by the fusion of the ventricular ends of the bulbar ridges with the interventricular septum. The bulbar ridges develop with a slight helical twist so that the resulting aortic and pulmonary trunks spiral round one another.

The heart valves develop simultaneously with the septa. The flaps which guard the entry of the inferior vena cava and the coronary sinus into the right atrium originate from the right-hand member of a pair of lips at the mouth of the sinus venosus. The mitral and tricuspid valves develop mainly from the atrioventricular endocardial cushions, while the aortic and pulmonary valves grow from a pair of *bulbar cushions* developing in the bulbar ridges.

The relevance of these structural features to the patterns of fetal and neonatal blood flow and to some developmental malformations are considered later in this section and in chapter 13.

By the fourth week the arterial system of the embryo consists of the arterial trunk emerging from the heart, several pairs of arterial arches which pass dorsally on each side of the foregut to enter the paired dorsal aortae, and the vitelline and umbilical arteries (see figure 9.10). In the human embryo six pairs of arterial arches develop but are not all present at the same time; the most anterior are formed first and disappear first, and only the third, fourth and sixth pairs are of any real importance as the origins of vessels present at birth.

The stages in development of the arterial pattern are indicated in figure 9.13 from which it is apparent that the third arch contributes to the common and internal carotid arteries on both sides, the fourth arch provides the aortic arch on the left and the proximal part of the subclavian artery on the right, and the sixth arch provides the proximal part of the pulmonary artery on both

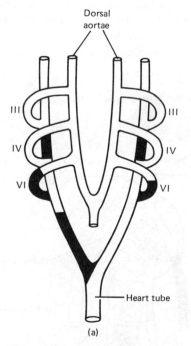

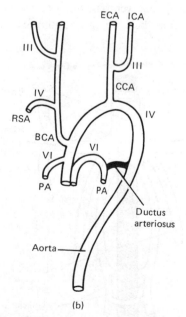

Figure 9.13   Fates of the arterial arches: (a) the third, fourth and sixth arches; (b) the same arches by the fetal period (PA, pulmonary artery; BCA, brachiocephalic artery; RSA, right subclavian artery; ECA, external carotid artery; ICA, internal carotid artery; CCA, common carotid artery)

sides and the *ductus arteriosus* on the left. This last vessel provides a route by which blood flowing through the pulmonary trunk can be diverted into the aorta without perfusing the lungs; the importance of this will be discussed later in the context of the fetal circulation.

Apart from the arterial arches the development of the arterial tree is simple. Fusion of the sections of the dorsal aortae caudal to the arches occurs at an early stage and leads to the formation of a single descending aorta which forks giving the common iliac arteries. The aorta gives rise to three sets of branches along its course through the thorax and abdomen: segmental somatic arteries (such as the intercostal arteries), paired arteries to organs arising in the intermediate mesoderm (kidneys, adrenals and gonads), and the large unpaired arteries of the gut (coeliac, superior mesenteric and inferior mesenteric arteries).

Development of the venous drainage is far more elaborate. By the fourth week three pairs of veins drain into the sinus venosus: the vitelline, umbilical and common cardinal veins – figure 9.14(a). The vitelline veins form a plexus round the midgut on their way to the sinus venosus, but between the gut and the sinus become interrupted by the

development of the liver – figure 9.14(b). The plexus round the gut becomes channelled to the liver through a single vessel, the portal vein. The proximal parts of the vitelline veins, between the liver and the sinus venosus, persist as the hepatic veins.

The umbilical veins which drain the placenta also become entrapped by the growing liver; the entire right vein and the proximal part of the left one are lost, but the blood flow through the left vein acquires a direct connection to the hepatic veins through the *ductus venosus*, thus bypassing the hepatic circulation – figure 9.14(b).

The common cardinal veins are short vessels formed by the union of an anterior and a posterior cardinal vein – figure 9.15(a) – which together drain the entire embryo apart from that part of the gut served by the vitelline veins. From the posterior cardinals develops a pair of more medially placed vessels, the subcardinals, which drain the same posterior abdominal region. The subcardinal veins enlarge at the expense of the posterior cardinals, which atrophy apart from their proximal portions. Anastomosis between the two subcardinal veins results in the diversion of their flow into the right subcardinal; the proximal part of the left

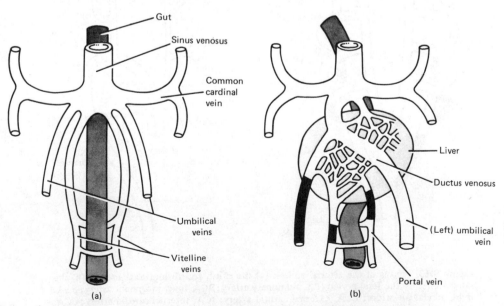

Figure 9.14   Effects of liver growth on the veins entering the sinus venosus

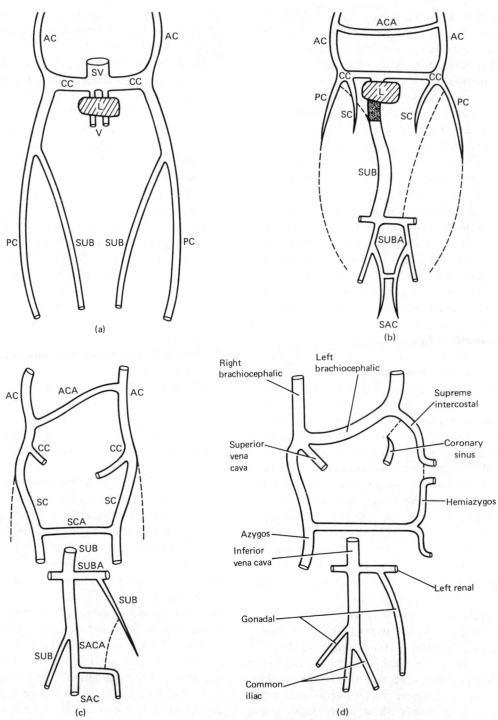

Figure 9.15   Four stages in the development of the venous system (SV, sinus venosus; CC, common cardinal; AC, anterior cardinal; PC, posterior cardinal; L, liver; V, vitelline; SUB, subcardinal; SC, supracardinal; SAC, sacrocardinal; ACA, anterior cardinal anastomosis; SUBA, subcardinal anastomosis; SACA, sacrocardinal anastomosis; SCA, supracardinal anastomosis)

subcardinal then disappears — figure 9.15(b). The enlarged left subcardinal then acquires a connection with the proximal part of the right vitelline vein and thus drains directly into the right horn of the sinus venosus. Having achieved this, the more roundabout drainage route through the right posterior cardinal remnant is gradually lost.

Thus return to the heart of blood from the abdominal wall and lower limbs is through a vessel derived principally from the right subcardinal vein and its branches and which terminates with the stump of the right vitelline vein; this composite vessel is the *inferior vena cava*. The terminal parts of the inferior vena cava and the common iliac veins are in fact derived from medial tributaries of the subcardinals, the sacrocardinal veins. The distal parts of the subcardinal veins lie lateral to these as the definitive gonadal (ovarian or testicular) veins. The large anastomosis between the sub-cardinals is preserved as the proximal part of the left renal vein — figure 9.15(b).

The regression of the major part of the cardinal veins would leave the thoracic wall without venous drainage. This deficiency is prevented by the out-growth of another pair of medial branches from the proximal parts of the posterior cardinals — figure 9.15(c). These vessels, the supracardinal veins, undergo a modification similar to that of the subcardinals, since an anastomosis develops between the two so that the main flow is directed into the right supracardinal, now recognisable as the definitive *azygos vein*. The reduced left supra-cardinal is interrupted, the larger portion becoming the hemiazygos vein which drains across the midline into the azygos vein. The smaller portion retains its connection with the stump of the left posterior cardinal and becomes the left supreme intercostal vein — figure 9.15(d).

The head, neck and upper limbs again demon-strate the principle of transference of the main venous flow to the right. The venous drainage is initially symmetrical through the anterior cardinal veins, but development of a transverse anastomosis between them shunts blood to the right, and is followed by atrophy of most of the proximal part of the left anterior cardinal vein. The trans-verse anastomosis becomes the *left brachiocephalic*

vein, whilst the isolated proximal stump of the left anterior cardinal becomes the *coronary sinus* — figure 9.15(a–d).

The main features of the circulation in the fetus are shown in figure 9.16. Special features of the fetal circulation are the presence of the large placental circulation and the effective bypassing of the lungs provided by the foramen ovale and ductus arteriosus. Oxygenated blood returns from the placenta through the umbilical vein but bypasses the liver through the ductus venosus to reach the inferior vena cava and thence the right atrium. Some of the blood leaving the right atrium enters the right ventricle and the pulmonary circuit, but most of it passes through the deficiency in the interatrial septum into the left atrium. Here it joins the small amounts of blood returning from the pulmonary circuit and enters the left ventricle and aortic trunk. Most of the blood entering the pulmonary circuit is returned to the aorta through the ductus arteriosus. The mechanisms by which this fetal pattern of blood flow is modified at birth are discussed in chapter 13.

In a developmental process as complex as that of the cardiovascular system occasional errors are bound to occur. These may range from trivial anomalies such as a displacement of the course of a minor artery to gross defects incompatible with life.

Septal defects are most commonly encountered in the interatrial septum. Since the initial closure of the septum is maintained by blood pressure a small degree of leakage is quite common in newborn infants; this normally disappears when the septum primum and septum secundum fuse together. A much more serious condition arises if the ostium secundum and foramen ovale are in line as a result of abnormal septal growth. Physiological closure of the septum then cannot occur so that shunting of blood between the pulmonary and systemic circuits continues after birth, thus considerably impairing blood oxygenation (see chapter 13).

Arch defects consist of an abnormal persistence or loss of one or more of the branchial arteries. For example, the aortic arch is sometimes double or only present on the right. Abnormal retention of arch arteries may cause problems through

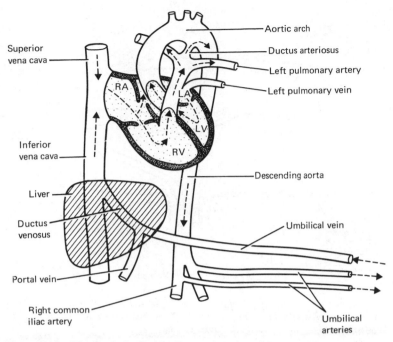

Figure 9.16   The fetal circulation. For explanation of the blood flow pattern see text (RA, right atrium; LA, left atrium; RV, right ventricle; LV, left ventricle)

pressure on adjacent organs such as the trachea or oesophagus. Congenital arterial defects need not involve complete absence of the vessel; for example narrowing or *coarctation* of a short segment of the aortic arch is a relatively common problem.

9.5   The alimentary system and its derivatives

The alimentary tract first becomes recognisable at the body fold stage (see section 8.14). The foregut and hindgut, respectively anterior and posterior to the yolk sac, are fairly well-defined endodermal tubes. The midgut, lying dorsal to the yolk sac, is ill-defined at first, but as the neck of the sac narrows to form the vitello-intestinal duct it becomes more evidently tubular. On each side of this tube lies one limb of the intraembryonic coelom; this subsequently becomes divided into the pleural (anterior) and peritoneal (posterior) cavities. In the abdominal region the gut is at first suspended between the right and left cavities by

both dorsal and ventral mesenteries, but subsequently the ventral mesentery is lost in all regions except the abdominal part of the foregut (figure 9.17). The vitelline arteries supplying the yolk sac reorganise to supply the abdominal part of the alimentary tract: the foregut by the *coeliac* artery, the midgut by the *superior mesenteric* artery and the hindgut by the *inferior mesenteric* artery.

The first conspicuous change in the foregut is a dilation in the region of the presumptive stomach. The anterior portion of the foregut which will form the oesophagus loses the cranial part of its dorsal mesentery as it approaches the dorsal wall. The heart is the most conspicuous structure derived from the preoral mesoderm (see section 8.11), but posterior to it lies an undifferentiated area called the *septum transversum*, through which the vitelline and umbilical veins enter the embryo. This septum is invaded by a ventral outgrowth of the posterior end of the foregut, the *hepatic outgrowth*, which crosses the ventral mesentery to proliferate within the septum. Eventually the growing liver takes over most of

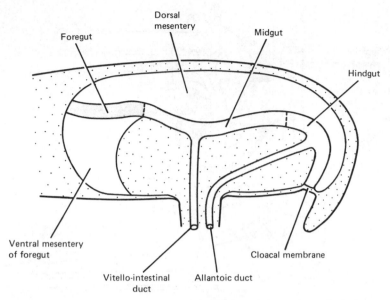

Figure 9.17   The embryonic gut, seen in left lateral view. The unshaded areas
are mesenteries attaching the gut tube to the dorsal body wall and the septum
transversum

the septum apart from a thin anterior layer which separates it from the pericardial cavity and which contributes to the diaphragm (figure 9.18). The pancreas originates from two caudal foregut outgrowths into the dorsal and ventral mesenteries. The ventral pancreatic outgrowth subsequently swings round the gut towards a dorsal position, eventually fusing with the dorsal outgrowth to form the definitive pancreas. This dual origin explains the existence in man of a main and an accessory pancreatic duct.

The development of the liver splits the ventral mesentery into dorsal and ventral parts; these are the *lesser omentum* and the *falciform ligament* respectively. Those structures which connect the liver to the gut and the dorsal wall of the abdomen must therefore run within the lesser omentum, and in fact the common bile duct, hepatic artery and portal vein are all found in its free caudal edge. The dorsal mesentery of the foregut bulges to the left to form a recess, the *lesser sac* of the peritoneal cavity, lying dorsal to the stomach. The spleen develops within the thickness of the dorsal mesentery and splits the mesentery into a dorsal part, the *lienorenal* ligament, and a ventral part, the *gastro-*

splenic ligament (figure 9.19). The lesser sac has a large caudal diverticulum, the *greater omentum*, which enlarges during the fetal period (figure 9.20).

The midgut lacks a ventral mesentery but greatly extends its dorsal one by developing a large, ventrally directed loop which protrudes through the ventral abdominal wall into the umbilical cord. This midgut herniation is then drawn back into the abdomen, at the same time undergoing a 90-degree anticlockwise twist around the superior mesenteric artery (figure 9.20). The proximal parts re-enter the abdomen first, so that the duodenum becomes attached to the dorsal wall in a curve round the right side of the superior mesenteric artery. The rest of the small intestine remains free, its line of mesenteric attachment extending rightwards to the point of termination of the ileum. When the hindgut re-enters the abdomen it is initially suspended from the dorsal wall by a mesocolon, but parts of this become fused to the dorsal wall so fixing the position of the colon. The caecum initially lies just below the liver, but with subsequent growth migrates to its definitive position in the right iliac fossa. The ascending and descending colons lose their meso-

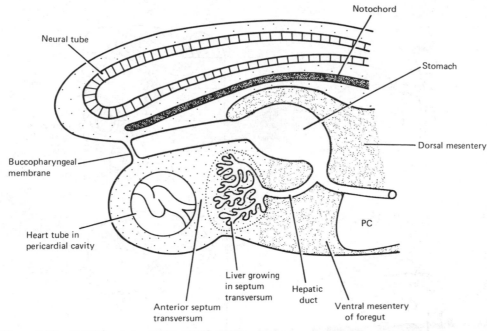

Figure 9.18 Relations between heart, liver and septum transversum. The cardiac mesoderm and septum transversum are derived from preoral mesoderm folded beneath the foregut during headfold formation (PC, peritoneal cavity)

colons to become retroperitoneal, but the sigmoid colon retains the primitive dorsal mesocolon. The transverse mesocolon fuses with the underside of the greater omentum as shown in figure 9.20.

The complexity of the anterior end of the embryo is reflected in the gut. Between the branchial arches described in section 9.2 lie out-pocketings of the endodermal lining of the gut, the pharyngeal pouches (figure 9.21). The first pair retains its connection with the pharynx,

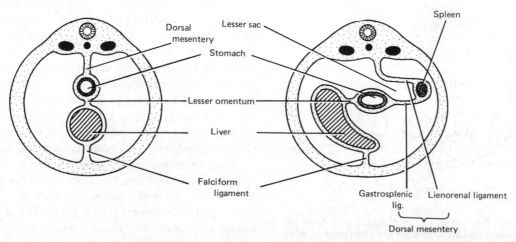

Figure 9.19 Development of the foregut mesenteries. Transverse sections in anterior view

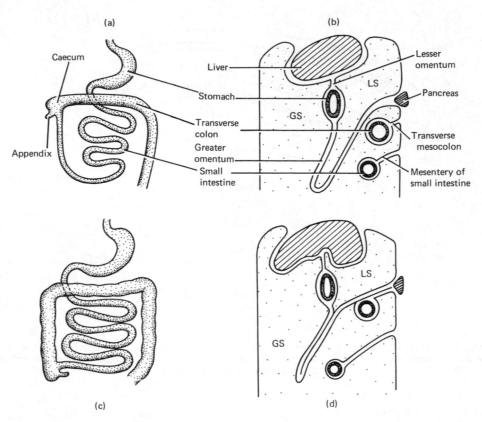

Figure 9.20   The effects of gut rotation: (a) and (c) show two stages of gut repositioning in ventral view; (b) and (d) are left views of transverse sections at the same stages to show the arrangement of the mesenteries (GS, greater sac of peritoneal cavity; LS, lesser sac of peritoneal cavity

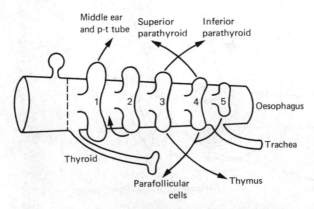

Figure 9.21   Derivatives of the pharynx, seen from the left. The numbered structures are the pharyngeal pouches of the left side

becoming the cavities of the middle ear and the pharyngotympanic tube. The ventral part of the second pair gives rise to the tonsils, while the dorsal parts of the third and fourth pouches give rise to the inferior and superior parathyroids respectively. The ventral parts of the third pouches fuse to form the thymus; both the thymus and tonsils are therefore epithelial structures which subsequently become colonised by lymphocytes.

Apart from these paired structures derived from the pharyngeal pouches, the oropharyngeal region has three unpaired midline outgrowths, one dorsal and two ventral (figure 9.21). The dorsal outgrowth, *Rathke's pouch*, arises from the ectoderm just anterior to the buccopharyngeal membrane and grows dorsally toward the forebrain. Its presence induces the downgrowth of a pouch from the floor of the diencephalon, the *neurohypophysis*. Rathke's pouch normally loses its connection with the oral cavity; it lies anterior to the neurohypophysis, its anterior wall thickening to become the pars distalis of the adenohypophysis while the posterior wall, in contact with nervous tissue, becomes the less conspicuous pars intermedia. The brain downgrowth retains its stalk, becoming the pars nervosa and the pituitary stalk.

The anterior ventral outgrowth arises at the level of the first pharyngeal pouch but grows caudally forming the bilobed thyroid gland at its end. The thyroid lies ventral to the more caudal pharyngeal outgrowth, the trachea. The tracheal rudiment starts as a groove in the pharyngeal floor but becomes cut off from the gut except at its cranial end. The blind caudal end bifurcates, each tip growing into the splanchnopleuric mesoderm and bulging into the pleural cavity to form a lung. Growth and branching of the airways continue so that by about 30 weeks the development of alveoli and capillaries is potentially sufficient to support the respiratory needs of the newborn (see chapter 13).

One of the most serious congenital malformations of the alimentary tract is failure of development of the lumen in a short segment of gut. Such *atresias* most commonly occur in the oesophagus, duodenum and rectum. Conversely the lumen of the vitello-intestinal duct may fail to close completely. This is serious if the gut lumen remains in communication with the umbilical cord, but usually only a short segment extending a few centimetres from the ileum remains patent (Meckel's diverticulum); this is usually symptomless. The process of herniation and rotation of the midgut sometimes deviates from normal. If the hernia is incompletely reduced it may persist until after birth and require surgical correction. Abnormal rotation leads to various unusual arrangements such as high caecum or left—right transposition of the large intestine. These abnormalities are in themselves unlikely to cause symptoms, but may create difficulties in diagnosis or confusion during surgery.

9.6   The genital and urinary systems

These two systems have a closely intertwined developmental origin, and remain closely joined in the male but less so in the female. Three main components contribute to their development: the intermediate mesoderm described in chapter 8, the endoderm of the allantoic duct, and the primordial germ cells which probably enter from the yolk sac.

The main features of development of the urinary tract are similar in both sexes. Starting in the cervical region, the intermediate mesoderm differentiates into epithelioid cells which form tubules. The cervical mesoderm on each side gives rise to a transient structure called the *pronephros* (figure 9.22) which degenerates after the fourth week of development. A similar process subsequently occurs in the thoracic and lumbar mesoderm and leads to the formation of a quite recognisable kidney called the *mesonephros* (figure 9.22). The mesonephric tubules link up on the lateral border of the mesonephros to form a longitudinal tube on each side of the body, the *mesonephric* (wolffian) *duct*, which develops an opening into the allantoic duct near its junction with the lowest part of the the hindgut, the *cloaca*. In spite of its extensive development, there is no evidence that the human mesonephros ever excretes urine, and it degenerates in the last part of the first trimester. It is replaced by the definitive kidney or *metanephros*, which develops from the caudal part of the intermediate mesoderm. Unlike the mesonephros, the metanephros does not develop its own duct but awaits the arrival of the *ureter*, which grows out as a branch from the lower part of the mesonephric duct (figure 9.22). In the female, the main part of the mesonephric duct degenerates, but in the male it is preserved as the main genital duct, the *ductus deferens*.

The lower part of the urinary tract is derived mainly from the cloaca and its outgrowth, the allantoic duct. It is divided into a ventral part, the *urogenital sinus*, and a dorsal part, the *anorectal canal*, by the development of a mesodermal *urorectal septum* which grows down from the angle between the allantoic duct and the hindgut to fuse

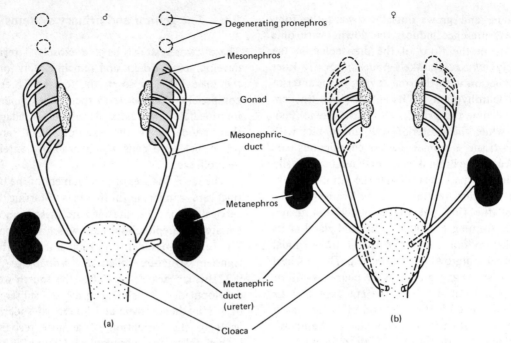

Figure 9.22   Urinary system development. Two stages in the replacement of the mesonephros by the metanephros

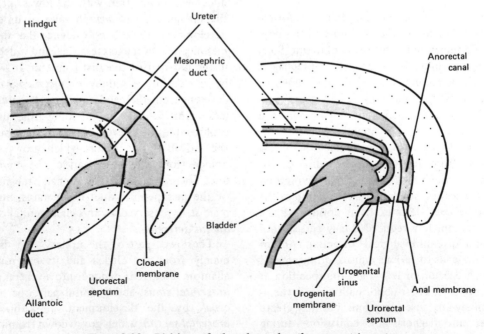

Figure 9.23   Division of the cloaca by the urorectal septum

with the cloacal membrane (figure 9.23). The urogenital sinus gives rise to much of the urethra in both sexes, and to the vestibule in the female. The urinary bladder develops as an expansion of the lower part of the allantoic duct; the upper part or *urachus* narrows, loses its lumen and becomes the median umbilical ligament. At this stage the mesonephric duct opens near the junction of the urogenital sinus and the allantoic duct. The lower end of the mesonephric duct and the lower part of the ureter become absorbed into the bladder so that the two ducts open separately, the ureters into the bladder and the mesonephric ducts into the upper urethra (figure 9.24). The triangular area of bladder wall between the ureteric and urethral orifices is thus of mesodermal rather than allantoic origin, and is known as the *trigone*.

Early development of the gonads follows a similar course in both sexes. The intermediate mesoderm medial to the mesonephros proliferates to form the genital ridge. The connective tissue of this ridge is subsequently invaded by cords of epithelioid cells derived from the lining cells of the coelom which form the covering of the ridge. The germ cells then migrate into the ridge as already indicated. In the male the germ cells develop into the seminiferous tubules of the testis while the cord cells differentiate into the sustentacular and perhaps the interstitial cells (see chapter 3). In the ovary the germ cells cluster in the outer part and become surrounded by cord cells which differentiate into follicular cells as described in chapter 2.

The origin of the duct system through which the gametes pass differs according to sex. In the male the seminiferous tubules establish a connection with the adjacent mesonephric tubules and thus with the mesonephric ducts; the latter become the ducti deferentes as shown in figure 9.24. In the female the major part of the mesonephric ducts degenerates, and oocytes are carried in the *paramesonephric* (mullerian) *ducts* (figure 9.24). The paramesonephric ducts fuse caudally to form the uterus, through which a connection with the urogenital sinus is established. The sinus is partitioned into a ventral channel destined to become the urethra and a dorsal channel which develops into the vagina.

The development of the external genitalia is complex and the reader is advised to consult one of the comprehensive embryology texts mentioned in the bibliography. However, the sex difference in

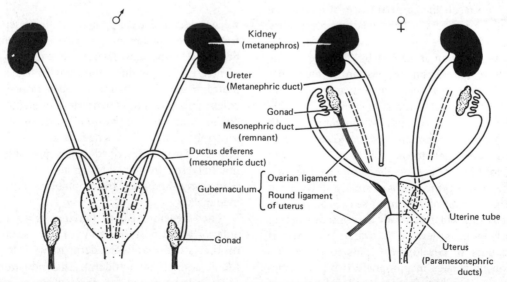

Figure 9.24 Urinary system, genital ducts and gonads in both sexes. In the female diagram (right) one side of the bladder has been omitted to show the relationship between the paramesonephric duct and the gubernaculum

the final position of the gonads deserves brief mention. In both sexes a column of mesenchyme develops into a ligament extending from the gonad to the connective tissue of the presumptive external genitalia (figure 9.24). As the embryo grows this ligament, the *gubernaculum*, fails to keep pace with it so that the gonad is drawn relatively closer to the caudal end of the embryo. In the male this process continues until the testes leave the abdominal cavity through the inguinal canal to reach a subcutaneous position in the scrotum. In the female the gubernaculum becomes attached to the paramesonephric ducts, being divided at the point of attachment into the *ovarian ligament* and the *round ligament of the uterus*. Growth of the latter structure almost keeps pace with that of the embryo as a whole, so the ovaries and upper uterus only descend as far as the pelvis (figure 9.24).

Various structural anomalies of the urinary and genital passages are occasionally encountered. Kidneys may be malpositioned, abnormal in form or congenitally absent, and the ureters may be partially or entirely duplicated. The urachus may remain patent so that urine leaks from the umbilicus, or short segments of it may persist as urachal cysts. Incomplete development of the urorectal septum can result in the persistence of a common cloaca-like opening to the vagina and alimentary tract.

Much confusion is caused by the use of the term 'hermaphroditism' in relation to anomalies of development of the genital system. Strictly defined, an hermaphrodite is an individual capable of full reproductive function as a member of both sexes. Although common in some lower animals this has never been recorded in man, so we will make no further use of the term. In the first instance, phenotypic sex is normally determined by the possession of XX or XY sex chromosomes, since it is this which generally determines whether the early gonads develop as ovaries or testes. If some failure of development leads to the differentiation of gonads inappropriate to the chromosomal sex, then the subsequent development of the duct systems and other sexual characteristics generally follows the gonadal rather than the

genetic sex. This occurs because such differentiation is determined by whether or not the gonads secrete testosterone during a crucial part of the fetal period; the production of testosterone commits the reproductive system to a male pattern of development. In the absence of such a stimulus the female pattern of development is followed (see section 11.13).

Inversion of sex characteristics may be incomplete, particularly if the sex chromosome constitution is abnormal with surplus or missing chromosomes or if the gonads themselves are intermediate between male and female types. These abnormalities cause a wide range of intersex conditions ranging from the trivial to the very severe. In addition maldevelopment of the genital ducts or external genitalia can produce apparent intersexual features in the absence of any chromosomal or gonadal abnormality. Apart from these physical variants, it is evident that other factors including upbringing can influence behaviour and sexual attitudes so as to produce a continuous range between the male and female stereotypes in people of either physical sex.

9.7   Limb development

We consider the development of limbs separately from the rest of locomotor system differentiation because it is the most thoroughly explored experimental model for differentiation in higher vertebrates. Much of the work has been carried out on chick embryos since their development is well documented and rapid, and surgical access is relatively simple. The evidence suggests that the general features described below probably apply not only to birds but also to all vertebrates with pentadactyl limbs, i.e. the amphibians, reptiles and mammals.

Limb development is initiated when both an anterior and a posterior zone of the somatic layer of the lateral plate mesoderm induce changes in the adjacent flank ectoderm. This induction leads to the development of a longitudinal ridge of thickened ectoderm along the margin of the limb mesoderm known as the *apical ectodermal ridge*.

This ridge in turn exerts an inductive influence on the underlying mesoderm which initially shows itself by proliferation of the committed limb mesoderm to produce a *limb bud* (figure 9.25). Outgrowth and maintenance of the limb bud mesoderm only occurs in the presence of the apical ectodermal ridge; its surgical removal leads to its replacement by ordinary ectoderm and cessation of limb bud development. It has recently been proposed that the apical ectodermal ridge not only maintains bud growth but has a crucial role in the specification of the proximodistal sequence of limb structures.

It is suggested that the mesodermal cells underlying the ridge are in a state of developmental plasticity in which their prospective fate changes with time. This zone of plasticity, called the *progress zone*, has a boundary across which mesoderm cells spill as mitosis leads to overcrowding of the zone. Any cell leaving the zone becomes 'frozen' in the state of commitment that it has reached. It is proposed that the progress zone

'clock' starts at proximal (limb girdle) positional values and runs to more distal values with time. Thus the first cells to leave the progress zone become limb girdle, the next become humeral or femoral region and so on down to digital structures last of all (figure 9.25). This sequence specification from the distal end contains the prediction that the grafting of a young bud apex on to an older bud deprived of its apical region will result in duplication of some limb segments (figure 9.26). By contrast, if the sequence were specified from the bud base no duplication would occur after such a graft. Most evidence thus far favours the progress zone model, and experiments on the chick wing bud give the expected duplications. Conversely transplantation of an older apex on to a younger bud results in the omission of some structures from the resulting limb (figure 9.26).

This model accounts for the specification of the proximodistal axis. The mechanism of specification of the anteroposterior axis has also been studied but is rather different. In this case the

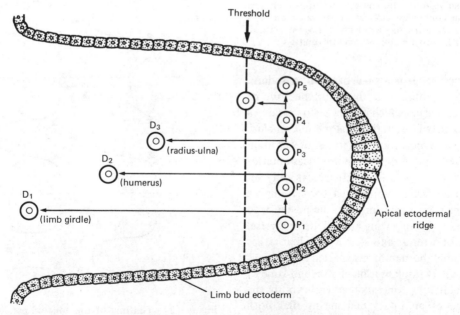

Figure 9.25 A model of limb bud pattern specification. Cells in the progress zone (to the right of the dotted line) pass with time through a series of positional values P_1–P_5. Cells crowded out of the zone while at value P_1 become fixed at that value and so differentiate to level D_1 (limb girdle) structures. Cells leaving later become fixed at value P_2, and so on. The proximodistal sequence is thus correctly ordered

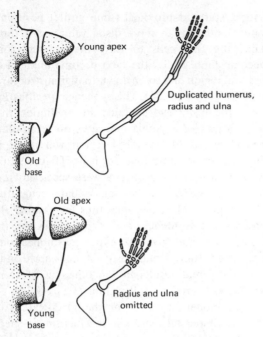

Figure 9.26 **Evidence supporting the progress zone concept. Grafting of a younger apex on to an older bud base introduces a progress zone containing cells still at the upper arm value, so causing duplication of humeral and radio-ulnar regions. The converse experiment grafts a progress zone containing cells at carpal value on to a base surface committed to form humeral level structures. The radio-ulnar region is therefore omitted**

crucial axis polariser is a small patch of mesoderm at the posterior border of the limb, the *zone of polarising activity*, which appears to create a developmental field dictating that mesoderm close to it forms the posterior structures of the limb whereas more remote mesoderm produces anterior parts. The zone of polarising activity can only act on mesoderm already committed to becoming a limb; thus its transplantation from the posterior to the anterior border of a wing bud results in reversal of the anteroposterior axis so that the ulnar rather than the radial border forms the leading edge – figure 9.27(a). Transplantation of a second zone of polarising activity from another embryo to the leading edge of an intact bud means that both borders are signalled to become posterior; thus a symmetrical limb with two posterior borders and no anterior borders develops – figure 9.27(b). Grafting of a second zone of polarising activity

into the apex of an intact bud leads to a more complex result because the grafted tissue has limb mesoderm both on its anterior and posterior surfaces. As predicted by the model the bud forks to produce two limb outgrowths with the symmetry patterns indicated in figure 9.27(c).

Specification of the dorsoventral limb axis has received less attention that the other two; it appears that specificity is determined by the ectodermal cap rather than by the mesoderm.

Although limb pattern formation has been discussed in terms of three axes, it will be evident that what has really happened is that each cell has been assigned a unique positional value within the limb bud. Currently the view is favoured that the cell positions are specified by three morphogen gradients acting approximately at right angles to one another, but such an interpretation may not explain all the experimental evidence and other mechanisms have been proposed.

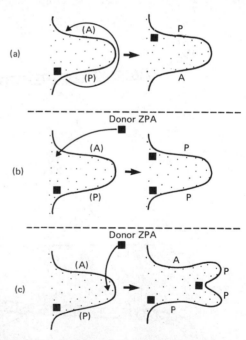

Figure 9.27 **Grafting of the zone of polarising activity (ZPA) – see text for explanations of these results: (a) transfer of ZPA from posterior to anterior border of the same wing bud; (b) graft of a donor ZPA into the anterior border of an intact wing bud; (c) graft of a donor ZPA into the apex of an intact wing bud**

During the development of the limb buds the muscles appear first as masses of myoblasts arranged around the cartilaginous elements which condense from mesenchyme. Until recently it was generally believed that the myoblasts of the limbs differentiate locally from limb mesenchyme, but recent experiments suggest that their origin is probably from the myotome component of the somites, like most of the other skeletal muscles in the body. The differentiation of the myoblasts into the characteristic muscle arrangement of the limb appears to be dependent on local positional information and occurs in the absence of any growth of nerves into the limb. The mechanism by which ingrowing nerves form synapses with the right muscles is not understood. However, one plausible view is that growing axons reach the correct area by 'following' a chemical gradient, perhaps on cell surfaces, but require a specific target receptor in order to establish the final close synaptic contacts with the muscle.

The process of specific, synchronised cell death described in section 8.8 is a conspicuous feature of limb development. Sharply defined patches of dying cells are seen at the sites of developing large joints, and another example occurs at the site of the zone of polarising activity well after its inductive influence has ceased. Among the best studied examples are the patches of dying mesenchyme that form at the sites of the prospective interdigital spaces. Initially the hand or foot develops as a paddle-shaped structure (figure 9.28) and digit separation results from death of the interdigital mesenchyme followed by phagocytosis of the dead cells. Species such as the duck, which retain interdigital webs, show much less cell death at these sites than free-toed species like the chicken.

It is of interest that tissue from the fore-limb bud is capable of differentiating in response to positional information intended for the hind-limb as it suggests that homologous structures retain similar pattern-forming signals. Since the transplanted fore-limb bud cells have already been programmed before excision to give rise to fore-limb structures, such a graft will produce a fore-limb structure of the type appropriate to the positional signals available at the hind-limb site to

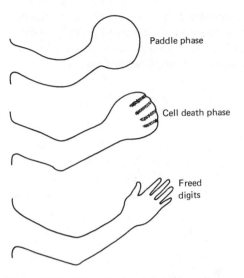

Paddle phase

Cell death phase

Freed digits

Figure 9.28   Three stages of digit formation

which it has been moved. Likewise grafted tissue seems to have a considerable capacity to respond to the positional information available in the homologous region of a different species, implying that the morphogens or other positional signals used in particular areas may have changed little during evolution.

Our present understanding of development in limbs is still rudimentary, but is none the less based on more experimental evidence than in any other part of the body. However, it is sufficient to permit us to speculate about the mechanisms underlying some of the congenital limb malformations seen in human infants. A relatively minor malformation is the presence of an extra finger or toe. Extra digits are also seen in a mutant strain of chicken and are probably caused by the development of an excessively long apical ectodermal ridge, which presumably leads to division of the underlying mesenchyme into an excessive number of digital fields. The limb malformations produced by the drug thalidomide are much more disabling. The most characteristic malformation is *phocomelia* or flipper limbs, in which intermediate limb elements are absent or reduced and the distal limb extremity may be directly attached to the trunk (see section 10.3). Although there is no explanation of how the drug produces this malformation, it is reminiscent of the effect of grafting an older limb-bud on to a younger base in the chick progress zone experiments discussed above.

Further reading

Balinsky, B. I. (1965). *An Introduction to Embryology*, Saunders, Philadelphia

Barr, M. L. (1974). *The Human Nervous System: An Anatomical Viewpoint*, Harper and Row, Hagerstown, Maryland

Beck, F., Moffat, D. B. and Lloyd, J. B. (1973). *Human Embryology and Genetics*, Blackwell, Oxford

Fitzgerald, M. J. T. (1978). *Human Embryology*, Harper and Row, Hagerstown, Maryland

Garrod, D. R. (1973). *Cellular Development*, Chapman and Hall, London

Hamilton, W. J., Boyd, J. D. and Mossman, H. W. (1962). *Human Embryology*, Heffer, Cambridge

Langman, J. (1969). *Medical Embryology*, Williams and Wilkins, Baltimore

10

Reproductive Failure and Wastage

10.1 Introduction

We are all well aware of imperfections and wastage in the human reproductive process such as the pregnancy which ends in a miscarriage or a still-birth and that tragically embodied in the child who suffers a major deformity or permanent handicap. These distressing outcomes of pregnancy are reminders that human reproduction is fallible and that conception does not automatically result in the birth of a live and healthy infant. The causes of failure and the inefficiencies of the human reproductive process are discussed in this chapter, with special emphasis on those developmental errors which give rise to abnormalities of the newborn.

About 10—15 per cent of all marriages are infertile, usually because one partner is sterile or of low fertility. Infertility of the husband accounts for about 30 per cent of cases. Fertility in women declines to zero at the menopause but in men fertility may persist into old age (chapter 15). Failure to produce gametes is the most fundamental cause of sterility and it may arise for an anatomical reason or because the ovaries or testes do not receive adequate hormonal support. Sterility may also result from extrinsic causes such as injury to the gonads or reproductive tract, castration or sterilisation. In addition, some marriages may be infertile because of imperfect understanding of necessary sexual technique or for cultural, nutritional or psychological reasons.

The most obvious physiological limitation to the successful outcome of coitus is clearly its timing, since it has been calculated that the fertile period only lasts 40—60 hours in each menstrual cycle. This value is based on estimates of the times for which spermatozoa and ova remain viable within the female reproductive tract. In some cases fertilisation may be compromised by the poor quality of the male gametes: for example some human ejaculates show a large proportion of morphologically abnormal (figure 10.1) or non-motile spermatozoa. Infertility may result when fertilisation is persistently hindered by the presence

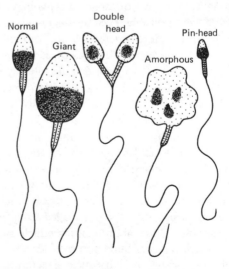

Figure 10.1 Some examples of misshapen spermatozoa (Redrawn from Evans, T. N. (1971). *Textbook of Obstetrics and Gynaecology* (ed. Danforth, D. N.), Harper and Row, New York)

of thick, impenetrable cervical muscus which prevents access of the sperms to the uterus and uterine tubes. Such conditions normally occur in the progesterone-dominated phase of the menstrual cycle or when the progestogen minipill is being taken (chapter 6).

Following fertilisation, failure may occur if the uterine environment is unsuitable for implantation, as for example it generally would be if oral contraceptives were being taken. Sometimes the fertilised egg does not reach the uterus, but instead is carried elsewhere and implants and develops at an unusual site (ectopic pregnancy) as discussed in chapter 5.

There is recent evidence that a high proportion of total reproductive wastage occurs soon after fertilisation or implantation. At implantation, pregnancy has begun (in the technical sense at least) and embryonic loss after this stage is therefore called *spontaneous abortion*. It is probable that most post-implantation losses occur because of defects in the genetic constitution of the zygote which are incompatible with the survival or correct development of the embryo, and which result in the spontaneous termination of the pregnancy. However, in some cases genetic defects are compatible with survival and result in the birth of a baby suffering from a congenital defect. This abnormality may be of organ morphology, and therefore often visible (i.e. a *congenital abnormality*), or of biochemical function (an *inborn error of metabolism*). Both types of genetic-based congenital defect are of considerable interest with regard to their medical and social importance, not least because they illustrate the importance of biochemical genetics in the study of human disease. In this context it is worth noting that the word 'congenital' means 'existing from birth', and does not necessarily imply 'of genetic origin'. Thus some abnormalities of the fetus which are caused by the action of external factors such as disease or drugs can also be called congenital abnormalities. Those abnormalities which are of genetic origin are heritable and may therefore be passed from parents to subsequent generations, or recur in other children of the same parents.

Fetal development and the outcome of pregnancy may be adversely affected by external factors acting on the mother or the fetus or on both. Fetal damage is manifested in its mildest form by retardation of growth. A fetus which is much smaller than is normal for its gestational age, but which otherwise appears to be fully developed, is said to be *small for dates*. These babies are often less healthy than their peers of equal gestational age and their perinatal mortality is higher. It is often difficult to pinpoint the reasons for the small size of many of these babies but it is thought that maternal malnutrition may account for some of them. Sometimes growth retardation may be due to inadequacy of the placenta, most usually of its capacity to support sufficient exchange of blood gases and nutrients. It is probable too that the well-established link between heavy maternal smoking and low-birthweight, high-risk babies resides in the effects of cigarette smoke or its constituents on placental function. Recent findings suggest that the nicotine absorbed from cigarettes causes constriction of placental blood vessels, thus diminishing the normal oxygen supply to the fetus. It is also possible that carbon monoxide in cigarette smoke might decrease the oxygen carrying capacity of the red cells of the mother and fetus.

In its worst form, fetal damage is expressed by the production of abnormalities or by death. In general those factors which cause growth retardation also increase the frequency of fetal death and stillbirth. Similarly, agents which produce fetal malformations often cause fetal death if applied in larger amounts or for longer. Although it is known and accepted that injury, infection and disease can all sometimes cause stillbirth or early fetal death and spontaneous abortion, it is perhaps much more important to remember that such factors can occasionally cause congenital abnormalities. This was vividly illustrated in the mid-twentieth century by the consequences of epidemics of german measles (rubella) and by the thalidomide disaster. The virus and the drug are both capable of causing major structural abnormalities of the fetus by interfering with its correct embryological development. These abnormalities are often not fatal; instead they result in severe and permanent handicap.

10.2 Congenital abnormalities

A congenital abnormality is a morphological abnormality present from birth. Other synonyms commonly used to describe such conditions include 'birth defects', 'developmental errors', 'fetal deformities' and 'congenital malformations'. Together these terms correctly imply that the structural abnormality originates because of an error in the embryonic development of the fetus and results in functional impairment which may prejudice health or survival. The range of congenital abnormalities described in humans and in other animals is wide and the following discussion is not intended to be comprehensive but seeks to underline some important general principles.

Congenital abnormalities are caused by impairment or interference with the usual correct sequence of embryological development of the organ concerned and are often caused by the slowing down or cessation of growth of one part of the embryo relative to the rate of development and differentiation of the rest. The impairment may be due to expression of an abnormal genetic component of the fetus, or be caused by some adverse external influence on a fetus which would otherwise be normal. The production of congenital abnormalities by external agents is known as *teratogenesis* and is discussed separately in a later section. Congenital abnormalities may thus not always have a genetic basis but those which have may be heritable. For example, some anomalies such as polydactyly (presence of extra fingers or toes) and cleft palate recur in successive generations, and sometimes several members of the same family show the same rare defect. There are also examples where a woman has given birth to several deformed children by one man but to healthy children by a second.

Nevertheless, the exact cause of most congenital abnormalities is still obscure. It has been estimated that 25 per cent may be ascribed to genetic causes or to gross chromosomal errors, about 2–3 per cent to maternal infection or to the ingestion of harmful drugs or environmental pollutants, but the causes of the remaining 60 per cent are still undefined. Moreover, it is likely that the majority of congenital malformations arise from interactions between as yet undetermined environmental factors and complex polygenic elements, involving several different gene loci.

Table 10.1 shows the eight most common congenital malformations which occur in Britain with an incidence of at least 1 per 1000 total births. The list illustrates the wide range of systems that can be affected by malformation and includes well-recognised defects of the central nervous, cardiovascular, musculoskeletal and alimentary systems. In addition, defects may occur in the genito-urinary system and in the eye and ear, as well as in several systems at once. The type of defect and its morphological characteristics can generally be interpreted in terms of interference with normal ordered organogenesis at a specific time during pregnancy.

Cleft palate is a condition in which the embryonic pharyngeal cavity does not undergo partition into oral and nasal cavities because the palatal shelves fail to fuse. A similar condition can be induced in mice by the injection of several teratogenic chemicals, including high doses of the hormone cortisone, between days 11 and 14 of gestation. In this species palatal fusion occurs by day 13–14. In man cleft palate has been well studied because it is a relatively common abnormality and cases are well documented because it is repaired surgically in hospital. It is thought that the error in embryological programming of the palate arises from two mutant genes, one a sex-linked recessive and the other an autosomal dominant.

Unlike cleft palate, congenital pyloric stenosis is not immediately recognisable at birth. Identifiable symptoms due to faulty digestion and consequent failure to thrive become recognisable a few weeks after birth and the condition may be alleviated by operating to divide a band of hypertrophied muscle which prevents the stomach contents from emptying properly into the duodenum.

The two examples quoted above and the others in table 10.1 illustrate that congenital abnormalities range from conditions such as clubfoot, congenital hip dislocation, hernias and cleft palate, which after appropriate treatment are not clinically

Table 10.1   Congenital abnormalities with incidences of at least 1 in 1000 total births in Great Britain

Abnormality	Incidence/1000	Sex ratio (male : female)
Down's syndrome (mongolism)	2	1.0
Cleft lip (± cleft palate)	1	1.8
Pyloric stenosis	3	5.0
Clubfoot	3	2.0
Congenital hip dislocation	1	0.2
Spina bifida	2.5	0.8
Anencephaly	2	0.4
Congenital heart defects	4	1.0

(From Carter, C. O. (1969).*British Medical Bulletin*, **25**(1), 52–57)

serious in terms of threat to life (although they may produce some degree of handicap), to those which cannot be treated effectively and which may be rapidly fatal. An example of the latter type is anencephaly — the complete absence of the forebrain and its replacement with spongy vascular tissue. This occurs when the neural plate fails to develop correctly at its rostral end (see chapter 9). Fortunately the defect is so severe that these appallingly malformed infants die within a few hours of birth.

Other neural tube defects are well known in both the human and other vertebrates and include several types of spina bifida which arise from varying degrees of failure of the lower part of the neural plate to fold and close into a tube during the fourth week of pregnancy. Advances in surgical treatment and in the prevention of infection using antibiotics allow doctors to keep alive many babies born with spina bifida. However, the treatment of many of them involves exceptional effort and a large share of special medical resources and there is a growing feeling that this cannot always be fully justified, particularly for those patients who can only be subsequently maintained under constant intensive care and who show gross mental retardation and complete lower body paralysis.

The incidence of human congenital abnormalities has been measured in several surveys which

show that one or more identifiable abnormalities occur in about 2–6 per cent of total births. About one-sixth of these babies show a serious handicap later in life. The frequency of abnormalities is much higher among infants dying in the first few weeks of life (10–20 per cent) since congenital abnormality makes a significant contribution to infant mortality. In fact it is noteworthy that the proportion of neonatal deaths due to congenital abnormality relative to the total number has risen over the last few years because other causes of death have been reduced by better perinatal care (chapter 13). A still higher frequency of abnormalities (20–40 per cent) is observed in those fetuses which die during pregnancy. Nevertheless, a large number of fetuses showing major abnormalities still survive, causing considerable grief and burden to individual parents as well as great expense to society.

The figures for the incidence of congenital defects are complicated by a number of factors. There are considerable regional and racial differences which may reflect both genetic and/or environmental variables such as diet or chemical contaminants. For example, anencephaly occurs at frequencies (per thousand total births) of 4.1 in Northern Ireland but only 0.4 in India and the USA. Polydactyly occurs at frequencies of 6.2 in South Africa but 0.5 in Northern Ireland and the

USA. In the UK spina bifida is three times more common in the Welsh mining valleys than in the nearby coastal region. In other cases variation in the statistics may reflect differences in the classification of congenital abnormalities or difficulties in their exact diagnosis. The frequencies may be underestimated because many defects of the special senses, such as auditory, visual or mental abnormalities, and some structural defects of internal organs, e.g. the presence of bicuspid aortic valves or of hernias, may not be immediately recognised. It is estimated that about 60 per cent of all abnormalities may be missed in the immediate postnatal period. In theoretical terms, the incidence of an abnormality in a human population must be the product of the mutation rate at the relevant genetic site(s) and of the frequency with which the abnormal fetus survives through pregnancy to term.

Some congenital abnormalities arise from gross chromosomal errors which can be recognised cytologically. In the human, as with other animals, but in marked contrast to some plants where polyploidy is relatively common, duplication of chromosomes has deleterious structural and functional consequences for the phenotype. Deletions of autosomes are rarely compatible with survival.

The condition of mongolism is characterised by eyelid abnormalities, stunted limb growth and mental retardation, and is often accompanied by abnormal muscle coordination and other major abnormalities. It is a relatively common condition (see table 10.1), and was first described accurately in the nineteenth century, for example by Down in 1866. It is now possible to prepare karyotypes in which the chromosome pairs are identified and placed in order by photographing the nucleus of cultured leucocytes during mitosis arrested in metaphase, and it was noted in 1959 that children suffering from Down's syndrome possess an extra chromosome, almost certainly that of pair 21 (figure 10.2). The extra chromosome arises in most cases from non-disjunction at the first meiotic division in the oocyte. It is thought that the probability of this type of meiotic error increases with advancing maternal

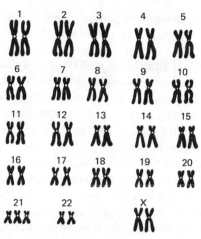

Figure 10.2 Karyotype of a female with Down's syndrome (mongolism) showing three 21 chromosomes (Redrawn from Strickberger, M. W. (1968). *Genetics,* **Macmillan, New York)**

age as the interval lengthens between the start of this first division (which occurred before birth) and its completion just before ovulation. Such reasoning may explain why the incidence of Down's syndrome (also called trisomy 21) is so much greater amongst children born to older mothers (figure 10.3) but not to older fathers.

Several other rare congenital defects are now known which result from gross autosomal errors, such as Edwards' syndrome (trisomy 18), Patau's syndrome (trisomy 13), and various conditions caused by partial deletions of chromosomal material. Generally these abnormalities are associated with a whole constellation of phenotypic

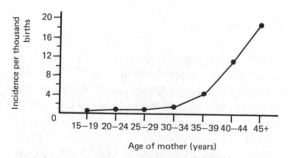

Figure 10.3 Incidence of Down's syndrome in the children of mothers of different ages (Redrawn from Strickberger, M. W. (1968). *Genetics,* **Macmillan, New York)**

alterations and each condition is therefore described as a 'syndrome', and often named after its discoverer.

There are also several well-recognised defects of the sex chromosomes such as Turner's and Klinefelter's syndromes, beside many others. Turner's syndrome (also called gonadal dysgenesis) is shown by phenotypic females who possess only a single X chromosome instead of XX and who therefore only possess 45 chromosomes instead of 46. These women lack gonads and usually appear as short of stature with a webbed neck and often mentally retarded, as well as showing a range of more variable malformations. It is estimated that only about 3 per cent of zygotes with the X0 genetic constitution reach term, the others ending in spontaneous abortion.

By contrast, Klinefelter's syndrome involves one, two or three extra X chromosomes in a phenotypic male. These patients are also infertile and do not have functional gonads but are often very tall and sometimes show mental deficiency. It is of interest that the XYY condition has also been described. These males usually have a normal phenotype and fertility but are frequently aggressive and often behave antisocially. The extra sex chromosomes characterising all these conditions probably arise from non-disjunction during either the first or second meiotic division of the developing gamete. Y0 zygotes are not viable, because the X chromosome (unlike the Y chromosome) carries many vital genes for somatic functions, for example the glucose-6-phosphatase gene.

10.3   Teratogenesis

Certain congenital abnormalities may arise from the action of external factors on the fetus. The environmental agent which causes the malformation is known as a teratogen, from the Greek word meaning a monster, and its effects depend upon the selective disruption of the patterning, differentiation or morphogenesis of the embryo. Technically the term teratogenesis refers to the production of malformed liveborn progeny but teratogenic agents usually also increase the propor-tion of fetuses dying *in utero* and the number of stillbirths, depending on the dose and timing of administration of the teratogen.

Interest in teratogenesis was forcibly stimulated by the thalidomide catastrophe which resulted in the birth of several thousand severely malformed babies to mothers who had taken this sedative drug during early pregnancy. There are fortunately no other known examples of common drug-induced malformations, and the use of thalidomide has been discontinued, but it known that other external agents may also cause abnormalities of the developing human or mammalian fetus. They include infective agents, certain toxic chemicals and drugs, nutritional imbalances, radiation and certain types of physical trauma.

The first evidence that abnormalities of the fetus, or 'monstrosities', might result from interference with the normal process of embryonic development, rather than as a result of witchcraft or an act of the Devil as had been popularly believed during the Middle Ages, was provided in the early nineteenth century. It was shown that mechanical trauma applied to hens' eggs frequently resulted in the birth of deformed chicks.

Despite this early start, there is still very little known about the exact cellular and molecular mechanisms that underly mammalian teratogenesis. In most cases teratogenic malformations do not involve any chromosomal changes, but are caused by selective interference with the biochemical expression of a normal genotype in such a way as to impede the organised development of certain localised groups of cells. Thus teratogenic effects are not heritable and affected animals may themselves produce quite normal progeny. However, in many cases this is purely theoretical since reproductive capacity or opportunity is often diminished by the abnormalities themselves.

At the time of its introduction, thalidomide appeared to be a valuable new drug since it could be used as a sedative and hypnotic without dangers of overdosage or addiction. Thus it was promoted vigorously as a favoured alternative to the barbiturates which possess both of these risks. Indeed, in West Germany thalidomide was freely available without prescription, even in some supermarkets, and its manufactured output and sales rose dramatically between 1958 and 1961. At about this time there was a rapid increase in several countries of the incidence of a condition greatly resembling *phocomelia*, a previously very rare congenital malformation (figure 10.4).

Phocomelia is a striking abnormality of limb development in which the limbs fail to grow normally and may be replaced by flipper-like appendages. The drug-induced condition was often accompanied by defects of the ears and internal organs. A link between thalidomide and phocomelia was established in Germany and Australia by carefully questioning mothers about their drug-taking habits during pregnancy. It is now known that the risk of malformation may approach 50 per cent if the drug is used at therapeutic doses during the critical period of organogenesis between 35 and 50 days following the last menstrual period.

Thalidomide is selectively toxic to the fetus and does not have adverse effects on the mother. It is particularly dangerous because there is a wide range of teratogenic doses below those large enough to kill the embryo altogether. By contrast, for most teratogens there is usually considerable overlap between teratogenic and embryotoxic doses.

There are marked species differences in sensitivity to thalidomide (the necessary daily doses for teratogenic effects in milligrams per kilogram body weight are approximately 1 in man, 10 in monkey, 30 in rabbit and more than 4000 in rat), and in common with other chemical teratogens, the timing of administration is critical in all species for optimal teratogenic effect. The differences in species sensitivity have prompted the suggestion that a metabolite unique to the human might be the teratogenic agent rather than the parent molecule itself, but of course this cannot be tested experimentally. Alternatively, species variations might relate to differences of penetration of drug to the fetus or to biochemical differences between species. Although there is still much uncertainty about the exact cellular site of action of thalidomide despite a large body of experimental work, it seems probable that the drug prevents the correct growth of cartilage by interfering with the mobilisation of glycogen in chondrocytes.

A large number of drugs and chemicals are thought or known to be teratogenic in animals or man. Many of these substances are known to be toxic in other ways to living organisms on account of their extreme reactivity (e.g. dyes), general effects on metabolism (e.g. heavy metals) or interference with fundamental biochemical processes (e.g. actinomycin, which inhibits RNA synthesis). In many cases, their danger to the fetus is assumed and they would never be knowingly administered to pregnant women. In some cases epidemics of accidental poisoning have contributed teratological examples, such as 'Minemata disease' in Japan, caused by eating fish contaminated with methylmercury from an industrial effluent. Certain occupations also appear to carry risks of teratogenesis. For example, large-scale surveys in the USA have revealed a higher incidence of congenital abnormalities and spontaneous abortion as well as increased risk of cancer among personnel working in operating theatres.

It is perhaps surprising that an excess or deficiency of hormones and vitamins can lead to embryonic malformation. One celebrated example discovered many years ago concerns vitamin A deficiency in pigs. This vitamin is incorporated into the visual pigment rhodopsin and its complete absence from the porcine diet caused microphthalmia and other eye defects in newborn piglets. The

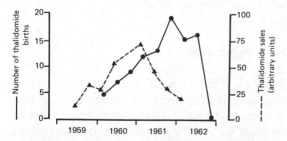

Figure 10.4 **Relation of the incidence of thalidomide births in England and Wales to the sales of thalidomide. Note that the highest incidence of the malformation occurred about 9 months after the sales of the drug had reached their highest point** (Redrawn from Saxen, L. (1975). *Methods for the Detection of Environmental Agents that Produce Congenital Defects* (eds. Shepard, T. H., Miller, J. R. and Marois, M.), North-Holland, Amsterdam)

abnormality was shown to be somatic and not genetic since the piglets themselves produced normal progeny even when inbred.

In many cases the supposed teratogenicity of certain drugs has not been proven beyond doubt in man. Since the frequency of fetal malformation is very low in most human populations and most abnormalities are probably genetic in origin, it is obviously very difficult to determine causation. Retrospective questioning is likely not to be very objective and many factors may plausibly be implicated as teratogens. Two illustrations serve to make this point.

The first concerns the unusually high incidence of babies with cleft palate and other congenital abnormalities born to mothers taking diphenyl-hydantoin or trimethadione for the control of epilepsy. It is not yet resolved whether the drugs themselves are teratogenic or whether the genetic factors which predispose to epilepsy also increase the chances of fetal malformation. Nevertheless, it is probably wise to use an alternative anti-epileptic drug which is not suspected as a teratogen.

The study of the geographical and social distribution of spina bifida in the UK led to the interesting idea that it might be caused by eating blighted potatoes. The idea received support from experiments using marmosets which showed that extracts of blighted potatoes caused malformations, possibly on account of the presence of fungal antibiotics such as cytochalasins in the blight. However, evidence from other countries with either high spina bifida incidence and low potato consumption, or high potato consumption and low spina bifida incidence, does not support the theory. Finally, a recent prospective trial in Belfast showed no difference in the incidence of the defect between a group of pregnant women who rigorously excluded potatoes from their diet and a control group who ate them as much as they liked.

Considering the vast exposure of human populations to active chemicals including drugs and environmental contaminants there is a very meagre harvest of established human teratogens. This is reassuring and suggests that the fetus is well protected from chemical insult.

The suffering caused by thalidomide focused attention on the possible dangers of drugs, and the damage and cost to the victims and their families and to society proved sufficient to ensure legislation in the major drug-producing and drug-consuming countries for the testing of new therapeutic substances. Small laboratory mammals are used as teratological models because they are relatively cheap, easy to house and reproduce rapidly. Substances under test are administered at various dose levels and at different times during pregnancy and the toxicological results evaluated in terms of fetal death and malformations. Yet this elaborate procedure is of uncertain predictive value since some substances are teratogenic in some species but not in others. For example, aspirin and pheno-barbitone are teratogenic in certain strains of rat but apparently not in man.

The toxicological evaluation of drugs is expensive and time-consuming and delays the introduction of new therapeutic agents. Many people believe that we have over-reacted to the possible dangers of drugs and that too much is expected of toxicological testing. In the long run it may be disadvantageous since the costs and the fear of expensive litigation following accidents when drugs are used over long periods may discourage the development of new drugs, except for those which have large and potentially profitable markets. Clearly we must recognise practical realities and there must be a proper balance between caution and progress.

Viral teratogenesis

Association between a viral infection during pregnancy and fetal abnormality was first suggested after an epidemic of german measles (rubella) in Australia in 1941. In a study of 130 children born to mothers who had rubella in the first trimester of pregnancy, 111 had impaired hearing and auditory defects, 38 congenital heart defects, 23 cataracts and most babies were mentally subnormal. The pattern of defects that follows rubella infection is variable, but is primarily dependent upon the time of infection, with the greatest risk of severe malformation in the first trimester. Fortunately the rubella syndrome is now rare because women can be safely immunised against german measles.

There is only one other virus (cytomegalovirus) which has an established teratogenic effect in man, although several others have been implicated. Several viruses have been shown to be teratogenic in domestic animals but they do not infect humans.

Bacterial and viral infections may also harm the fetus in other ways. Some adversely affect the rate of growth or increase the frequency of stillbirths. Other infective agents may cross the placenta and persist after birth in the tissues (for example, syphilis or rubella) thereby leading to later disease or disability. Despite this, it seems that the placenta probably provides an effective barrier to most invading microorganisms, especially later in gestation. Fetal damage caused by infective agents is comparatively rare despite the fact that many women (at least 5 per cent) catch infectious diseases during early pregnancy. Once in the fetus, however, the organism finds an environment favourable for multiplication: many tissues contain rapidly dividing cells and fetal immune defence systems are poorly developed.

10.4 Inborn errors of metabolism

The term 'inborn error of metabolism' was originally coined by Garrod in 1909 to account for certain diseases in which there appeared to be genetic-based defects in specific metabolic pathways. Garrod was particularly interested in the clinical condition of alkaptonuria, in which there is a life-long excretion of large amounts of homogentisic acid in the urine. The urine darkens on exposure to air since this acid is easily oxidised to the black pigment alkapton. Homogentisic acid is not normally found in the urine and it was suggested that the condition arises because of a defect in the normal metabolism of this compound. This rare disease also has a characteristic familial distribution: sometimes two or more siblings show it, even though it may not be observed in their parents or other relatives.

We now know that alkaptonuria is caused by an heritable chromosomal error which results in faulty production of the polypeptide chain of the enzyme homogentisic acid oxidase. Although neither the identity of the abnormal human chromosome nor the molecular nature of the miscoding in the nucleic acid sequence has been determined, it is understood that the defect represents a recessive allele of the normal gene which has arisen by mutation. Thus an individual who is homozygous for this allele will exhibit defective homogentisic acid metabolism, whereas his parents (assumed to be symptomless carriers, each heterozygous for the aberrant gene) appear to be normal. Furthermore, the defective gene may be passed from generation to generation.

Something like 1000 inborn errors of metabolism have now been described and they range in clinical severity from conditions which are essentially harmless to those which are permanently disabling or rapidly fatal. On the face of it they are more difficult to recognise than the congenital abnormalities of organ structure since the defect is at the subcellular level.

Each disease in this varied collection may be characterised in terms of the defective production of a single specific peptide chain. Most of them involve defects in enzymes and well-known examples that are discussed comprehensively in textbooks on biochemical genetics include the families of glycogen and lysosomal storage diseases, albinism, phenylketonuria, galactosaemia and cystic fibrosis. Some other important groups of hereditary metabolic diseases involve defects in proteins with non-enzymatic functions. For example, there are a number of conditions caused by defects in proteins necessary for membrane transport or absorption of solutes. Other inborn errors of metabolism involve defects in structural proteins or in those concerned with transport functions such as haemoglobin.

It is obvious then that the symptoms of disease may result from a variety of causes. In the case of the enzyme defects the symptoms often result from a deficiency of a necessary biochemical intermediate that cannot be furnished by another route or because of the accumulation in abnormal quantities of a toxic intermediate. For example, untreated phenylketonuria results in permanent brain damage in early life, probably because of defective myelination of neurones in the central nervous system. It is believed that this occurs as a consequence of the accumulation of excess phenylalanine, and in some patients the damage can be avoided by the careful preparation of a special diet from which this amino acid is rigorously excluded. However, in most inborn errors of metabolism the exact causes of the pathological effects have not been satisfactorily explained and it is consequently much more difficult to devise appropriate treatments.

Some individuals may be especially sensitive to the actions of certain drugs because they lack the normal amounts of enzyme responsible for their metabolism. This is known as pharmacogenetic sensitivity. For example, about one person in every 3000 shows abnormal responsiveness to the muscle-paralysing action of succinylcholine because of a genetically determined deficiency of the enzyme plasma cholinesterase.

In about 100 of the inborn errors of metabolism the identity of the defective enzyme or protein has been established. In some of these conditions this permits assessment of the disease by means of an *in vitro* assay, such as measurement of the rate of an enzyme catalysed reaction. Sometimes the assays are sufficiently precise to distinguish not only the normal and homozygous states but also the heterozygous 'carrier' condition. For example, the carrier may show an intermediate enzyme activity. Thus it is possible in some cases to determine whether the brothers and sisters of a person suffering from an inherited metabolic abnormality are themselves carriers of the defective recessive allele. If they are, they can be advised about the risks of passing the defective gene on to their own children ('genetic counselling').

In about 40 of the better-characterised inborn errors of metabolism, the enzymatic defect can also be measured in cultured cells taken from the fetus *in utero* by amniocentesis (see section 10.6). To date, prenatal diagnosis of an inborn error of metabolism has been made successfully in some dozen or so different conditions in which genetic

disease was suspected from the parents' family histories and the results confirmed using material taken from the fetus following therapeutic abortion.

In most populations, inborn errors of metabolism are extremely rare and figures for the incidence of each of the many known conditions are usually of the order of 1 in 10^5 to 1 in 10^6. Most of these metabolic abnormalities, particularly those involving defective enzyme activities, are autosomal recessive. A few others are recessive sex-linked. This means that the incidence of the rogue mutant allele is probably much higher than the disease frequency would suggest. For example, if the frequency of the disease is 1 in 10^5, then 1 person in 160 must be a carrier of the recessive gene, assuming random cross-breeding. Furthermore, if the defective gene is recessive, then this implies that it will gradually be lost in the course of time, since only half of the offspring of each carrier will inherit the gene. The dilution by successive generations will probably result in the elimination of the gene in 10—20 generations, provided family size is not large and that inbreeding does not occur.

These calculations can be grossly upset in certain special cases of socially dictated inbreeding or where pioneers have ventured to form isolated communities in which inbreeding and large families may occur, thus concentrating the prevalence of an otherwise rare recessive gene. Good examples of this effect are the high frequencies of albinism in the Trobriand Islanders in Australasia, hereditary tyrosinaemia in an isolated French-Canadian population living in Quebec, and drug-induced acute porphyria among Afrikaaners of Dutch origin. In the latter two cases, painstaking study of family histories and church records has enabled medical 'detectives' to identify the original ancestors who first brought the defect into the community.

Another mechanism which favours the survival of a defective recessive gene occurs when the heterozygous condition possesses some advantage which is favoured by natural selection. An outstanding example is provided by sickle cell anaemia (also discussed in section 10.6): although the homozygote sickle genotype is fatal in infancy, the heterozygote appears to offer some protection against malaria – perhaps because the partially defective red cell no longer provides an optimal metabolic environment for the protozoal parasite. This explanation has been given as the reason for the widespread prevalence (5–40 per cent) of the heterozygote sickle gene in those areas of African tropical rain forest where malaria is endemic (see figure 10.8).

10.5   Spontaneous abortion and fetal losses

In previous sections of this chapter it was mentioned that grossly abnormal embryos and those damaged by external agents or injury are often aborted spontaneously during pregnancy. Spontaneous abortion is defined as the spontaneous termination of a pregnancy before the fetus is viable. In Britain, this is usually considered to be prior to the 28th week of gestation, although very occasionally fetuses expelled before this time have survived. Abortion, or miscarriage, may also occur later in pregnancy: the term 'late abortion' is used to describe abortions occurring in the third trimester.

Spontaneous abortions in early pregnancy may or may not be accompanied by the visible expulsion of the uterine contents. In rodents, spontaneous abortion is not normally accompanied by expulsion: instead the uterine contents are resorbed, thereby providing some measure of nutritional conservation. Resorption may occur in very early pregnancy in primates and man, too. This means that it is very difficult to make an accurate estimate of the frequency of spontaneous abortion in humans, since the woman may not realise she has been pregnant if the invisible termination of pregnancy occurs within four weeks of conception, that is after the first missed menstrual period, but before the second.

A survey of the outcome of pregnancy carried out on a large number of women who had their pregnancies confirmed after the first missed menstrual period showed that spontaneous abortions apparently occurred most frequently between 8 and 12 weeks of gestation. Thereafter the incidence of spontaneous abortions declined. Since the peak frequency of spontaneous abortions occurs at a time when human chorionic gonadotropin and progesterone are being secreted (chapters 5 and 7), it is possible that the abortions are due to failure of adequate hormone production. This plausible explanation could be tested by measuring hCG and progesterone levels in pregnancy in a prospective survey to check for any association between low hormone levels and ensuing spontaneous abortion in the first trimester. As described in chapter 7, hCG is secreted by the conceptus from the first days of pregnancy onwards, and is important for the self-maintenance of the feto-placental unit as it provides a luteotropic stimulus for continued steroid production from the corpus luteum.

The comments about spontaneous abortion made in the preceding paragraph were concerned with abortions which occur after the fourth week, but in fact it is highly probable that the largest proportion of fetal losses occurs before this time. Figure 10.5 shows an estimate of true fetal losses throughout pregnancy, taking into account the large number of losses at the very beginning of pregnancy which are either not detected at all or not reported. The graph traces the fate of 100 potential pregnancies starting with the contact of spermatozoa with that number of freshly ovulated eggs. The figure shows clearly that almost 60 per cent of potential embryos are lost during the first two weeks, either because of failures of fertilisation or at the pre-implantation and implantation stages. Possible reasons for failure at these stages are discussed elsewhere, but we should note that they occur so early that the aborted pregnancy does not even disturb the menstrual cycle. Most of them probably occur because of genetic abnormality in the fertilised zygote incompatible with survival. The larger proportion of these abnormalities comprises gross chromosomal errors, resulting from a failure in the meiotic divisions of either male or female germ cells. The others are genetic abnormalities which produce a structural malformation or biochemical inadequacy of the embryo sufficient to prevent its early development.

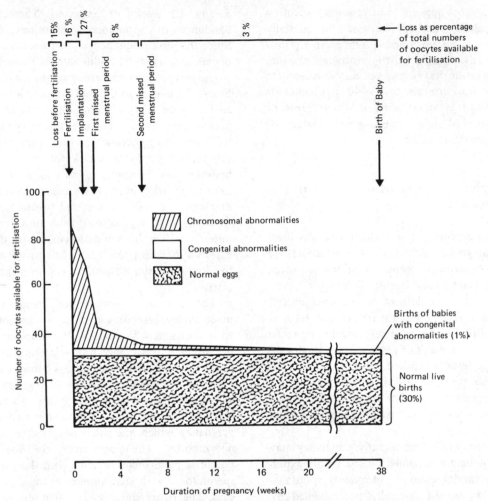

Figure 10.5   The estimated extent and characteristics of fetal losses during early development in man. The graph shows the fate of 100 oocytes and illustrates the large losses that occur in early pregnancy (i.e. before the second missed menstrual period). Note that 15% loss occurs before fertilisation and another 43% before implantation. Most of the losses are due to major structural chromosomal abnormalities, but some are due to congenital abnormalities incompatible with fetal survival that are not associated with visible chromosomal abnormalities. About 30% of oocytes are normal. At term, about 1 per cent of the oocytes result in detectable congenital abnormalities; that is about 1 in 30 of all live births (Redrawn from Witschi, H. P. (1970). *Proceedings of the Third International Conference of Congenital Malformations* (eds. Fraser, F. C. and McKusick, V. A.), Excerpta Medica, Amsterdam)

These conclusions are based on two findings. First, fetuses aborted in early pregnancy show a high proportion of major chromosomal disorders. Second, more than 40 per cent of implanted ova recovered up to 14 days after ovulation from normally fertile women awaiting hysterectomy showed major disturbances of differentiation of the embryonic disc or implantation of the trophoblast incompatible with further development.

It is also possible to calculate a theoretical value for fetal loss based on a comparison of the observed and expected numbers of births. Estimates are used for coital frequency and the use of contraceptives, and an arbitrary value of 50 per cent is taken as the chance of successful fertilisation if coitus occurs on the two out of 28 days of the cycle when the egg is viable. These rather crude calculations yield a theoretical birth rate which is far higher than is observed and it is thought that the difference might be accounted for by fetal losses of 50 per cent or more.

The preceding comments suggest that spontaneous abortion serves as a fortunate natural means of eliminating abnormal zygotes. This idea is strongly supported by a comparison made in Japan of the frequency of some selected congenital malformations in spontaneous abortions and in live births (table 10.2). The prevalence of the abnormalities is much greater in the abortions, showing that most are eliminated *in utero*. Nevertheless, a few survive to term, accounting for the small but important proportion of infants possessing congenital defects. It is possible that geographical or racial variations in the frequencies of certain congenital abnormalities (see section 10.2) may be due to differences in the frequencies with which they are recognised *in utero* and spontaneously aborted. Spontaneous abortions occur with much greater frequency in older mothers, e.g. 30 per cent of pregnancies in the age group 40–44 years end in abortion, probably because at this age there is a much higher incidence

of genetic abnormalities in the zygote for the reasons outlined previously.

Second and third trimester fetal loss accounts for a much smaller contribution to total fetal wastage (figure 10.5). In the second trimester, most spontaneous abortions occur because of inadequate placental support. This is usually manifested by low maternal plasma levels of progesterone, oestrogens and human placental lactogen (hPL) which are essential for pregnancy. The measurement of hPL has diagnostic value, since if plasma levels at week 14 are very low there is a high probability of subsequent spontaneous abortion due to placental insufficiency. Intermediate values of hPL predict some degree of placental insufficiency which might lead to complications in the third trimester calling for caesarean section or other special handling of delivery. Human placental lactogen measurement cannot be used to detect a dead or malformed fetus as in these cases the placenta may produce normal amounts of hormones.

Spontaneous abortion sometimes results from maternal disease or a structural abnormality of the female reproductive tract. Abortion is much more common in women suffering from moderate to severe hypertension, hyperthyroidism or from uncontrolled diabetes, and in these women it generally occurs late in pregnancy. Interestingly, there is evidence that in some cases of chronic

Table 10.2 Prevalence of selected malformations in embryos and fetuses taken at spontaneous abortion compared with prevalence at birth

| Type of malformation | Prevalence/1000 | | Wastage |
	abortions	births	(%)
Neural tube	13.1	1.0	92
Cleft lip and palate	21.4	2.7	87
Polydactyly	9.0	0.9	90
Cyclopia and cebocephaly	6.2	0.1	98

(From Nishimura, H. (1970). *Proceedings of the Third International Congress on Congenital Malformations* (eds. Fraser, F. C. and McKusick, V. A.), Excerpta Medica, Amsterdam)

maternal disease fetal lung maturation accelerates faster than usual in the third trimester, almost as if the premature birth is expected.

Several structural abnormalities of the female reproductive system are prejudicial to the satisfactory outcome of pregnancy. Two examples which usually result in spontaneous abortion are cervical incompetence and bicornuate uterus. Cervical incompetence occurs when the cervix is flaccid and cannot contain the pressure of the growing conceptus. The uterine contents prolapse through the cervix but can be retained by partially suturing the cervix until the time of delivery.

There are several types of bicornuate uterus. These congenital abnormalities occur when the fusion of the two mullerian ducts during embryological development is incomplete. These morphological abnormalities are very rare and can be detected by pelvic X-ray, although this should not be attempted during early pregnancy. The lumen of a bicornuate uterus is inadequate for the growing fetus and spontaneous abortion generally occurs.

Very rarely abortion may result from an immunological assault by the mother on the fetus. The mechanisms for the immunological protection of the fetus from the mother (or for its breakdown) are not fully understood (see chapter 5). There is some evidence that women who repeatedly abort in this way may be unusually sensitive to certain tissue antigens possessed by their husbands, as evidenced by the rapid and vigorous rejection of skin grafts taken from their spouses. Infertility may also result from another type of immunological rejection by the mother. In a small number of instances it has been shown that women possess antibodies to the antigens found on the egg surface; this would clearly result in infertility by destruction of the egg, either before or after fertilisation, and might indeed represent a novel approach to contraception.

10.6 Prenatal diagnosis of fetal abnormalities

Several techniques and methods can be used to detect abnormalities of the fetus while still *in utero*. Therapeutic abortion (see chapter 12) can be offered to mothers when a firm diagnosis of severe abnormality has been made before the 20th week of gestation. The ultimate aim is to reduce the incidence of serious congenital abnormalities, thereby reducing perinatal mortality and the number of severely handicapped children.

Ultrasonography (or sonar) is used widely in obstetrics to study the development and position of the fetus and placenta and is a useful recent diagnostic technique. Directionally focused sound waves of wavelength shorter than audible sound are passed from an emitter into the organ under study. Part of the beam is reflected back when it passes an interface between two structures or organs differing in their physical properties. The beam is thus attenuated and continues until partially reflected at deeper interfaces. The reflected signals, which are Doppler shifted, are detected by a receiver crystal which converts them to electrical signals for display on an oscilloscope. The apparatus can be used to scan organs, giving a two-dimensional picture of the anatomical arrangement of internal structure within the field of view (the B scan), as well as to measure time-dependent changes such as fetal heart rate and ventilatory movements.

The placenta can be localised with accuracy and fetal growth may be charted by measuring the biparietal diameter of the skull (figure 10.6). Using ultrasound, it is possible to detect gross skeletal or central nervous system abnormalities such as anencephaly (before the 20th week) and hydrocephalus.

Ultrasonography is completely safe and is now used in preference to (or at least before) radiology for most obstetric applications, as X-rays are known to be harmful to the developing embryo and fetus.

Amniocentesis can be used routinely to detect a host of genetic disorders and other defects in the fetus. It is performed by inserting a cannulated needle through the abdominal wall into the amniotic cavity after local anaesthesia of the overlying surface. The placenta (localised by ultrasound) should be avoided. Ten to 15 mℓ of amniotic fluid are aspirated and centrifuged. The

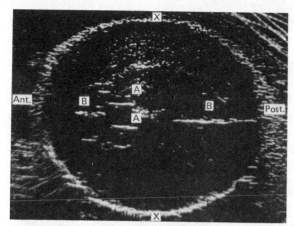

Figure 10.6 Ultrasound scan of fetal head in correct plane for measurement of the biparietal diameter (Ant., anterior; Post., posterior; A, third ventricle of brain; B, midline echo produced by the interhemispheric fissure). The biparietal diameter is measured across the width of the head, x–x (Photograph courtesy of Professor S. Campbell)

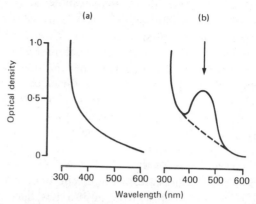

Figure 10.7 Spectrophotometric analysis of amniotic fluid, showing the normal pattern (a), and a case of severe rhesus haemolytic disease of the newborn (b). There is a large peak at 450 nm due to bilirubin (Modified from Freda, V. J. (1965). *American Journal of Obstetrics and Gynaecology*, **92**, pages 341–352)

supernatant may be used for biochemical tests and the cells for subsequent cell culture. Sufficient amniotic fluid is present by about the 15th week and amniocentesis may be performed thereafter until the end of pregnancy. In experienced hands there appears to be little hazard of mortality due to the procedure but amniocentesis is none the less not performed unless there are strong indications. These include advanced maternal age (giving a high risk of chromosomal abnormalities), known family history or previous child with abnormality, or a parent suspected of carrying a damaging recessive gene.

Two important tests using amniotic fluid are for the presence of haemoglobin degradation products and for α-fetoprotein. Rhesus haemolytic disease of the newborn causes the destruction of fetal red cells, thereby producing bilirubin and related pigments. The presence of bilirubin may be detected in amniotic fluid by spectrophotometric analysis: fluid containing these pigments absorbs strongly in the region 375–525 nm, and the optical density at 450 nm can be used as an index of the severity of the condition (figure 10.7).

α-Fetoprotein is the major fetal plasma protein produced by the liver and can be measured by radioimmunoassay. Normally it is restricted to the fetal cardiovascular system but also passes into the cerebrospinal fluid because the blood–brain barrier is poorly developed in the fetus. In cases where the spinal cord is imperfectly developed, most notably in spina bifida, α-fetoprotein escapes into the amniotic fluid. High levels are diagnostic of spina bifida, anencephaly and other related congenital malformations. More recently it has proved possible to diagnose spina bifida accurately by the 18th week by measuring α-fetoprotein in maternal blood, thereby considerably simplifying prenatal diagnosis of this condition. Confirmation of diagnosis requires amniocentesis. The method is simple and inexpensive enough to provide the basis for a screening programme aimed at the reduction of spina bifida.

Several other biochemical tests on amniotic fluid may be used for the diagnosis of fetal abnormalities. For example, recent work on the estimation of creatine kinase in amniotic fluid in the second trimester of pregnancy suggests that elevated levels of this enzyme may be a reliable marker for Duchenne muscular dystrophy, carried by a sex-linked recessive gene.

The detection of chromosomal abnormalities and inborn errors of metabolism in the fetus requires the collection and culture of cells of fetal origin obtained at amniocentesis. Most of the cells are dead but some may be cultured with difficulty under optimal conditions. This usually takes about 2—5 weeks of culture before sufficient cells are obtained. They can then be used for karotyping (as in figure 10.2) or for biochemical analysis. About 60 inborn errors of metabolism can now be detected by measuring enzyme activities in the cultured cells, although few of these tests are available routinely.

New methods for the detection of fetal haemoglobin abnormalities are of considerable importance since the various haemoglobin disorders, such as α- and β-thalassaemia (Cooley's anaemia) and sickle cell anaemia, are probably the most serious genetic diseases in many parts of the world. They have a widespread distribution and high incidence, especially in Africa (figure 10.8) and the Mediterranean region. Both β-thalassaemia and sickle cell anaemia are autosomal recessive conditions; the

homozygous condition is fatal without heroic repeated transfusion. In both conditions the heterozygous carrier can be recognised easily and therefore the disease incidence could theoretically be much reduced by population screening and genetic counselling.

Prenatal diagnosis of both of these diseases is now possible, although expensive, and is available in specialised centres where the biochemical methods are being developed. The techniques require collection of reticulocytes from the fetal blood circulation and involve the culture of these cells and analysis of the globin chains that they manufacture. Although fetal red cells contain mainly fetal haemoglobin, which possesses γ- instead of β-globin chains, there is sufficient adult haemoglobin A (about 5—10 per cent from the eighth week of gestation) for the purpose of the tests.

Fetal blood may be obtained by inserting a needle into the placenta or by using a fetoscope to locate a specific placental blood vessel. In both cases, samples of fetal placental blood are aspirated and the reticulocytes cultured for several weeks. At present these techniques are difficult and dangerous and the sampling carries a risk of about 15 per cent fetal mortality.

Both β-thalassaemia and sickle cell anaemia result from errors in the expression or sequence of the gene coding for the β-globin chain. Sickle cell anaemia is caused by the mutation of an adenine to uracil residue in the base triplet coding for amino acid in position 6 of the β-chain. This results in the substitution of valine for the usual glutamic acid, causing a damaging change in the solubility properties of the haemoglobin molecule. Such globin variants can be detected *in vitro* by carboxymethylcellulose column chromatography. In β-thalassaemia no β-chain is produced at all (although the correct gene coding for it is still present); the abnormality is detected as a very much lower than usual ratio of β- to γ-globin chains in the culture system.

If a fetal homozygote is detected the pregnancy may be terminated if desired, provided that the diagnosis is made soon enough to avoid substantial maternal risk.

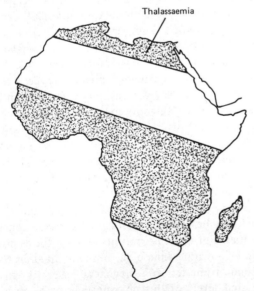

Figure 10.8   **Map of Africa showing the distribution of areas with high frequency of sickle cell anaemia and thalassaemia. The sickle cell trait has an incidence of as much as 40 per cent in parts of Africa, with an average in the shaded area of about 10 per cent** (Redrawn from Burnet, M. (1971). *Genes, Dreams and Realities*, MTP, Aylesbury)

Further reading

Catalano, L. W. and Sever, J. L. (1971). 'The role of viruses as causes of congenital defects', *Annual Review of Microbiology*, **25**, 255

Emery, A. E. H. (ed.) (1973). *Antenatal Diagnosis of Genetic Disease*, Churchill Livingstone, London

Harris, H. (1975). *The Principles of Human Biochemical Genetics*, North-Holland, Amsterdam

Mirkin, B. L. (ed.) (1976). *Perinatal Pharmacology and Therapeutics*, Academic Press, London

Raivio, K. O. and Seegmiller, J. E. (1972). 'Genetic diseases of metabolism', *Annual Review of Biochemistry*, **41**, 543

Scrimgeour, J. B. (ed.) (1978). *Towards the Prevention of Fetal Malformation*, Edinburgh University Press

Wilson, J. G. (1977). 'Teratogenic effects of environmental chemicals', *Federation Proceedings*, **36**, 1698

Berry, C. L. (ed.) (1976). 'Human malformation', *British Medical Bulletin*, **32**(1), 1–89

Maternal and Fetal Physiology

11.1   Introduction

Numerous adaptive physiological changes occur in the pregnant woman to support the growing conceptus within the uterus. These can occur either within the mother as a homeostatic response to the additional metabolic load imposed by the growing conceptus or as a direct result of the actions of fetoplacental hormones on maternal physiology.

The fetus is very largely dependent upon the mother for homeostasis through the placental exchange mechanisms described in chapter 7, but as growth and development occur its own physiological control mechanisms differentiate and its capacity for autoregulation increases. However, it should be appreciated that in all stages of pregnancy there is a dynamic interaction between mother and fetus which optimises fetal development and growth.

11.2   Maternal weight gain and nutrition in pregnancy

One of the most obvious changes in the pregnant woman is her gain in weight. In spite of the simplicity of this statement it is surprisingly difficult to determine an average figure for weight gain in a normal pregnancy because there are a number of variables which have not been adequately controlled in many studies. Examples include socioeconomic, nutritional and genetic factors. For European and North American mothers an average weight gain of 12.5 kg is taken as the norm but the figure varies widely and gains in weight from 6 to 17 kg during normal pregnancy have been recorded. However, the pregnancies of mothers showing such extremes of weight gain would be carefully monitored.

Figure 11.1 shows a graph of gain in weight plotted against gestational age in primigravidae, and shows that the increase really gets under way only after the first trimester. During the next 28 weeks the increase in maternal weight is about 450 g per week. In the early weeks of pregnancy some women may even lose weight because nausea

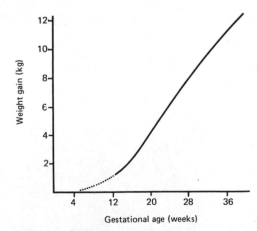

Figure 11.1   Gain in weight during pregnancy. Curve based on data from 3000 normal first pregnancies (Redrawn from Hytten, F. E. and Leitch, I. (1971). *The Physiology of Human Preganancy*, **Blackwell, Oxford)**

Table 11.1   Components of the weight gained during pregnancy*

Component	Increase in weight (kg)	Non-pregnant weight (kg)
Fetus	3.3	–
Placenta	0.7	–
Amniotic fluid	0.8	–
Breasts	0.4	0.3–0.4
Uterus	0.9	0.1
Blood (plasma)	1.3	3.9
Extracellular– extravascular water	1.2	9.7
Maternal stores	4.0	–
Total weight gain	12.6	

* The data give average figures for the changes in a first pregnancy.

(morning sickness) which may be produced by altered hormonal balance often reduces appetite.

The increase in body weight during pregnancy is not due solely to growth of the conceptus because there is an increase in mass of several maternal tissues (table 11.1). About 50 per cent of the weight gain at term results from growth of the conceptus and the rest from an increase in maternal mass. This includes an increase in total maternal body water of about 7–8l.

One interesting point is that this increase in body mass during pregnancy decreases with parity: the mean weight gain in *multigravidae* (women who have had more than three pregnancies) is some 900 g less than for primigravidae. Furthermore, the infant's weight at birth tends to increase with parity, so it appears that in subsequent pregnancies a mother can produce a larger baby with a smaller total weight gain.

Part of the increase in maternal mass is due to accumulation of protein and fat. The mother gains about 1 kg of protein during pregnancy., one half of which is in the fetus and placenta, and about 3.5 kg of fat, of which 450 g is in the fetus and placenta and the rest in her own fat depots. Most of the additional maternal protein is incorporated into the breasts, uterus, blood proteins and red cells.

Although the uterus grows considerably in mass, the growth of the conceptus within it is such that it becomes stretched, and the myometrium thins from about 2.0 to 0.6 cm.

The increase in mass and growth of tissues during pregnancy is supported by a larger calorific intake resulting from an increased appetite. The additional dietary calorific requirement for an average pregnancy is estimated at about 70 000 kcal, nearly all of which is assimilated in the second and third trimesters. During this period the mother requires an extra 300–400 kcal per day. In the average Western diet the specific nutritional requirements of pregnancy are usually met with something to spare, and sometimes the increased appetite causes obesity. Excessive weight gain and obesity in pregnancy should be controlled by dietary means because overweight women are more likely to suffer complications of pregnancy. By contrast, it is well established that many babies are born underweight in regions where malnutrition is common and the calorific value of the diet is low. Even so, in cases of maternal malnutrition fetal growth is maintained as far as possible at the expense of the mother.

A balanced diet satisfies all the nutritional requirements of pregnancy with the possible exception of iron. The state of iron balance of a non-pregnant woman is sometimes delicate (chapter 2) and in pregnancy actual iron deficiency may result. The total iron requirement of pregnancy is 350 mg for the fetus and 600 mg for the mother, in both cases mainly needed for haemopoiesis. Maternal stores of utilisable iron can provide about 100–200 mg and the rest must be provided by the diet. For this reason, most pregnant women are advised to take supplementary iron tablets. In spite of popular belief, fetal demand for calcium is relatively low because most ossification takes place postnatally, and the 350 mg per day which are necessary can be supplied by 200 ml of milk.

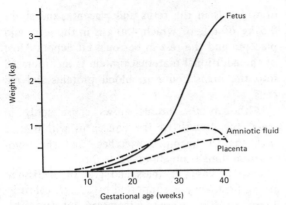

Figure 11.2   Increase in mass during pregnancy of fetus, placenta and amniotic fluid (Redrawn from Hytten, F.E. and Leitch, I. (1971). *The Physiology of Human Pregnancy***, Blackwell, Oxford)**

11.3   Fetal growth

The overall pattern of growth in weight of fetus, placenta and amniotic fluid is shown in figure 11.2. Up to 10 weeks of gestation, fetal growth is slow and placental growth is rapid. Embryogenesis is almost complete by 10 weeks, and thereafter fetal growth involves a large increase in mass. The rate of fetal weight gain increases from week 10, reaching a maximum at 28 weeks which is maintained until 36 weeks, after which the rate falls.

Protein accumulates in the fetus throughout gestation and during the third trimester is synthesised at a rate of about 5 g per day. Most of it is derived from amino acids that are transported across the placenta, and in animal experiments radioactively labelled amino acids injected into the mother are rapidly incorporated into fetal protein. In early pregnancy most protein synthesis is directed towards structural protein and plasma proteins other than gamma globulins.

Catabolism of proteins may also contribute to the pool of free amino acids available for protein synthesis, and in the adult accounts for about one-half of the free amino acid pool. It is possible that this also is an important source of amino acids for the fetus, especially in early pregnancy, because many cells are actively broken down during early embryonic development.

The formation of fetal adipose tissue is slow until the 28th week of gestation, after which fat is laid down rapidly in subcutaneous and intra-abdominal stores (figure 11.3). Lipids are trans-

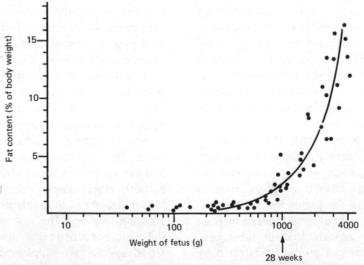

Figure 11.3   The formation of fat in the fetus as a proportion of total fetal weight. Note that the growth of the fetus is plotted in terms of fetal weight rather than age, and that the scale is logarithmic (Redrawn from Hytten, F. E. and Leitch, I. (1971). *The Physiology of Human Pregnancy***, Blackwell, Oxford)**

ported across the placenta in the form of free fatty acids (see chapter 7) and are rapidly taken up by the fetal liver and adipose cells and added to the triglyceride stores. Fetal hepatocytes and adipocytes are also able to synthesise free fatty acids from glucose, amino acids, ketones and pyruvate and this contributes further to the production of adipose tissue. Babies born to mothers who have uncontrolled diabetes are generally large and have generous deposits of adipose tissue because of the conversion in the fetus of excess glucose to fat. Since fat has a high calorific value relative to protein or carbohydrate, the adipose tissue of the normal neonate constitutes an important energy store for early life. Because fat storage occurs relatively late in development, pre-term babies and some growth-retarded babies have little stored fat and are at a disadvantage.

Fetal water content as a proportion of body weight falls steadily during gestation in step with protein accumulation; at 20 weeks of gestation the water content is 88 per cent of total fetal weight, falling to 79 per cent at 30 weeks and 71 per cent at term.

The factors influencing fetal growth are complex and are of two types: fetal genetic constitution and maternal factors. The genetic constitution of the fetus determines the maximum potential growth rate that the fetus could attain assuming no external constraints. These fetal genetic factors act at many levels to influence the organisation of the fetus and placenta and are inherited from both parents. Maternal factors that influence fetal growth largely relate to the mother's ability to meet the fetal demand for nutrients dictated by its genetic constitution.

The fetal genes influencing growth rate and ultimate birth weight function independently of maternal size and nutrition; they do not operate by altering gestational length. In man there are clear genetically determined differences in the mean birth weights of babies of different races. For example, the average birth weight of North American Indian babies is about 3.6 kg, that of European babies about 3.2 kg and of Indian babies about 2.9 kg, even with optimal maternal nutrition.

Placental weight is related to fetal weight and may be genetically determined; thus a small fetus generally has a small placenta. However, it is not possible to distinguish whether the fetus is small because its growth is limited by placental insufficiency, or whether the smallness of both is determined by the same genetic factors. In some cases, for example where there is a large area of infarcted placenta or other abnormality, the reduction in placental exchange area can clearly be held responsible for fetal growth retardation.

The most important maternal factors influencing fetal growth concern the mother's ability to sustain fetal demand for nutrients by sufficient perfusion of the uterus and intervillous space. Figure 11.4 shows typical fetal growth curves between 28 and 40 weeks of gestation for both singleton and twin pregnancies of Caucasoid mothers, upon which is superimposed an extrapolated curve showing how the fetal growth weight would increase if growth did not slow down towards the end of pregnancy. In twin pregnancies, where the individual birth weights are smaller than for singletons, the fetal growth curve slows at 30 weeks when the com-

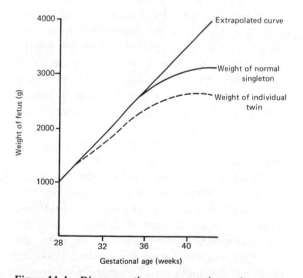

Figure 11.4 Diagrammatic representation of relation between gestational age and birth weight for singleton and twin pregnancies. The graph also shows an extrapolated curve assuming no reduction in fetal growth towards term (Modified from Gruenwald, P. (1975). *The Placenta* (ed. Gruenwald, P.), MTP, Lancaster)

bined fetal weight is equivalent to that of a single-ton fetus at 36 weeks.

The reduction in fetal growth rate towards term is thought to occur because the fetus outgrows the ability of the placenta and its maternal blood supply to support its rate of increase in mass. The placenta becomes senescent at term and its efficiency as an exchange organ decreases (chapter 7). Thus it is unlikely that a fetus ever expresses its full genetic potential for growth and it seems that in late pregnancy the growth of the fetus is actually held back or limited. A further observation that supports this concept is that the growth rate increases postnatally and for a few weeks reaches the same rate as achieved maximally during gestation. This is particularly marked in babies whose growth *in utero* was limited by placental insufficiency: they usually show a faster rate of growth after birth when food is plentiful and rapidly catch up with their fellows.

Thus in summary the actual growth rate of a fetus is determined by an interaction between maternal and fetal factors. An impressive demonstration has been provided by the technique of ovum transplantation. If the fertilised eggs of a normal-sized pig are placed in the uterus of a dwarf sow the piglets born are about half the size of normal piglets. If the experiment is reversed and dwarf zygotes are placed in a normal pig the piglets produced are twice the size of usual dwarf piglets, although they are still smaller than normal piglets. After birth the piglets show a growth pattern appropriate to their genetic constitution. Clearly dwarf piglets have a lesser potential for fetal growth than normal piglets but their fetal growth is retarded even further by maternal factors when they develop within dwarf mothers.

Until the advent of ultrasonography, longitudinal studies of human fetal growth were difficult to perform since the use of X-rays to measure fetal dimensions carries unacceptable risks and cannot be adopted for routine studies. However, the alternative methods of assessing fetal growth by palpation or by measuring maternal weight gain and increase in girth are not sufficiently accurate.

Ultrasonography (see chapter 10) provides an accurate means of assessing fetal growth through measurements of biparietal diameter or head circumference and circumference of the fetal abdomen. The biparietal diameter or head circumference shows a very good correlation with gestational age (figure 11.5) and allows an accurate estimate of gestational age to be made by comparison with this standard reference curve. It is of interest that ultrasound measurements have revealed that in fetuses with growth retardation, for example due to placental insufficiency, cephalic growth and dimensions tend to be spared but the abdominal circumference is greatly reduced due to impairment of liver growth.

11.4   The maternal cardiovascular system

The reflexes which regulate the cardiovascular system so as to ensure adequate perfusion of organs operate in the same way in pregnancy as at other times. In the first 10 weeks of pregnancy the cardiac output rises from 4.5 l/min to 6.0

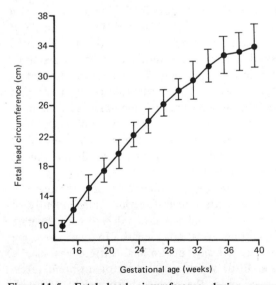

Figure 11.5   Fetal head circumference during normal pregnancy measured by ultrasound scanning. Values show mean (± two standard deviations) and are based on 400 measurements (Redrawn from Campbell, S. (1976). *Fetal Physiology and Medicine* **(eds. Beard, R. W. and Nathanielsz, P. W.), Saunders, London)**

l/min and remains high until parturition, thereafter returning to normal during the puerperium. The reasons for the increased cardiac output are not known, but it is probably under hormonal control because the return to normal after parturition occurs gradually over a few days rather than immediately. The increase in cardiac output occurs while the weight of the uterus and its contents is still relatively small. As the amount of blood perfusing the uterus continues to rise in the second and third trimesters, it cannot be argued that the increased cardiac output occurs solely to provide for additional uterine flow. It is probably a response reflecting generalised vasodilation, with the uterus receiving a larger proportion of the cardiac output as pregnancy progresses. The marked cutaneous vasodilation in pregnancy probably serves to dissipate heat generated by the mother's increased metabolic rate.

Early investigations suggested that the cardiac output falls in the third trimester. These results were misleading because the measurements were made with the mother lying on her back so that the gravid uterus pressed on the inferior vena cava, thereby reducing venous return and cardiac output. This artefact is removed if the subject lies in a lateral position. The reduction in venous return in the supine position can be so marked in late pregnancy as to make many women feel unwell if they lie on their backs.

The rise in cardiac output during pregnancy is produced by increases in both heart rate and stroke volume. Mean heart rate rises from a basal 70 to 85 beats per minute at term, with most of the increase in the first trimester. Stroke volume increases from 64 to 71 ml per beat.

Regular measurements of blood pressure during pregnancy are of great importance, but their interpretation is complicated by variations between individuals and with age. Both systolic and diastolic pressures fall in the first half of pregnancy but begin to rise in the third trimester. This effect is more pronounced for the diastolic pressure, and typical blood pressure and peripheral resistance values for a young woman before and during her first pregnancy would be as tabulated below.

The reduction of blood pressure in the sitting position results from venous pooling, and this is more pronounced during pregnancy as a result of decreased tone in the superficial veins.

The fall in blood pressure that occurs during pregnancy indicates that vasodilation must more than offset the increased cardiac output. Generalised oedema and vasodilation of the uterus occur after treatment with steroid hormones, especially oestrogens. The hyperaemia of skin and dilation of superficial veins are thought to be effected principally by progesterone.

The increase in systemic blood pressure observed towards term probably results from increased resistance in the degenerating maternal vessels supplying the intervillous space. The effect is more marked in older mothers, especially if it is their first child. Excessive increases in blood pressure during pregnancy and associated complications can threaten the lives of both mother and fetus.

Pulmonary arterial pressure does not change in pregnancy because the pulmonary vascular bed has a great capacity for autoregulation and can accept increases in blood flow without changes of pressure.

There is little change in venous pressure during pregnancy except in the leg veins. Femoral venous pressure may rise to 25 mmHg during gestation because the growing uterus presses on the iliac veins and the inferior vena cava. This effect is most marked in the standing or supine position. Obstruction of the venous return from the legs is partially relieved by shunting of blood through portal-

	Non-pregnant	Mid-pregnant	Late pregnancy
Lying lateral	118/69	112/60	115/68 (mmHg)
Sitting	110/70	103/60	108/68 (mmHg)
Peripheral resistance	1740	980	1240 dyn/(s · cm^{-5})

systemic anastomoses, thus bypassing the inferior vena cava. The femoral venous pressure rises continuously during pregnancy in step with increasing uterine size and falls as soon as delivery is completed. The raised venous pressure contributes to oedema of the legs which is common and may lead to varicosity of the superficial veins.

The maternal cardiovascular responses to exercise are not altered in pregnancy. However, in severe exercise uterine perfusion is reduced as demand by the skeletal muscles increases, and this can lead to fetal distress.

11.5   The fetal cardiovascular system

A circulatory system is established early in embryogenesis and a heart beat is present by 4—5 weeks of gestation. The fetal heart rate is at first slow, about 65 beats per minute, rises until mid-gestation and then later declines. The definitive fetal circulation develops by the 11th week of gestation; this ways illustrated earlier in figure 9.16 and is schematised in figure 11.6.

Oxygenated blood in the upper part of the inferior vena cava is about 70 per cent saturated with oxygen; it enters the right atrium where it mixes with deoxygenated blood returning from the head and upper limbs via the superior vena cava. The blood entering the heart from the inferior vena cava has a lower oxygen saturation than that in the umbilical vein as it is mixed with the deoxygenated venous blood returning from the lower parts of the fetus.

About 40 per cent of the venous return entering the right atrium passes through the foramen ovale into the left side of the heart and is pumped into the systemic circulation (figure 11.6). The arrangement of the septum secundum and septum primum ensures that the blood passing through the foramen ovale is almost entirely derived from the inferior vena cava and thus a further fall in oxygen saturation is avoided (figure 11.7). The remainder of the venous return is pumped by the right ventricle into the pulmonary artery whence it may pass either through the lungs or into the aorta via the ductus arteriosus. The amount of blood that passes through the lungs is small because the collapsed lungs of the fetus present a great resistance to flow, and represents only about 20 per cent of the total venous return. The rest of the blood, about 40 per cent of the venous return, enters the

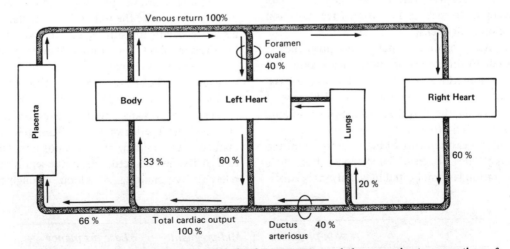

Figure 11.6 Diagram representing the fetal circulatory system, and the approximate proportions of blood flowing through its various elements. Note that much of the venous return bypasses the right heart direct to the left heart via the foramen ovale and that most of the right heart blood bypasses the lungs by flowing through the ductus arteriosus. Both of these bypass routes close after birth, thus establishing the mature circulatory system. The ductus venosus has been omitted for clarity, but see figure 9.16

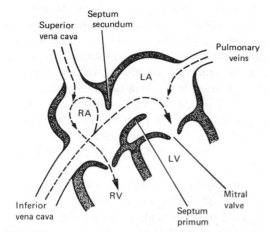

Figure 11.7   Diagram of the great veins and atria in the fetus which shows how oxygenated blood returning via the inferior vena cava divides into two streams at the septum secundum

aorta from the left pulmonary artery through the ductus arteriosus and mixes with the output of the left side of the heart. As the brachiocephalic, carotid and subclavian arteries leave the aorta proximal to the entry of the ductus arteriosus the upper limbs and the head receive the better oxygenated blood from the left ventricle with only a minimal further dilution by deoxygenated blood from the pulmonary circuit. However, the rest of the fetus is perfused with blood of relatively low oxygen content, and the oxygen tension can be measured in the umbilical arteries which are branches of the aorta and contain blood of identical composition. At the usual umbilical arterial oxygen tension of 24 mmHg the fetal blood would be 60–65 per cent saturated.

Thus all fetal organs including the brain receive oxygen at a very low tension compared with the adult state. To meet the metabolic requirements of the tissues, the fetal circulation must be able to deliver a large volume of blood to them so that they receive enough oxygen. In fact, fetal tissues are extremely well perfused because cardiac output is high in relation to tissue mass. Fetal cardiac output is 200 ml/kg body weight per minute, compared with 80 ml/kg body weight per minute in the adult. This high output is maintained at a low systemic blood pressure of 70/45 mmHg, indicating that peripheral resistance is low. Fetal

tissues are also richer in capillaries than adult tissue and this reduces diffusional distances thus helping to maintain adequate intracellular oxygen tension.

The control of cardiac output in the fetus differs from that of the adult and the full complement of cardiovascular responses is probably not developed until after birth. For example, in the adult stroke volume falls as heart rate increases and conversely cardiac output can be maintained during bradycardia by increasing the stroke volume. However, in the fetus cardiac output is determined solely by the heart rate as the stroke volume does not change if the heart speeds or slows.

Autonomic control of the heart and blood vessels becomes effective during the third trimester. The heart rate rises from its initial low rate to a maximum of about 160 beats per minute at 15 weeks of gestation and then falls to approximately 140 beats per minute at term during the period when parasympathetic vagal tone is established. As the heart rate slows, fetal systemic blood pressure rises due to the establishment of peripheral vascular tone. These changes probably coincide with the functional development of the carotid and aortic arch baroreceptors.

Some chemoreceptor activity develops by the third trimester since fetal hypoxia causes bradycardia and a rise in blood pressure due to vasoconstriction and reduction in peripheral blood flow. This maintains perfusion of the brain and placenta. It is thought that the aortic chemoreceptors are more important for this response than the carotid or central chemoreceptors because in experimental animals the effect is abolished by vagal nerve section.

11.6   Maternal blood and body fluids

The maternal net water gain during pregnancy is between 7 and 8 l as mentioned previously. Only a small fraction of this is intracellular water used for maternal tissue growth as 6.5 l lie outside the maternal cellular compartment. Much of this consists of maternal plasma, amniotic fluid and fetal tissue water. However, a litre or so cannot be accounted for in this way and appears to result from generalised maternal oedema due to water retention. This tendency to retain water is especially marked during the third trimester and depends on endocrine and renal changes as discussed later. Sometimes water retention is excessive; marked oedema is a common complication of pregnancy and excessive water retention exacerbates any existing tendency to hypertension.

Maternal plasma volume increases by about 40 per cent during pregnancy (figure 11.8). The red cell volume also increases by some 250 ml. The maximum plasma expansion is attained by about 34 weeks of gestation, after which it falls slightly until term. The form of this rise and fall in plasma volume largely determines many of the changes seen in the composition of maternal blood during gestation. Thus as the plasma volume increases some blood constituents show a relative dilution and then concentration near term.

Plasma concentrations of sodium, potassium and chloride fall slightly but significantly during pregnancy by about 5 mmol/kg of water but remain within the normal range. Total plasma protein decreases from 7 to 6 g/100 ml and this is largely due to a reduction in albumin with little change in the amount of globular proteins. In pregnancy the synthesis of albumin by the liver appears to be insufficient to compensate for the increased plasma volume. As a result there is a fall in plasma osmolarity from 290 to 280 mosmol within the first 8 weeks of pregnancy and this is maintained until term. Blood coagulability increases considerably due to elevation of plasma fibrinogen from 200 to 600 mg/100 ml, together with a decrease in fibrinolytic activity. This is of obvious advantage for haemostasis at the vulnerable placental site but together with the reduced rate of flow in the leg veins probably accounts for the increased incidence of thromboembolism in pregnancy.

Erythropoiesis is stimulated during pregnancy as a result of the expanding plasma volume but does not keep pace with it. As a result, by term the haematocrit falls from 40 to 33 per cent and the blood haemoglobin from 13.5 to 11.5 g/100 ml. Both changes are most pronounced at about 34 weeks of gestation and constitute the so-called anaemia of pregnancy. The mean corpuscular haemoglobin content and red cell volume do not change unless there is a marked iron deficiency. The dilution of the blood during pregnancy reduces its viscosity and thus probably limits any rise in blood pressure associated with the raised maternal cardiac output. Red cell fragility also increases due to the fall in colloid osmotic pressure of the plasma. This causes water uptake by the cells and the red cell electrolytes are thus diluted.

The white cell count rises in pregnancy from about 7000 to 10 500 per mm^3, largely due to an increased number of neutrophils. The mechanism and significance of this are unknown.

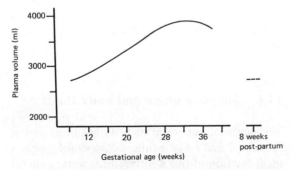

Figure 11.8   Rise in plasma volume during pregnancy compared to the volume post-partum. Graph shows average values for women in their first pregnancy (Redrawn from Hytten, F. E. and Leitch, I. (1971). *The Physiology of Human Pregnancy*, Blackwell, Oxford)

11.7   Fetal blood and body fluids

The water content of the fetal body declines during gestation (see section 11.3). This is due to reduction of the percentage of extracellular water as a fraction of body weight; by contrast the percentage of intracellular water increases. This redistribution of water suggests that cellular growth in the fetus occurs at the expense of extracellular space. At term extracellular fluid comprises some 45 per cent and intracellular fluid 30 per cent of the total body weight. This is very different from the adult where the values are 23 per cent and 40 per cent respectively, so the relative reduction of the extracellular space evidently continues after birth.

The amniotic fluid is probably mainly of fetal origin although several sources may contribute components to it. Its ionic composition is similar to that of extracellular fluid, as shown in table 11.2, but it only contains a little protein. Amniotic fluid also contains a large number of desquamated fetal cells in suspension and these may be cultured for analysis after collection by amniocentesis (see chapter 10); also present is other fetal debris such as particles of vernix (fetal sebum) and hairs.

The volume of amniotic fluid increases during pregnancy and reaches a maximum between 30 and 37 weeks of gestation (figure 11.2). During the last few weeks of pregnancy its volume declines rapidly from about 800 to 400 ml. This reduction in volume may assist the engagement of the fetal head prior to parturition. The fetus is able to move freely within its private pond when the amniotic fluid is abundant in relation to its size, but as fetal growth continues its freedom of movement becomes restricted. An important function of the amniotic fluid is to protect the fetus from mechanical trauma or from pressure which might affect its development. Any force applied to the surface of the uterus is spread evenly over the fetal body as the amniotic fluid pressure rises. The efficiency of this protective mechanism is such that fetuses may not be injured by falls that kill their mothers.

There is a rapid turnover of amniotic fluid and it is calculated that the water is replaced every three hours and the electrolytes every 15 hours. It is not known exactly how this is achieved but both the fetus and mother contribute to this turnover. During early gestation the amniotic fluid could be regarded as an extension of the fetal interstitial fluid, but as the integument develops the possibility of significant exchange across fetal skin declines.

Transfer of substances across the avascular amnion is possible and exchange of water and electrolytes may occur as well as of some maternal macromolecules. The amnion has a high rate of metabolism and oxygen consumption. Both the amnion and amniotic fluid contain large amounts of prolactin which influence water movement across the amnion, although it is not known whether the amnion synthesises or merely binds the hormone.

The fetal kidneys begin to form hypotonic urine from mid-gestation onwards; by late gestation this contributes an estimated 500 ml to the amniotic fluid each day and for this reason levels of creatinine and urea in amniotic fluid rise during gestation. In human fetuses with renal agenesis there is a marked reduction in the volume of amniotic fluid.

Injection of radio-opaque materials into the amniotic cavity shows that the fetus swallows about 500 ml of fluid per day. Any imbalance is made up by movement of water across the placenta. By contrast, amniotic fluid volume is excessive in fetuses with oesophageal atresia or with inoperative swallowing reflexes due to anencephaly. However, an imperforate anus has no influence on the volume of the amniotic fluid.

The protein and bilirubin contents of amniotic fluid decline during gestation as a result of fetal swallowing and absorption. The fact that lack of swallowing or urine production can influence amniotic fluid volume so considerably suggests that they are important mechanisms for regulating its volume, particularly in late gestation. In early gestation, when urine production and the swallowing reflex are absent, production by the amnion may be more important.

The fetal lungs also contribute to amniotic fluid and there is a continuous production of lung

Table 11.2   Composition of amniotic fluid compared with other extracellular fluids

Fluid	Protein (g/100 ml)	Ionic composition (mmol/kg water)			
		Na^+	K^+	Cl^-	HCO_3^-
Amniotic fluid	0.10	113	7.6	87	19
Lymph	3.27	147	4.8	107	24
Plasma	4.09	151	4.8	106	26
Fetal lung fluid	0.03	150	6.3	157	2.8

(From Adamson, T. M., Boyd, R. D. H., Platt, H. S. and Strang, L. B. (1969). *J. Physiol. Lond.*, **204**, 129.)

fluid, the importance of which is discussed below.

The affinity of fetal haemoglobin for oxygen and the haematological indices of fetal blood were discussed in chapter 7. The sites of erythropoiesis in the fetus alter as development progresses. Megaloblastic erythroblasts first appear in the blood islands of the yolk sac and embryo at 23 days menstrual age and disappear by 11 weeks of gestation when the fetal pattern of circulation is established. At 8 weeks of gestation secondary megaloblastic erythroblasts begin to appear, largely in the liver but also in the yolk sac, spleen and bone marrow. These cells persist throughout fetal life and finally disappear in the first few weeks after birth. The definitive normoblastic erythroblasts appear in the bone marrow at the beginning of the second trimester and become the principal source of erythrocytes by the third trimester.

The haemoglobin molecule is composed of four subunits each consisting of a globin chain and a haem group. There are five types of globin chain: alpha, beta, gamma, delta and epsilon. In the assembly of the haemoglobin molecule two identical chains plus attached haem groups associate to form a dyad and then two dyads combine to form the haemoglobin molecule. The two dyads that combine may have identical or differing globin chains and thus a variety of haemoglobin molecules can be constructed. Normal adult haemoglobin consists of two alpha and two beta subunits and fetal haemoglobin (HbF) has two alpha and two gamma chains.

Each of the erythropoietic sites mentioned above has the genetic potential to produce all five globin chains although the actual ratios produced vary from site to site as a result of gene regulation. This explains why the dominant haemoglobin type changes during gestation as the main site of erythropoiesis shifts. Figure 11.9 shows the relative proportions of different globin chains produced during gestation and early life. The blood islands of the embryo and yolk sac produce mainly epsilon chains and the liver and spleen mainly gamma chains. The rise in proportion of beta globin chains is associated with the onset of erythropoietic activity in the bone marrow. All sites produce alpha chains and these therefore

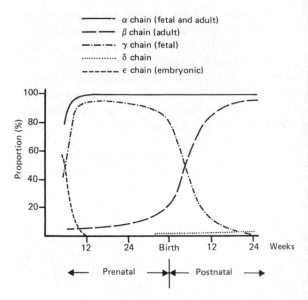

Figure 11.9   Changes in the proportions of the different haemoglobin chains produced at different stages of development (Redrawn from Strickberger, M. W. (1968). *Genetics*, Macmillan, New York)

appear early in gestation. Delta chains never appear in large quantities but can be detected postnatally. In the early embryo the haemoglobin may comprise epsilon chains alone or a combination of epsilon and alpha chains. Although embryonic haemoglobin uncontaminated with maternal blood cannot be obtained in any quantity, such experiments as have been performed suggest that these haemoglobins have a higher affinity for oxygen at a given partial pressure than HbF.

Little is known about the development of white cells in the fetus. At birth the white cell count is high, about 18 000 cells per mm³, but declines to the adult level in early postnatal life. The high fetal count is largely due to a raised proportion of polymorphonuclear cells. In pre-term babies the white cell count is low, suggesting that leukocytes develop relatively late in gestation, whereas the red cell count and blood haemoglobin is often higher in the pre-term than the term baby.

The principal plasma protein in the fetus is α-fetoprotein which during development is replaced by albumin. Thus the concentrations of α-fetoprotein and albumin in the fetal circulation are inversely related.

α-Fetoprotein is synthesised in the fetal liver, with probably a small contribution from the yolk sac early in gestation, and reaches a maximum concentration in fetal plasma of 3–4 mg/ml between 12 and 15 weeks of gestation. At this time it comprises one-third of the total plasma protein of the fetus. After this the levels decline to term when it is present at about 1 per cent of the peak value. α-Fetoprotein also appears in the maternal circulation from 10 weeks of gestation onwards and reaches a peak of 250 μg/ml at 30–35 weeks of gestation, that is after fetal levels have begun to decline. α-Fetoprotein in the maternal circulation probably originates from small lesions in the chorionic villi which allow fetal blood to leak into the mother. The protein is normally found in amniotic fluid and its concentrations both here and in maternal plasma are of diagnostic value (see chapter 10).

The physiological significance of α-fetoprotein as a plasma protein distinct from albumin is not known. It is larger than albumin and, unlike albumin, contains 4 per cent of carbohydrate. Both proteins consist of a single polypeptide chain and show considerable homology in amino acid sequence, suggesting that they derive from a common ancestral molecule.

11.8 The maternal kidney

Some of the changes in maternal renal function during pregnancy are a direct consequence of increased renal plasma flow whereas others reflect changes in renal tubule function. Renal plasma flow rises from about 500 to 730 ml/min per 1.73 m^2 of body surface area (average human body surface area). This occurs at the same time as the increase in maternal cardiac output early in pregnancy.

Glomerular filtration rate increases in early pregnancy from 90 to 150 ml/min per 1.73 m^2 of body surface. As the effective filtration pressure in the renal corpuscle is given by the difference between the hydrostatic pressure of the perfusing plasma and the colloid osmotic pressure opposing it, the fall in plasma osmolarity during pregnancy (see section 11.6) also contributes to the increased glomerular filtration rate.

The glomerular filtration rate increases more than the renal plasma flow and so there is a rise in the proportion of plasma that is filtered (the filtration fraction). The renal clearance of several important excretory products from blood increases because of the increased glomerular filtration rate. For example, plasma levels of creatinine, uric acid and urea are reduced in pregnancy. Filtration of sodium and other ions also rises in step with the change in glomerular filtration rate. For sodium this increase is about 60 per cent, but most is resorbed by the kidney tubules.

The reduced plasma sodium concentration in pregnancy (see section 11.6) may lead to increased renin release by the juxtaglomerular cells of the kidney and a consequent rise in plasma aldosterone. In fact renin, aldosterone and angiotensinogen levels are all elevated during pregnancy but the relationship between the renin–angiotensin system, renal function and maternal body fluids is poorly understood. Although the raised plasma levels of aldosterone lead to increased tubular resorption of sodium, the actual plasma level of sodium falls and so the water retention of pregnancy is certainly not due simply to sodium retention.

It is interesting that the ability to excrete a water load alters during pregnancy. For the first two trimesters 1 l of water taken orally produces a diuresis which is usually greater than in the non-pregnant woman (figure 11.10). However, the rate of urine production with the same water load during the third trimester is well below that of non-pregnant controls. This inhibition of diuresis in late pregnancy may possibly be associated with changes in hypothalamic and posterior pituitary function or to the changes in hormone levels mentioned in the preceding paragraph. This phenomenon probably explains the tendency towards oedema commonly observed in late pregnancy. Many of these changes in renal function may be associated with the high levels of circulating progesterone and a similar but smaller water

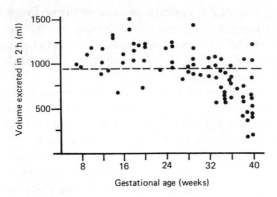

Figure 11.10 Renal function during pregnancy. The graph shows the amount of urine passed after drinking 1 litre of water, and compares water excretion with that of non-pregnant control women (dotted line). Diuresis in early pregnancy gives way to a marked antidiuresis towards term (Redrawn from Hytten, F. E. and Leitch, I. (1971). *The Physiology of Human Pregnancy,* **Blackwell, Oxford)**

retention is seen in the luteal phase of the menstrual cycle (see chapter 2).

Urinary levels of several substances, notably amino acids, glucose and vitamins, rise during pregnancy, probably because increased filtration of these substances exceeds the capacity of the tubules to reabsorb them. Many women show a marked glycosuria during pregnancy and may lose up to 1 g of glucose per day in this way. It has been suggested that this may be due to a decrease in the efficiency of tubular resorption of glucose. It is certainly very curious that important metabolites for which there is increased demand during pregnancy should be wasted in this way.

11.9 The fetal kidney

The embryological development of the kidneys is described in chapter 9. Functional renal corpuscles appear in the juxtamedullary region of the cortex of the metanephric kidney at 22 weeks of gestation and glomerular filtration begins. The renal corpuscles continue to differentiate from the deeper layers of the cortex outward. Nephrogenesis is usually complete by 36 weeks gestation but functional maturation of the kidneys continues after birth.

The glomerular filtration rate increases towards term partly because there are more glomeruli but also because of the increase in fetal blood pressure. Furthermore, the efficiency of ultrafiltration is increased by thinning of the glomerular membrane. In the fetus and neonate the glomerular filtration rate is directly proportional to the systemic blood pressure as the adult mechanisms for autoregulation of renal blood flow are not yet established.

As the glomeruli develop from deeper regions of the cortex outwards the pattern of blood flow in the fetal kidney alters so that most flow is diverted to the active glomeruli. However, in the fetus only about 2 per cent of the cardiac output perfuses the kidneys compared with 25 per cent in the adult.

The fetal renal tubules are probably capable of active transport even before any glomerular filtrate is received. Human metanephric tubules taken at the end of the first trimester have been shown *in vitro* to transport phenol red from the medium into the lumen. Thus some urine may be produced within the tubules by active secretion before glomerular filtration starts.

However, the efficiency of tubular reabsorption is low even when glomerular filtration occurs. A moderate rise in fetal plasma glucose from its normal value of 75 mg per cent (4.2 mmol/l) causes it to spill into the fetal urine and produce a diuresis. This occurs in the case of uncontrolled maternal diabetes. The urine of a normal fetus is glucose and protein-free and its major osmotic constituents are sodium and fructose, so the relatively large volumes of hypotonic urine that are produced must be the result of active resorption of solutes without isosmotic water absorption. Until renal blood flow is stable a countercurrent exchange mechanism for urine concentration cannot be established. It is obvious that these properties of the fetal kidney make the application of standard tests of kidney function to the fetus difficult to interpret.

Thus the importance of the fetal kidneys in fetal fluid balance is difficult to assess. In human renal agenesis it is possible for the fetus to survive until term and in such cases fluid balance has presumably been maintained across the placenta. There are probably species differences as chronic drainage of the ureters in the fetal sheep causes death whereas the fetus can survive if the urine is returned to the amniotic cavity.

11.10   The maternal respiratory system

The vital capacity of the lungs is not altered in pregnancy but the tidal volume rises continuously to a third trimester maximum some 40–50 per cent above non-pregnant levels. In certain body positions the uterus may restrict movement of the diaphragm and this is followed by a compensatory increase in the rate of ventilation so that the minute volume is maintained. Thus the minute volume may rise from non-pregnant levels of 7.2 l to as much as 11 l but falls again very rapidly after delivery. Since the dead space of the airways is constant an increase in the minute volume augments alveolar ventilation.

Inhibition of diaphragmatic respiration in late pregnancy leads to a compensatory increase in intercostal activity. Changes in the shape of the thoracic boundaries take place with the transverse diameter increasing by up to 2 cm and the dome of the diaphragm rising by about 4 cm. The lower ribs undergo an outward displacement and often do not return to their former state after pregnancy. These changes are not directly due to uterine enlargement as they occur fairly early in pregnancy.

The volume of oxygen consumed per minute rises by at least 50 ml during pregnancy. Some of this is used to satisfy the demands of the feto-placental unit (see table 7.2) and some to sustain the increase in maternal tissue mass and in cardiac and respiratory work. It can be calculated from the increase in cardiac output and blood volume that the volume of oxygen that is delivered to the tissues exceeds their oxygen demand. This may explain why there is a reduced arteriovenous oxygen difference during pregnancy. The minute volume increases more than is necessary to supply the additional oxygen required; in other words the pregnant woman hyperventilates. Hyperventila-

tion ensures not only that maternal arterial blood is always fully saturated with oxygen but also results in a fall in the partial pressure of carbon dioxide of about 6 mmHg in her arterial blood. This helps the fetus to eliminate carbon dioxide by increasing the partial pressure gradient across the placenta.

It is thought that hyperventilation results from a direct action of progesterone on the respiratory centres as similar but smaller changes in the alveolar carbon dioxide tension associated with hyperventilation occur in the luteal phase of the menstrual cycle. They can also be induced in men by injection of progesterone. Despite this hyperventilation many pregnant women experience shortness of breath, perhaps as a result of this increased hormonal drive on the respiratory centres.

11.11   The fetal respiratory system

The use of ultrasound for measuring fetal growth has already been mentioned. A modification of the technique using Doppler analysis of the reflected sound allows fetal movements, including those of fluids in the trachea, heart and major blood vessels, to be detected. These studies have confirmed the long-held view that the fetus performs ventilatory movements *in utero*.

Figure 11.11 shows a tracing of fetal breathing movements near term obtained by reflecting the ultrasound from the fetal thorax. This regular pattern of ventilatory movements is present from 34 weeks of gestation onwards and is due to activity in the intercostal muscles and diaphragm. These movements average about 40–60 per minute and are interspersed by frequent periods of apnoea lasting for a few seconds. Prior to this, from 24 weeks of gestation, the ventilatory movements are more rapid but less regular and the periods of apnoea are longer. The earliest that ventilatory movements have been detected is at 12 weeks of gestation. The establishment of regular breathing movements at 34 weeks is indicative of the maturation of respiratory centre activity.

The fetal breathing movements are relatively

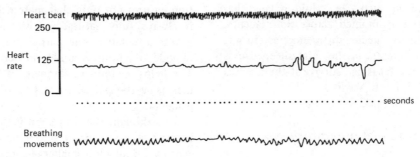

Figure 11.11 Ultrasound recording from a human term fetus. The record shows heart beat and heart rate as well as fetal breathing movements which are regular and of even depth but interrupted by a period of apnoea lasting about 5 s (Redrawn from Boddy, K. (1976). *Fetal Physiology and Medicine* (eds. Beard, R. W. and Nathanielsz, P. W.), Saunders, London)

shallow and do not aspirate amniotic fluid into the lungs. Occasionally the fetus shows 'gasps' or 'sighs' *in utero* when a larger flow of fluid is detectable in the trachea but even these augmented breaths are insufficient to clear the dead space and radio-opaque material injected into the amniotic cavity does not appear in the bronchial tree.

The pattern of fetal breathing movements shows circadian fluctuations and the duration of the apnoeic periods is longest in the early morning. During this period and during the 72 hours prior to labour, breathing movements occur less than 50 per cent of the time. Fetal breathing movements are also strongly suppressed after maternal fasting or the smoking of a cigarette.

Alterations in the pattern of fetal breathing movements have also been observed in response to changes in fetal blood gas tensions. Most of the experimental work has been conducted in the sheep although the results mentioned below have been shown to be applicable to the human fetus. Hypercapnia is a potent stimulus to fetal breathing: the depth of the movements and the frequency and duration of apnoeic periods are increased considerably, although the frequency of breathing movements within a period of activity is not affected. By contrast, hypoxia tends to reduce breathing movements and to increase the frequency and duration of apnoea.

This lack of reflex response to hypoxia is consistent with the view that the carotid bodies do not influence fetal ventilatory movements. Thus without this peripheral chemoreceptor drive

hypoxia causes a reduction in neuronal activity in the respiratory centres and a reduction in breathing movements. However, the activity of the central chemoreceptors at normal fetal oxygen tensions explains the potency of hypercapnic stimulation. It seems logical that the carotid body chemoreceptors should not be functional in the fetus because the low oxygen tensions normally present would cause continual stimulation if the receptors had adult sensitivity.

In severe asphyxia the regular breathing movements vanish but the incidence of gasping behaviour increases. This mechanism may be of importance in initiating the first breath at birth and is discussed in chapter 13. If uterine contractions in labour are of sufficient intensity and frequency to cause fetal asphyxia, fetal breathing movements stop altogether as the fetal heart rate slows (see chapter 12), and gasping behaviour predominates.

The bronchial tree is formed by the end of the first trimester and during the second trimester the respiratory bronchioles develop. Further development of the bronchioles and alveoli continues during the third trimester and after birth.

During fetal development the lungs fill with fluid secreted by the alveoli. The composition of fetal lung fluid was given earlier in table 11.2 and it should be compared with amniotic fluid and the others listed in the table. The chloride concentration in alveolar fluid is high; it is thought to be actively transported into the alveoli and followed passively by sodium, potassium and water. The bicarbonate concentration is low and so the alveolar fluid is acid. Lung fluid is formed at the rate of about 3 ml/kg fetus per hour, and at term the lungs contain about 40 ml. Excess lung fluid either passes into the amniotic fluid or is swallowed by the fetus.

There are two main types of alveolar epithelial cell: type I cells across which gaseous exchange occurs and type II cells which secrete phospholipid surfactant, essential to prevent collapse of the inflated lung. Fetal alveolar fluid is thought to be formed at the type I cells. Type II cells are particularly numerous in the alveoli of the term fetus and of the newborn. The two principal surfactants produced in the fetal lung are sphingomyelin and lecithin. The amount of lecithin rises rapidly from 26 weeks of gestation to term and its concentration in amniotic fluid relative to that of sphingomyelin is a useful indicator of the maturity of the fetal lung. This is an important consideration if the delivery is to be induced.

11.12   The fetal gastrointestinal tract

The functional development of the fetal gastrointestinal tract occurs rapidly. Mucosal glands appear at 16—20 weeks of gestation and by about 26 weeks it is capable of digesting milk. Although most digestive enzymes are present by 26 weeks amylase is not secreted until pancreatic exocrine function matures after birth. Pepsinogen (and perhaps also rennin) is present in the gastric mucosa by 20—24 weeks of gestation but the stomach contents are only just acidic until birth. However, the stomach contents acidify within 30 minutes of birth, probably because vagally-mediated gastric acid secretion occurs as a result of stress during delivery. Dipeptidases and tripeptidases are formed in the small intestine from 16 weeks of gestation and are followed slightly later by the disaccharidases which hydrolyse lactose and sucrose. Amino acid transport in the fetal gut is also established at about this time.

The fetus continually swallows amniotic fluid (see section 11.7) and radio-opaque material injected into the amniotic fluid is eventually propelled into the colon. Peristaltic gut movements begin at mid-gestation and become more coordinated towards term. Since the fetal gut has considerable digestive capacity in the third trimester the protein and cells in the swallowed amniotic fluid are broken down and form fetal faeces or *meconium*. Exfoliation of mucosal cells from the fetal gut also contributes significantly to the meconium which is a viscid material coloured greenish-black by bile pigments. The fetal gut is microbiologically sterile and so the meconium is unaltered by bacterial action.

Meconium accumulates in the fetal colon and rectum during gestation but is not normally voided into the amniotic fluid. Fetal asphyxia stimulates gut peristalsis, often causing the appearance of meconium in amniotic fluid; when this occurs the fluid becomes dark and turbid. This may sometimes be observed in amniotic fluid obtained by amniocentesis or seen during the second state of labour when the amniotic fluid is released. Such staining is a sure sign of fetal distress.

11.13   The fetal endocrine system

The fetal endocrine system plays a key role in the development of the fetus by influencing fetal homeostasis and by inducing specific developmental changes in a coordinated manner.

The placenta is impermeable to polypeptide hormones, but catecholamines, thyroid hormones and steriods may theoretically cross from the maternal blood stream to influence the fetus. However, catecholamines are prevented from reaching the fetus because the placenta contains large amounts of monoamine oxidase which breaks them down. The placenta is also rich in the enzyme which inactivates cortisol by conversion to cortisone and, unlike the adult, the fetus cannot reverse the reaction. Small but significant amounts of thyroid hormones enter the fetal circulation although placental permeability to them is relatively low. The only hormones that have an unrestricted passage across the placenta are the sex steroids and their precursors.

This extensive insulation from direct influence

by maternal hormones allows the fetal endocrine system to regulate growth, development and metabolism with a considerable degree of autonomy.

Growth hormone

Growth hormone has surprisingly little effect on fetal growth. In anencephalic fetuses in which the level of growth hormone may only be 20 per cent of that in normal fetuses, the birth weight is often within the normal range. In genetic growth hormone deficiency the fetus is still of normal birth weight but is often short in stature. Thus it appears that fetal growth hormone influences skeletal growth and development rather than increase of mass. Fetal levels of growth hormone are highest at mid-gestation and fall sharply until birth, but even then the amounts are considerably higher than in normal adults. Fetal growth hormone has a permissive role, increasing the sensitivity of the pancreas to glucose and promoting beta cell growth.

Insulin

Insulin is probably the most important 'growth hormone' of the fetus. The pattern of secretion of insulin and the demands on the pancreas differ from those of the adult because the supply of glucose to the fetus from the mother is relatively constant. In other words, the fetus does not have to arrange its secretion of insulin around meal times.

In mid-gestation glucose does not stimulate the release of insulin from the fetal pancreas although from this time until term the sensitivity of the beta cells increases. However, even at term the response of the fetal pancreas to glucose is sluggish and the slow, protracted release of insulin resembles that of a diabetic.

Although the fetal pancreas is not very responsive to acute fluctuations in blood glucose it responds to the chronic elevations that occur in uncontrolled maternal diabetes. The fetus of a diabetic mother has beta cell hyperplasia and its response to glucose is similar to that of an adult. Thus the chronically elevated glucose levels in the fetus accelerate functional differentiation of its pancreas.

Amino acids stimulate the release of insulin far more effectively in the fetus than glucose and this is consistent with the mainly anabolic and growth-promoting actions of this hormone in the fetus. Fetal insulin levels show a better correlation with birth weight than any other fetal hormone. Many term fetuses of low birth weight (1250–1800 g) are diabetic, whereas in maternal diabetes, where the fetal insulin levels are raised, the fetuses may have a birth weight of as much as 6000 g.

Thyroid hormones

The influence of thyroid hormones on human fetal growth and development appears to be more subtle than many animal experiments might have suggested. The fetal thyroid is active from an early stage of gestation and thyroid hormones are elaborated from 12 weeks of gestation onwards.

A fetus that is hypothyroid is usually of above average birth weight although the development of the central nervous system and the skeleton is retarded relative to other systems. The ratio of brain to body weight is normal and the brain has its normal complement of cells but is deficient in total RNA and protein.

Because the placenta is permeable to small amounts of maternal thyroid hormones, fetuses do not experience a total absence of these hormones even if fetal thyroid function is deficient. Thus the typical signs of cretinism due to thyroid deficiency are not pronounced at birth and only become easily recognisable in the neonatal period. However, the signs are obvious at birth if the mother is also hypothyroid, thus emphasising the importance of placental transfer of thyroid hormones. Fetal hyperthyroidism is usually associated with low birth weight.

The adrenal glands

The adrenal cortex first develops as the non-zoned *fetal cortex*, but at 5–6 weeks of gestation further proliferation of cells takes place at the surface of the fetal cortex and eventually forms the zoned *definitive cortex*. The cells of the medulla separate from the sympathetic ganglia at about 7 weeks of gestation and migrate between the developing cortical cells to produce a complete adrenal gland. The glands grow rapidly and reach their maximum size relative to other organs between 3 and 4 months of gestation when they are as big as the kidneys. Their growth rate relative to other organs then slows down but even at term they are 20 times larger in relation to body weight than in the adult. The mass of medullary tissue also increases steadily until term (figure 11.12).

Very little is known about the function of the adrenal medulla during development although in the late fetus it functions in an adult manner releasing catecholamines into the circulation if the fetus is stressed, for example by hypoxia.

The importance of the fetal cortex in providing precursors for the synthesis of oestrogens by the fetoplacental unit has already been discussed in chapter 7. The definitive cortex shows little synthetic activity for much of fetal life but has the capacity to convert placental progesterone to cortisol. During the last trimester this capacity increases enormously and fetal plasma cortisol levels rise as shown in figure 11.13. In the neonatal period the fetal cortex involutes rapidly, leaving the definitive cortex which then displays renewed growth (figure 11.12).

The rise in fetal plasma cortisol during the last trimester probably underlies several important changes in fetal physiology at this time. There is an important relationship between fetal cortisol and lung maturation because cortisol induces the enzyme which is rate limiting for lecithin synthesis and lecithin levels rise sharply (figure 11.13). This is accompanied by an increase in the number of type II cells in the alveoli. Cortisol also accelerates the functional differentiation of the liver and induces a number of liver enzymes including those stimulating glycogen synthesis (figure 11.13). The possibility that fetal cortisol release acts as a stimulus for parturition in the human is discussed in chapter 12.

The involution of the fetal zone of the cortex and the full functional development of the definitive cortex are dependent upon changes in the tropic activity of the pituitary. Endocrine activity in the definitive cortex is supported by the 39

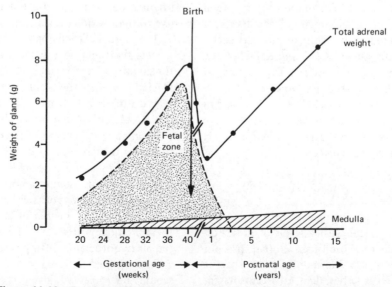

Figure 11.12 Development of the adrenal gland during the second and third trimesters of pregnancy and during the postnatal period. The graph emphasises the rapid growth and large relative size of the fetal zone of the cortex

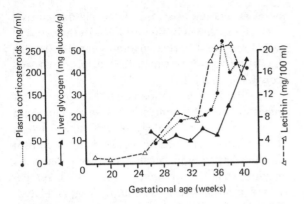

Figure 11.13 The time courses in human pregnancy of the concentrations of corticosteroids in umbilical cord plasma, of lecithin in amniotic fluid, and of glycogen in fetal liver (Redrawn from Liggins, G. C. (1976). *Fetal Physiology and Medicine* (eds. Beard, R. W. and Nathanielsz, P. W.), Saunders, London)

amino acid pituitary peptide corticotropin (ACTH), which is secreted at a low level for most of gestation. The fetal cortex is supported by two smaller tropic polypeptides: corticotropin-like intermediate lobe polypeptide (CLIP, which is composed of amino acids 24–39 of ACTH) and alpha-melanocyte stimulating hormone (αMSH, comprising amino acids 1–13 of ACTH). Involution of the fetal cortex and further development of the definitive cortex is associated with a shift of pituitary secretions from the fragments CLIP and αMSH to the single intact corticotropin ACTH. The anatomical origin of the three tropic hormones can also be distinguished: CLIP and αMSH are synthesised in the pars intermedia which is well defined in the fetus but much less so in the adult, whereas ACTH is synthesised in the pars distalis.

Sex steroids

The placenta is freely permeable to progesterone and oestrogens so fetal plasma levels of these hormones are similar to those of the mother. It is not known whether these hormones exert specific effects on the fetus other than as precursors for fetal steroidogenesis. The fact that they have free access to the fetus suggests that they do not regulate fetal development directly because the fetus can exert little control over their levels.

An important difference between male and female fetuses is the presence in the male of circulating testosterone. The relatively high levels of chorionic gonadotropin in the fetal circulation act on the interstitial tissue of the developing testis in an LH-like manner to promote the synthesis of testosterone. On the other hand, the developing ovary is not susceptible to this type of stimulus and does not manufacture steroid hormones. The sustentacular cells of the developing testis also produce a protein hormone called anti-müllerian hormone but its exact structure and function have still to be determined.

Sexual development in the embryo and fetus proceeds towards a female pattern unless actively opposed by specific masculinising stimuli. In the genotypically male fetus testosterone and anti-müllerian hormone are responsible for masculinisation. Testosterone induces the growth of all male structures whereas anti-müllerian hormone causes the regression of the müllerian ducts from which female structures are derived. A number of errors in the development of the urogenital tract arise if these masculinising hormones are not secreted in sufficient amount or at the appropriate time, or if the target structures are insensitive to their action (see chapter 9).

It is also believed that circulating testosterone affects the functional differentiation of the hypothalamus so as to cause the development of a mechanism for the tonic rather than cyclical release of gonadotropin releasing hormone. A tonic pattern of release is characteristic of the adult male (see chapter 3). If indeed the hypothalamus is masculinised in this sort of way in the human, then it must occur early on in gestation and require only minute amounts of testosterone. Furthermore the hypothalamus must then become refractory to any further influence. For example, there are no reported cases of masculinisation of the female hypothalamus in opposite sexed human twins with conjoined placental circulations although this would be expected given the theory discussed above. It should be remembered that testosterone is aromatised to oestradiol in the hypothalamus and it is probable that it exerts its masculinising effect as oestradiol. One might therefore expect placental oestradiol to exert an effect on the hypothalamus in both male and female fetuses but this does not occur because oestradiol is tightly bound to plasma proteins in the fetus and does not enter the hypothalamus.

The circulating oestradiol and progesterone exert effects on the mammary tissue of both sexes. At birth the glands may be hypertrophic and produce a watery secretion called 'witch's milk' (see chapter 14).

11.14 The fetal central nervous system

The fetal brain grows rapidly during the second and third trimesters and this is shown in figure 11.14 in terms of the *rate* of growth. The full complement of neurones, which must serve an individual throughout his life time, is reached by 8 months of gestation. However, functional maturation of the brain and proliferation of glial cells is far from complete and continues for many years after birth.

Before 10 weeks of gestation there is no myelin in the fetal brain and the fibre tracts progressively

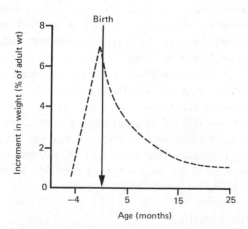

Figure 11.14 Rate of growth of the human brain in the fetal and postnatal period. The gain in weight is expressed as a percentage of the weight of the adult brain gained in each month (Redrawn from Davison A. N. and Dobbing, T. (1966). *British Medical Bulletin*, **22(1), pages 40–44)**

myelinate from this time onwards. This continues after birth and some important tracts do not complete the process until the end of the first postnatal year. The absence of myelin sheaths does not imply that the tracts are not functional: for example the optic nerves do not develop myelin sheaths until just before term but pupillary reflexes in response to light are present before this time.

At term the fetal brain is about one-quarter of the weight of the adult brain but its gross appearance is similar. As the cerebral cortex develops its surface complexity increases; fissures and sulci become visible at 20 weeks of gestation. At term, however, the cerebral cortex is still functionally very immature and most of the central nervous activity of the fetus and newborn occurs in the basal brain and spinal cord and is reflex in nature.

Reflex activity is first noticeable at 5–6 weeks of gestation in the area supplied by the trigeminal nerve and tactile stimulation produces a deflection of the fetal head away from the side of stimulation. At 8 weeks of gestation palmar and plantar reflexes have developed, and pupillary and blinking reflexes are evident by 28 and 30 weeks respectively.

Many of the fetal movements (*quickening*) felt by the pregnant mother are produced by reflexes of this sort. They are usually noticed by about 18 weeks of gestation but imperceptible movements occur long before this time. In subsequent pregnancies a mother often notices fetal movement at an earlier time than in her first pregnancy because she knows what to expect.

Fetal cerebrocortical activity can be detected from about 20 weeks of gestation onwards by electroencephalography (EEG) but is irregular and the traces show periods of relative inactivity. In older fetuses electrocortical activity similar to that of rapid eye movement sleep in adults has been observed and is associated with rapid eye movements in the fetus and with fetal breathing movements.

Fetal brain damage may occur in a number of ways but a full discussion of the causes would not be appropriate here. Poor fetal nutrition can cause intellectual impairment in later life and may arise from malnutrition of the mother or from inadequate placental function. Fetuses that show demonstrable growth retardation before 34 weeks of gestation often show impaired intelligence in later life. There are probably especially vulnerable periods during brain development and differentiation when damage can more easily occur, as is the case for the induction of malfunctions by the action of teratogenic agents during organogenesis. Hypoxia during the uterine or prenatal period is also an important cause of brain damage. The incomplete development of the blood–brain barrier in the fetus may increase its vulnerability to injurious agents.

11.15   Other metabolic changes in the mother during pregnancy

We have already discussed a number of important metabolic changes in the mother during pregnancy, but a few extra points need to be made. We have stressed that many of the changes seen in the pregnant woman are preparations for fetoplacental growth rather than responses to it. Some of these adaptive physiological changes occur in early pregnancy before the demands of the fetoplacental unit are significant.

The basal metabolic rate of a pregnant woman is about 15 per cent higher than the non-pregnant level as judged by oxygen consumption. It is not clear whether this is due to increased activity of the thyroid gland although its gross appearance and histology suggest this. The action of oestrogens on the liver increases the plasma concentration of thyroid hormone binding globulin; with the raised plasma volume this means that more thyroid hormone can be carried in the blood. However, plasma levels of free active thyroid hormones do not alter significantly, perhaps due to faster turnover. There is some immunological evidence that a TSH-like thyrotropic hormone is produced by the placenta, but it should be noted that the alpha chains of hCG and TSH are very similar (see chapter 7), and that hCG has a weak thyrotropic action, perhaps due to the beta subunit. The basal body temperature rises by about 0.6°C during pregnancy, as in the luteal phase of the menstrual cycle, perhaps because progesterone resets the hypothalamic thermoreceptors.

Plasma levels of free cortisol are very high in pregnancy and so contribute to the metabolic changes. Alterations in glucose metabolism are probably partly due to the gluconeogenic activity of cortisol working with the growth hormone-like action of human placental lactogen. Fat storage in pregnancy is probably also stimulated by the high levels of plasma cortisol. These high concentrations cannot be suppressed by steroid administration, a finding which has led to the suggestion that there is also a placental corticotropin. However, the evidence for such a hormone is scanty. Corticotropin-like immunological activity rises continuously throughout pregnancy and is responsible for the raised plasma cortisol and is also associated with the changes in skin pigmentation that occur. Cortisol binding globulin (transcortin) levels are also raised in the same manner as those of thyroid binding globulin mentioned above. As transcortin binds both progesterone and cortisol (see chapter 2) there is competition for the carrier.

Peristaltic activity of the mother's gastrointestinal tract is reduced during pregnancy so that the mean transit time increases. This is probably the main reason for constipation, which is common in pregnancy, and may be caused by progesterone. Gastric emptying is also delayed and stomach acidity reduced. The increase in transit time may be responsible for the observed increase in the efficiency of absorption of some nutrients, for example iron and some vitamins.

Levels of many blood metabolites change in pregnancy. Plasma concentrations of vitamins, free amino acids and glucose fall, the latter from 80 to 65 mg per 100 ml. It is interesting to recall that these same nutrients also spill over into the urine during pregnancy (see section 11.8). In contrast, levels of all major plasma lipids rise by 35–40 per cent during pregnancy.

Further reading

Beard, R. W. and Nathanielsz, P. W. (eds.) (1976). *Fetal Physiology and Medicine*, Saunders, London

Comline, R. S.,   Cross, K. W.,   Dawes, G. S.   and
Nathanielsz,   P. W.   (eds.)   (1973).   *Fetal and
Neonatal   Physiology*   (Barcroft   Centenary
Symposium). Cambridge University Press

Dawes, G. S. (1968). *Fetal and Neonatal Physiology*, Year Book Medical Publishers, Chicago

Hafez, E. S. E.   (1975).   *The Mammalian Fetus*,
Charles C. Thomas, Springfield, Illinois

Hytten, F. E. and Leitch, I. (1971). *The Physiology
of Human Pregnancy*, Blackwell, Oxford

12

The Initiation and Course of Labour

12.1 Introduction

In man, as with other mammals, the gestation period is remarkably constant, and has a duration of 40 ± 2 weeks (i.e. 10 lunar months) from the last menstrual period, with the majority of pregnancies lying between these limits. However, in extremely rare cases, normal babies have been born after as little as 32 or as much as 52 weeks of gestation. Gestational age is most often calculated from the first day of the last menstrual period which occurs 13–16 days before ovulation. This is termed *menstrual age*, and it is a useful measure since it is timed from an obvious and visible event which the mother is often able to date precisely. *Fetal age* is also commonly used to refer to the progress of gestation, and is defined as menstrual age minus two weeks. Because some women are unsure of the date of their last menstrual period, other methods may have to be used to determine how far pregnancy has advanced. These were discussed in chapter 10.

It is obviously important that the length of gestation and the timing of parturition be such that the infant is born at an optimal stage of development for its survival. If *term* is defined as 40 weeks of menstrual age, then even babies of 2.5 kg (which is widely accepted as a normal birth weight) show a significantly elevated perinatal mortality rate if they are born more than 2 weeks pre- or post-term. For this reason, many obstetricians prefer to induce labour artificially if it does not begin spontaneously once the expected date of delivery has passed.

The factors which trigger parturition are not yet understood but it seems that increasing placental inadequacy and the mechanical effects of the fully grown fetus on the uterus are both important. Nevertheless it is probably unwise to seek a single cause or trigger for parturition; rather it occurs because of an accelerating convergence of mechanical, electrophysiological, neural and endocrine signals of both fetal and maternal origin.

Uterine contractions occur spasmodically throughout the later part of pregnancy in preparation for parturition, but only become strong and coordinated as labour approaches. Thus there is a prelude of activity which precedes labour itself. Labour is conveniently divided into three stages: stage I – onset of coordinated powerful uterine contractions, leading to full cervical dilation; stage II – passage of the baby through the birth canal and its complete delivery; stage III – delivery of the placenta and membranes (afterbirth). These events and the use of drugs to expedite or ease labour will be discussed in more detail in subsequent sections. After childbirth, the mother enters the period of *puerperium* during which she recovers from the changes and stresses brought about by her pregnancy and delivery. The changes and adaptations of the newborn infant to extrauterine life after delivery will be discussed in chapter 13.

12.2 The uterus in late pregnancy

In the first months of pregnancy, the growth of the uterus outstrips that of the fetus (figure 12.1), but falls behind after the fifth or sixth month. During the final months of pregnancy the fetus grows rapidly, whereas there is very little further growth of the uterus. The fetus is accommodated by the continued stretching of the uterus which becomes thinner as its musculature is distended. The thinning of the uterine wall and consequent stretching of the smooth muscle fibres is most marked at the fundic (top) part of the uterus: this becomes more distended, whereas the caudal (lower) part of the uterus retains a smaller radius of curvature, merging at its lowest part into the thickened cylindrical ring of the cervix (figure 12.2). Thus at term, the uterus viewed from the side approximates in shape to an inverted pear.

One consequence of uterine stretching is to

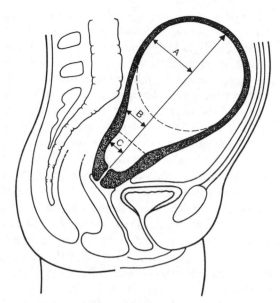

Figure 12.2   Illustration of the shape and curvatures of the gravid uterus

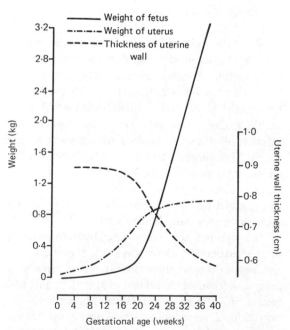

Figure 12.1   Growth of the fetus and uterus. Note that fetal growth overtakes that of the uterus after week 24, and that there is progressive thinning of the uterine wall after the 16th week (Redrawn from Gillespie, C. G. (1950). *American Journal of Obstetrics and Gynaecology,* **59, pages 949–959)**

increase excitability of the muscle layer. As the uterine contents expand, the stretching of the myometrium and its change of shape alter the relative disposition of the smooth muscle fibres. At the beginning of pregnancy the fibres lie obliquely to one another in a criss-cross arrangement; towards term, because of uterine expansion, their relative arrangement alters and becomes circular or spiral. This means that muscular activity originating in the fundus and spreading downwards tends to squeeze the uterine contents towards the cervix.

Animal experiments have revealed changes in muscle biochemistry in late pregnancy compatible with the idea that the myometrium is being prepared for sustained work. Thus the uterine contents of actomyosin, calcium-dependent ATPase, ATP, inorganic phosphate and phosphocreatine all increase towards term, although the concentrations of these substances are always much lower than in skeletal muscle. It is probable that these biochemical changes are dependent upon the presence of oestrogen, since their levels decline after ovariectomy but are restored after administration of oestrogen.

It has been known for more than a century that uterine contractions occur from mid-pregnancy onwards, and gradually become larger, more forceful and better coordinated as the onset of labour is approached. These are referred to as *Braxton Hicks contractions*. In mid-pregnancy and up to the middle of the third trimester, Braxton Hicks contractions are relatively feeble (generating intrauterine pressures of a few millimetres of mercury), and are very localised. In the last few weeks they become more forceful, and myogenic activity may be sufficient to cause larger, well-coordinated contractions which spread further over the uterus, involving more fibres. These labour-like contractions, although isolated, may be of sufficient intensity (generating from 20 to 50 mmHg pressure) to cause pain as well as awareness, but they occur irregularly and do not indicate the immediate onset of labour. The Braxton Hicks contractions tend to occur earlier and to be more painful in succeeding pregnancies, i.e. in *multiparous* women, but can be distinguished readily from true labour contractions since they are not regular.

Spontaneous activity of the myometrium occurs because of the inherent instability of certain focal pacemaker cells. The resting membrane potential of these smooth muscle cells is close to the threshold for depolarisation; further depolarisation due to inward leakage of sodium or other ionic movements may be sufficient to trigger an action potential which then spreads from the key cells to adjacent cells by myogenic conduction. In this respect, uterine smooth muscle behaves like a syncytium, especially at the very end of pregnancy. Stretching of the fibres, for example by fetal movements or distension by growth, also promotes spontaneous excitation.

Experiments in which ovariectomised laboratory mammals were treated with steroid hormones have shown that the spontaneous activity of myometrial smooth muscle is dependent upon endocrine influences. Thus the oestrogen-primed uterus is sensitive to externally applied uterine spasmogens (such as oxytocin, histamine, acetylcholine and prostaglandins), reflecting increased excitability due to alterations in resting membrane potential. By contrast progesterone treatment causes the myometrium to hyperpolarise and inherent myogenic activity and sensitivity to drugs decreases. It is believed that myometrial sensitivity in pregnancy is similarly influenced by exposure to circulating oestrogen and progesterone. Thus it is proposed that excitability during the first and second trimesters of pregnancy is inherently low because the uterus is dominated by progesterone, and shows little spontaneous myogenic activity. It is also relatively refractory to the action of smooth muscle agonists. As pregnancy advances towards term, oestrogen is secreted in increasing amounts relative to progesterone, and uterine excitability increases. There is some support for this idea in both man and animals, based on the measurement of oestrogen and progesterone levels in peripheral blood samples. Figure 12.3 shows the changing uterine sensitivity during pregnancy for a number of species: it should be noted that the time scale has been normalised for the purposes of comparison. It is interesting that myometrial sensitivity develops more gradually in man and the guinea-pig compared to the precipitous increase in the rabbit.

With the advent of synthetic radioactively labelled oxytocin the question of uterine sensitivity to this hormone can be investigated directly. In ovariectomised rats, treatment with the powerful synthetic oestrogen diethylstilboestrol leads within a day to an increase in the number and affinity of oxytocin binding sites present in the tissue. This suggests that oestrogen directly influences myometrial sensitivity by altering the number and nature of oxytocin receptors, either by stimulating their synthesis *de novo* or by unmasking previously hidden sites.

The myometrium is innervated by both divisions of the autonomic nervous system. Stimulation of the pelvic nerves which supply parasympathetic innervation causes the release of acetylcholine, and results in uterine contraction. Sympathetic innervation is provided by the inferior mesenteric and hypogastric nerves, arising from the lower thoracic and upper lumbar spinal cord segments, and stimulation of these nerves causes noradrenaline release which may result in either contraction or relaxation. The uterus contains both alpha

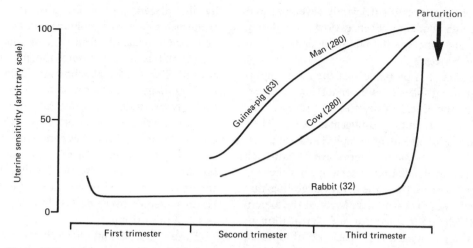

Figure 12.3   Diagram showing the changing uterine sensitivity to oxytocin during pregnancy in several species, plotted on a normalised scale. Figures in parentheses show actual gestation lengths

(excitatory) and beta adrenoceptors (inhibitory); the relative proportions of these receptor types, and hence response to catecholamines, depend on hormonal balance as well as species. Thus progesterone treatment tends to produce a predominance of beta adrenoceptors (at least in the rat and rabbit), and activation of these receptors by administration of adrenaline or nerve stimulation causes hyperpolarisation of the pacemaker cells. This results in relaxation of the muscle, or a reduction in spontaneous activity, via a mechanism involving the elevation of intracellular concentrations of cyclic AMP. By contrast, application of an agonist selective for alpha adrenoceptors causes contraction, especially in the oestrogen-dominated uterus or in the presence of a beta adrenergic antagonist. It is possible that the calcium-dependent changes causing depolarisation and muscle contraction may depend upon intracellular synthesis of cyclic GMP.

In spite of the sensitivity of the uterus to autonomic factors, it appears that myometrial activity in labour is largely independent of innervation. For example, uterine function in labour is adequate in paraplegic women. Nevertheless, beta adrenergic agonist drugs may be of some use in the treatment of threatened late abortion (i.e. premature labour) by directly inhibiting the spontaneous uterine

activity which threatens to develop into full-blown labour. The most useful drugs for this purpose are those which are selective for beta$_2$ adrenoceptors (which involve responses mediating dilation of blood vessels or relaxation of smooth muscle), thereby avoiding the stimulation of beta$_1$ adrenoceptors which would produce tachycardia and other undesirable symptoms. Salbutamol and ritodrine are two of the several drugs which have been suggested for this purpose and are reasonably effective in suppressing threatened labour if administered before too much cervical dilation has taken place. After dilation, intervention with drugs is generally ineffective. Administration of ethanol has also been proposed as a means of treatment, since ethanol inhibits the release of antidiuretic hormone and oxytocin from the posterior pituitary gland. Oxytocin is certainly released during labour, but it is not the sole humoral factor reinforcing uterine motility (see below), and this may explain why alcohol is not very effective for the treatment of threatened labour.

12.3   The initiation of labour

Parturition is the culmination of an orderly increase in myometrial excitability which is timed so as to occur when the fetus is sufficiently developed and ready for independent existence. How is the timing achieved, and what are the factors or signals which trigger the process?

On balance it is probable that the most important regulating signals are endocrine changes, notably in the levels of oestrogens, progesterone, cortisol, ACTH and prostaglandin $F_{2\alpha}$. Their interactions are extremely complex, and are determined by both fetal and maternal events, although there is now evidence that in some species the first signal of all comes from the fetus, suggesting that the fetus 'times' its own birth. Many of the experiments which are needed for the clarification of these hormonal mechanisms make use of repeated sampling of fetal and maternal blood, and of injections or selective ablations in the fetus. Clearly this is not possible in man, and for this reason our knowledge of the mechanisms of initiation of human parturition is not very advanced. Therefore it will be useful to consider what is known about initiation of parturition in the sheep, perhaps the best studied case, so as to illustrate some possible features of the process in man. Nevertheless, as usual there are important species differences which mean that it is unwise to extrapolate too freely to man.

As in man, maintenance of the fetus in the second and third trimesters of pregnancy in the sheep requires endocrine support from the placenta but is independent of ovarian function. This is also true in the horse and guinea-pig, and contrasts with pregnancy in the cow, pig, goat, rat, rabbit and hamster, all of which require a functional corpus luteum throughout pregnancy.

The most important hormonal changes in late pregnancy in the sheep are illustrated diagrammatically in figure 12.4. The maternal blood levels of oestrogen and progesterone can be measured by taking blood samples from a cannula implanted into the jugular vein; these measurements show that the maternal progesterone level declines gradually over the last few days of pregnancy, and that there is a very sharp increase in circulating oestrogens within the last 48 hours before delivery. These results reflect the changing steroid output of the placenta. Prostaglandin $F_{2\alpha}$ is also formed

by the placenta, most probably in the decidua (maternal side) from polyunsaturated fatty acid precursors released from membrane phospholipids, and is liberated into the maternal blood stream. Since prostaglandins are rapidly metabolised by many organs, especially by the lungs, they can only profitably be measured close to their site of release, in this case in the utero-ovarian vein which drains the uterus. Such experiments have shown that there is a large increase in prostaglanding $F_{2\alpha}$ output just before delivery. Finally, figure 12.4 shows that the level of cortisol in the fetal circulation increases over the last few days before the onset of parturition.

These observations have been combined in several ways, but one useful hypothetical scheme for the initiation of labour is set out here. It is supposed that an event of primary importance is the 'maturation' of the fetal adrenal cortex in the third trimester. It becomes more sensitive to ACTH, and responds by secreting larger amounts

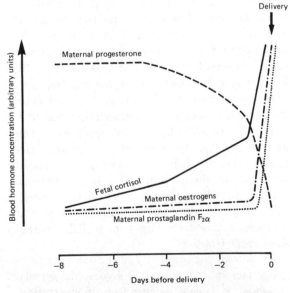

Figure 12.4 Hormones and parturition: a simplified diagram showing the changes in blood hormone levels in the pregnant sheep and fetal lamb in the days immediately preceding delivery. Blood taken from the maternal jugular vein for steroids or utero-ovarian vein for prostaglandin $F_{2\alpha}$, and from fetal umbilical vein for cortisol; all hormones measured by radioimmunoassays

of cortisol. Cortisol causes the redirection of placental steroid synthesis away from progesterone towards oestrogens. It is thought that the mechanism for this is by a cortisol-dependent increase in the amount of 17α-hydroxylating and 17-side-chain cleaving enzymes, which during pregnancy are not found in the placenta. This absence explains why the placenta cannot manufacture oestrogens directly from progesterone, as in the ovary, but can only aromatise dehydroepiandrosterone precursors which are made by the fetal adrenal cortex (see chapter 7). The change from progesterone to oestrogen dominance caused by this shift in placental steroid synthesis increases uterine excitability by removing the progesterone 'block' and possibly by increasing uterine sensitivity to oxytocin (see section 12.2).

Oestrogens also increase placental prostaglandin $F_{2\alpha}$ synthesis and release. Prostaglandin $F_{2\alpha}$ is a potent direct myometrial stimulant, and increases uterine responsiveness to other smooth muscle spasmogens such as oxytocin. Prostaglandin $F_{2\alpha}$ also depresses progesterone synthesis by a luteolytic action, which has been particularly well demonstrated in the sheep (see chapter 2). Finally, myometrial contractions elicit reflexes which cause the pulsatile release of oxytocin from the neurohypophysis. Oxytocin further increases myometrial contractility.

This working hypothesis concerning the initiation of labour in the sheep draws together some previously antagonistic theories, particularly those concerning the importance of the fetal pituitary—adrenal axis for the initial stimulus, the theory concerning the importance of progesterone withdrawal, and that proposing a fundamental role for the prostaglandins. However, our understanding of parturition in the sheep is still incomplete since we do not know how the maturation of the fetal hypothalamo—pituitary—adrenal axis is controlled. In addition, neural factors are probably also involved but these have not yet been clearly defined. For example, it is thought that light may influence integration of the events of parturition, because some species usually deliver during daylight hours, whereas others deliver at night.

To complete this discussion it is appropriate to see how far such ideas can be applied to man. It should be stressed that as yet there is little good evidence of altered placental hormone metabolism during human labour. Fetal corticosteroids may be important, since the gestation of anencephalic fetuses (lacking a fully developed pituitary, and hence showing marked adrenal hypoplasia) is sometimes very prolonged and the precision of the timing of parturition is lost. There is some evidence for a rise in fetal cortisol levels before the onset of labour, but the administration of glucocorticoids does not induce premature labour. Prostaglandins have potent effects on human myometrial contractility and are used clinically for the induction of labour and for therapeutic abortion in the second trimester (see later). They also appear to sensitise the human uterus to the effects of oxytocin.

In a retrospective study it was found that prolonged treatment of women suffering from rheumatoid arthritis with aspirin-like drugs (which inhibit prostaglandin biosynthesis) was associated with prolonged gestation. Plasma levels of prostaglandin metabolites rise during labour.

Oxytocin does not appear to be indispensable to human labour, since women suffering from diabetes insipidus (caused by posterior pituitary failure) come to term satisfactorily, even though labour may be prolonged.

In summary, we can only conclude that human labour, like that in other mammals, results from a complex interplay of endocrine signals. The unravelling of these signals promises to remain an absorbing study.

12.4   Mechanisms and progress of labour: events leading to the first stage

At the onset of labour, the Braxton Hicks contractions become coordinated and more forceful, generating intrauterine pressures of 50 mmHg or more. They may occur once every 10—30 min, becoming more frequent as labour approaches, but do not usually become painful until just before stage I labour begins.

The coordinated muscular contractions originate from the uterine fundus; these tend to pull the

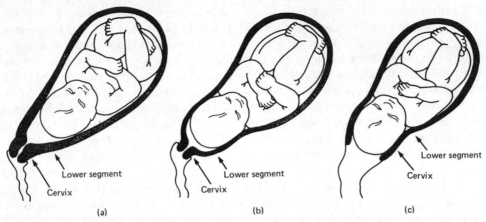

Figure 12.5   Uterine and cervical changes during stage I of labour: (a) before engagement of the head, the lower uterine segment is narrow and thick-walled; (b) during engagement the lower segment expands and elongates to surround the head; (c) cervical effacement – the cervix thins and moulds round the head, and appears merged with the lower segment of the uterus, and the vagina is shortened and dilated

lower parts of the uterus upwards. The muscle fibres not only shorten during each contraction, but also progressively alter so that they become shorter and fatter while at rest between contractions. The lower part of the uterus between the cervix and the fundus thins as it is pulled upwards, and this creates the *lower uterine segment* (figure 12.5). At the same time, myometrial contractions begin to force the fetus downwards so that it settles into the pelvis with its presenting part, usually the head, coming to lie against the thinner wall of the lower uterine segment. The entry into the pelvic inlet is called *engagement*, and the whole settling process is known as *lightening*.

In the final weeks before delivery the cervix softens and thins (*cervical effacement*). In part, the thinning results from the traction from above which pulls the cervix up towards the uterine fundus (figure 12.5). However, effacement cannot occur without radical changes in the mechanical properties of the cervix which is normally firm and cannot be widely dilated because of the tightly cemented bundles of collagen in its connective tissue. Prior to labour the cement appears to break down so that the fibres slide past each other. The cervical canal begins to dilate during the preliminary phase of labour, and usually reaches a diameter of 2–3 cm.

12.5   First stage of labour

It is often difficult to determine the precise onset of stage I labour because there is a gradual transition between the events preceding labour and labour itself. The onset is marked by the beginning of progressive cervical dilation. The uterine contractions become smooth, well coordinated and regular, and accelerate in frequency from once every 10–15 minutes at the beginning of labour to once every 3–5 minutes at full cervical dilation. They generally last about 1 minute and gradually increase in intensity, generating pressures of 30–50 mmHg or more. There are occasional contractions of greater force.

Uterine contractions can be measured externally or internally. The simplest method (*tokodynamometry*) is to apply a pressure-sensitive transducer closely to the abdomen. Alternatively, catheters at the tip of which are small distensible balloons may be passed transabdominally or vaginally. Changes of pressure are detected by pressure-sensitive transducers and displayed on a pen recorder. Figure 12.6 shows a record of typical intrauterine pressure changes during the stages of labour, illustrating the transition into stage I.

The purpose of the first stage of labour is to achieve complete cervical dilation of approximately

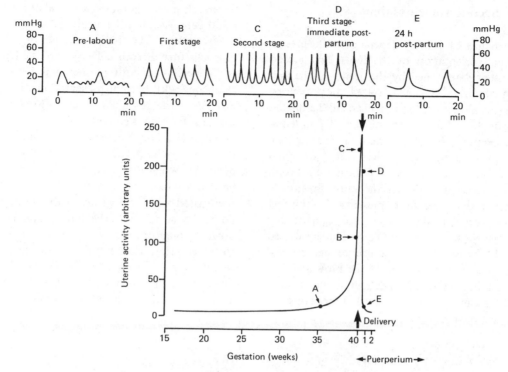

Figure 12.6   Uterine activity and characteristics of uterine contractions before, during and after labour. The uterine activity is calibrated using an arbitrary scale which takes into account both the force and frequency of contractions (Redrawn from Llewellyn-Jones, D. (1977). *Fundamentals of Obstetrics and Gynaecology*, vol. 1, Obstetrics, Faber & Faber, London)

10 cm. This requires strenuous muscular effort as the uterine fundus pulls the softened cervix outwards and upwards. The uterus contracts powerfully against its taut ligamentous supports which are anchored to the skeleton (see chapter 2). This anchorage limits upwards traction of the cervix and lower uterine segment, and further contractions serve to expel the fetus in the downwards direction.

The pain of labour is usually most intense during the dilation at the end of stage I. It is probably provoked as a result of stretching and distension of soft tissues, especially the cervix, and because of pulling on the ligamentous supports. It may also be caused by ischaemia resulting from the compression of blood vessels during contractions. Pain may be relieved with analgesics or local anaesthetics as discussed in section 12.9. More rarely, general anaesthetics may be used, particularly if there are

complications of delivery.

The time taken to achieve full cervical dilation is variable. In primigravid women, stage I is usually completed within 8–12 hours, but is almost always shorter in subsequent deliveries.

The forceful uterine contractions may threaten the welfare of the fetus if they are too frequent or prolonged, since they may arrest uterine and placental blood flow. The fetal heart rate sometimes slows during the forceful contractions (see section 12.12). This effect is probably due to an increase in vagal tone following compression of the fetal head, and can also be demonstrated in the newborn by gently squeezing its head. Clearly, then, it is important that uterine contractions should be directional and transient, so as to propel the fetus through the birth canal, rather than repeatedly compressing it.

12.6   Second stage of labour

The mechanics of delivery depend upon the presentation and orientation of the fetus, and are to some extent determined by the events of the first stage of labour. At the end of stage I, the presenting part of the fetus is closely applied to the dilated cervix. In about 95 per cent of cases the presentation is cephalic, in which the head (usually the occiput) lies above the pelvic inlet. Occipital presentation occurs when the neck is well flexed, chin on chest, and this is the most favourable orientation since the head presents the shortest effective diameter, the suboccipitobregmatic diameter, as shown in figure 12.7. The head also forms the most effective wedge to aid cervical dilation in this presentation. In the brow and face presentations (figure 12.7) labour is much more difficult as the presenting head dimensions are larger.

Breech presentation occurs in about 5 per cent of all deliveries, but the incidence is higher if birth is premature. The baby presents upside-down, buttocks first. Breech delivery carries a higher risk of mortality to both mother and fetus than is associated with occiput presentations. In very rare instances, the shoulder comes first, and such labour is hazardous and difficult.

Stage II labour begins when complete cervical dilation is achieved and ends when the baby is delivered. When the cervix is fully dilated and the head has descended into the pelvic canal a reflex is initiated which brings about the desire to 'bear down' so as to push the fetus from the uterus, down through the cervix and pelvic outlet and so to the exterior. The reflex originates from stretch receptors in the cervix. Bearing down is a Valsalva manoeuvre, in which expiration is made against a closed glottis so that intra-abdominal pressure is raised.

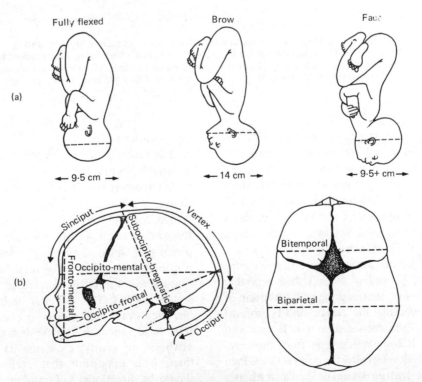

Figure 12.7   (a) Three types of cephalic presentation — the diagrams show that the presenting diameter varies according to the degree of flexion of the neck; (b) the diameters of the fetal head

The conscious effort of the mother to bear down amplifies the intrinsic expulsive mechanisms, but it may be weakened or abolished by analgesic and anaesthetic procedures, most notably after blocking spinal cord nervous traffic by epidural analgesia or in general anaesthesia. By contrast, the mother usually must be restrained from bearing down if her efforts tend to expel the fetus at such a rate as to damage it or her own soft tissues.

The stretching of the cervix also initiates a powerful local positive feedback effect to enhance myometrial activity, and initiates the Fergusson reflex which results in the secretion of oxytocin from the posterior pituitary. Oxytocin has direct contractile effects on the myometrium, and it is possible that it may also trigger the release of prostaglandins from the endometrium, thereby increasing the local concentration of smooth muscle spasmogens even further.

The amniotic membranes normally rupture spontaneously during the first or second stages of labour, releasing a gush of amniotic fluid. If this does not happen, the progress of labour may be retarded, and artificial 'rupture of the fore-waters' is usually performed by puncturing the membrane (*amniotomy*). It is not clear why the sudden reduction in uterine volume and tension should enhance spontaneous contractility of the uterus, but this is generally observed.

The transit of the baby through the birth canal is determined by size and spatial relationships, and is assisted by the midwife or medical attendant. The different fetal presentations have been mentioned above; another important determinant of the course and conduct of labour is the size and shape of the maternal pelvis. The most usual pelvic type has a large round inlet with a spacious and well-curved arch and is called *gynaecoid*. When the inlet arch is more triangular and narrow from front to back, with a narrow fore-pelvis, the pelvis is said to be *android*, since it somewhat resembles the shape found in men. An average-sized or large baby would only pass through such a pelvic inlet with considerable difficulty.

In the usual labour with a cephalic presentation and an adequate gynaecoid pelvis, the head engages transversely, most commonly with the fetal occiput to the mother's left, and descends into the midpelvis as stage II labour commences (figure 12.8). Thus the head fits the pelvic inlet most advantageously, with the biparietal diameter at right angles to, and the suboccipitobregmatic diameter parallel to, the transverse diameter of the inlet. The head then rotates to achieve the occiput–anterior position, so that the ischial spines are avoided—figure 12.8(b–d). The head advances as the hindparts of the fetus are squeezed down by frequent upper uterine contractions, and negotiates the pelvic curve by neck extension—figure 12.8(d) and 12.8(e). It gradually moves downwards, distends the vulva and appears at the introitus (*crowning*). The neck is examined to check that the umbilical cord is not wrapped around it. The shoulders traverse the pelvis in an oblique orientation without rotation, figure 12.8(f), and the head turns to take up its correct orientation to the trunk as it is delivered (*restitution*).

The shoulders, arms, trunk and legs usually follow without difficulty as support is given to the baby and gentle traction applied. After birth, the baby is heid up for a moment by its feet so that secretions can drain and be cleared from its nose and mouth, and the umbilical cord is then clamped.

Sometimes there is a danger that the soft tissues in the vulval region may tear as the head squeezes through. This can be prevented by cutting the perineum with a short posterior incision (*episiotomy*), which is repaired soon after delivery of the placenta.

Figure 12.9 shows the head of a newborn baby at birth and three days later. The changes in shape which take place on engagement and transit through the birth canal are termed *moulding*, and they help to reduce the cross-sectional size of the head and therefore aid its delivery. Moulding of the head is possible because the bones of the vault are not fused, and may overlap under compression. Normal cranial shape is restored during the first few days of life.

The birth process described above generally takes about 50 minutes in a primigravid woman, and about 20 minutes if she is multiparous. Stage II labour lasting longer than two hours must be completed by active medical intervention because both mother and fetus are endangered.

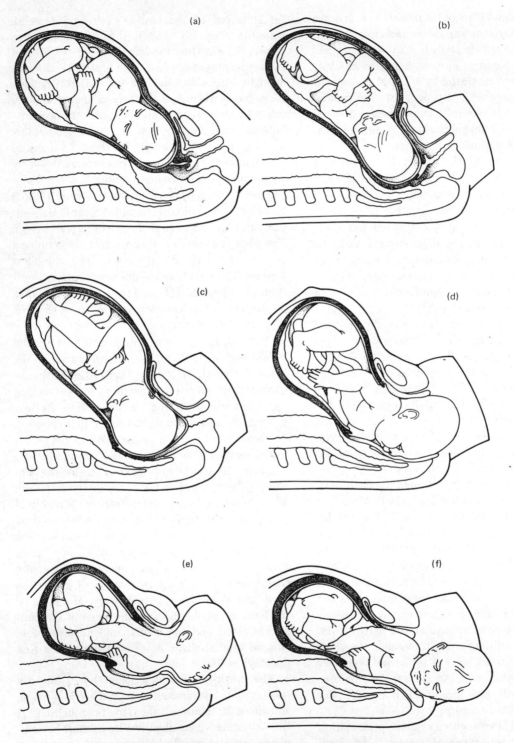

Figure 12.8   The second stage of labour. The diagrams show the descent, rotation, expulsion and restitution of the head, as described more fully in the text

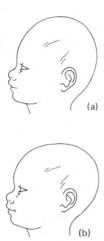

Figure 12.9 **(a) A typical well-moulded head of a new-born baby; (b) the same head three days later, showing that it has regained its normal shape**

12.7   Third stage of labour

Stage III labour comprises the delivery of the placenta and membranes. Although it usually lasts for a few minutes only, this is potentially the most hazardous part of labour from the point of view of maternal morbidity and mortality. The dangers arise because of the possibility of extensive post-partum haemorrhage during placental separation.

After the expulsion of the fetus and amniotic fluid, the volume of the uterine contents is reduced by about seven-eighths. This means that uterine muscle contractions can generate much higher pressures. The contractions occur less frequently than at the end of the second stage but manometric measurements show that pressures of up to 250–300 mmHg are generated, although remarkably little pain is experienced. This shows that the pain of labour cannot simply be due to the force of uterine contractions alone, or to uterine ischaemia during periods of compression.

These contractions reduce the size of the uterus considerably and the decrease in surface area of the part in contact with the relatively incompressible placenta causes the two to shear apart. When this happens, blood flows out of the severed uterine spiral arteries, and there is a transient increase in blood passed vaginally. If all is well, successive contractions of the uterus compress the spiral arteries so that blood loss is minimised. Oxytocic drugs are often administered to promote uterine contractions so as to reduce post-partum bleeding. Average blood loss is of the order of 350 ml, of which about 250 ml represent the maternal placental blood volume.

After separation of the placenta, further uterine contractions expel it. This is assisted by gentle traction on the umbilical cord. The fetal side of the placenta usually appears first; it has a shiny surface because it is covered by the amniotic membrane. The maternal surface is uneven and is covered by torn tissues and blood clots. It is important to verify by inspection that the entire placenta has been delivered.

Oxytocic drugs are usually administered by intramuscular injection late in stage II so as to ensure adequate uterine muscular activity in stage III labour. Oxytocin and ergometrine are used for this purpose. Ergometrine is one of the alkaloids found in the ergot fungus of rye, and has been widely used in obstetrics since the early nineteenth century. It has a specific stimulant action on uterine smooth muscle, as well as being a weak vasoconstrictor, and both effects are of value for the control of post-partum haemorrhage. The duration of action of ergometrine is much longer than that of oxytocin since it is very slowly broken down; it also tends to produce a sustained contracture of the myometrium, and for this reason is not suitable for the induction of labour. The selective action of ergometrine on uterine smooth muscle and the relative absence of vasoconstrictor and alpha adrenoceptor antagonist properties distinguish ergometrine from other clinically important ergot alkaloids.

The severance and expulsion of the placenta removes the source of the four major hormones of pregnancy at a stroke. Maternal plasma levels of progesterone, human chorionic gonadotropin and human placental lactogen decline rapidly as these hormones have short biological half-lives. The level of oestrogen declines more slowly since it is not metabolised so quickly. Thus the ratio of oestrogen to progesterone increases and therefore uterine excitability is favoured.

12.8   The puerperium

The puerperium is the time during which maternal recovery and repair takes place, and normally occupies the first six weeks following delivery. Most evident of the important changes which affect the uterus during this time is the marked reduction in its size towards its previous non-pregnant dimensions (*involution*). The endometrial lining is gradually autolysed and there is marked tissue invasion by leukocytes. The products of autolysis are released over a period of 3—4 weeks as a vaginal discharge called *lochia*. At first it is bloodstained, but later becomes straw-coloured, reflecting the presence of serum and white cells. Meanwhile, the inner layer of the endometrium becomes covered by regenerating epithelium.

Before the advent of antibiotics and strict attention to antiseptic precautions in obstetrics, puerperal fever was a much-feared and common cause of maternal mortality in the postnatal period. This may occur if bacteria in the lower genital tract are transferred to the uterus, which at this time provides an exceptionally favourable environment for bacterial multiplication.

At term, the uterus weighs about 1000 g; the reduction in its mass after delivery is initially rapid, the uterus weighing about 500 g at the end of the first week post-delivery, shrinking to between 50 and 70 g at the end of the puerperium, by which time it lies once more within the pelvis.

The abdomen, vagina and pelvic floor are stretched and extended greatly during the course of pregnancy and labour. They too return towards their previous size during the puerperium. The vagina often does not recover its exact former dimensions, but the abdominal wall and pelvic floor usually regain good muscular tone, especially if assisted by correct exercise.

It is believed that many of the changes discussed above occur as a result of progesterone removal. This also explains the marked diuresis which occurs 2—4 days post-partum, and which results in a considerable reduction in extracellular fluid and a consequent increase in the haematocrit. Fluid loss may amount to more than 3 l per day. Abrupt endocrine changes may also underlie some of the marked psychological symptoms, such as postnatal depression and rapid changes of mood, which are often experienced in the puerperium.

Lactation is described in chapter 14; it is appropriate here to note that it begins very shortly after delivery. The decline of oestrogen levels probably triggers increased prolactin release, and this initiates the production of colostrum and milk. Lactation may suppress ovarian function during and after the puerperium by inhibiting hypothalamo—pituitary—ovarian function as described in chapter 14. If the mother does not breast feed, ovarian function generally returns within 8—12 weeks and cyclical ovulation and menstrual activity is re-established. Ovulation may even occur during lactation, and thus lactational amenorrhoea is not a completely reliable contraceptive mechanism for the spacing of births.

12.9   Analgesia and anaesthesia in labour

The aim of analgesic and anaesthetic therapy in labour is to reduce pain and distress felt by the mother without prejudicing the welfare of the fetus. The pain of labour varies considerably and is rarely predictable. It is dependent upon emotional and psychological variables, as well as purely physical factors, so it is important to minimise anxiety and to build up confidence in the mother during her prenatal instruction.

Prior to labour or during early stage I, it may be of benefit to administer a sedative drug, such as a benzodiazepine, to reduce apprehension and thereby to diminish pain. If stage I labour is very prolonged opiates (e.g. morphine) can be used for pain relief and to facilitate sleep.

Drugs can no longer be given orally in late stage I labour and after because gastrointestinal activity is inhibited and absorption is very poor. For analgesia in late stage I the synthetic narcotic analgesics pethidine or meperidine administered intravenously provide good relief from pain without causing excessive respiratory depression of the fetus. In both cases, concurrent administration of a tranquilliser, such as a phenothiazine, reduces the required dose of analgesic.

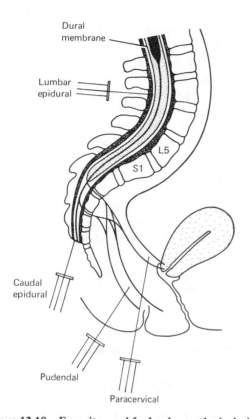

Figure 12.10   Four sites used for local anaesthesia during labour. An epidural injection is made into the space outside the dural membrane, and the words 'caudal' or 'lumbar' describe the level of the spinal column at which the injection is made (Redrawn from Beischer, N. A. and Mackay, E. V. (1976). *Obstetrics and the Newborn*, Saunders, London)

Local anaesthetics are widely used to relieve pain in stages I and II of labour and the several sites where they may be injected are shown in figure 12.10. They can be used to produce paracervical or pudendal block. In the former case this abolishes pain originating from the uterus but not that due to distension of the perineum, which requires pudendal block. Total relief from pain in labour has now become a reality with the development of techniques for caudal or lumbar epidural block. These procedures abolish sensory nerve conduction within the spinal canal.

Epidural analgesia has become very fashionable in recent years because the technique provides complete pain relief without loss of consciousness or drowsiness. It requires infiltration of the local anaesthetic into the epidural space, entered by a catheter inserted between two of the mid-lumbar vertebrae. Although stage I labour is not prolonged, the mother loses much of her ability to exert voluntary 'bearing-down' effort as motor control is severely impeded; thus stage II is lengthened, and frequently requires forceps assistance. With epidural block there is relatively little fetal depression.

Inhalation anaesthetics also have a very important place for the relief of pain in labour. Three agents are particularly important: nitrous oxide in 50 per cent mixture with oxygen, trichloroethylene and methoxyfluorane. Nitrous oxide is administered to the conscious mother through a face mask which she operates herself when she feels the onset of a particularly powerful uterine contraction. Although she becomes drowsy, she can still bear down and participate actively in labour.

In certain cases it is necessary to administer a general anaesthetic for caesarean section or obstetric complications. Halothane, nitrous oxide/ oxygen and cyclopropane all have advantages and disadvantages depending on the circumstances. However, it is now considered that the use of a general anaesthetic is a rather extreme (as well as relatively dangerous) means of reducing pain in normal childbirth since the active participation of the mother is lost, thereby greatly prolonging labour. There is also often quite marked depression of the fetus because anaesthetics readily cross the placenta. Yet is is worth remembering that the introduction of anaesthetics from the mid-nineteenth century onwards was the first effective method for the reduction of pain during childbirth and was an important milestone in the history of medicine.

12.10   Induction of labour

The direct myometrial stimulant action of oxytocin and prostaglandins may be exploited therapeutically to induce or assist labour so as to accelerate delivery. Amniotomy, performed by rupturing the amniotic membrane, may also be used to induce labour as described in section 12.6. Induction can only be attempted when there is sufficient evidence that the uterus is primed, that labour is imminent and that the cervix is ripe for dilation.

Considerable experience has been acquired over the past 25 years in the use of oxytocin, first obtained from extracts of cattle posterior pituitaries and now available as the synthetic polypeptide. Because it is a peptide it is virtually inactive by mouth, and its short biological half-life of a few minutes dictates that it must be administered by the inconvenient procedure of a constant intravenous infusion. Normally it is infused at increasing rates (by using a carefully monitored drip or infusor pump) until satisfactory contractions become established. Larger doses may cause dangerous overstimulation with maintained uterine contracture and fetal hypoxia so the drug should be administered under close supervision.

There is much less experience with prostaglandins because they have only been available for trials for a decade or so, but it is clear that they are versatile and can be administered by a number of routes, for example by intravenous infusion, intra-amniotic and extra-amniotic injection or infusion, and even orally or intravaginally. The biological half-lives of the naturally occurring prostaglandins are very short, due to rapid metabolism, and so repeated administration near to the site of action (e.g. into the amniotic cavity) is advantageous, since it maximises the useful effect of the dose and reduces the amount reaching other parts of the body. This is important because prostaglandins have many other actions, and side effects such as gastrointestinal upsets, pyrexia and changes in blood pressure are often troublesome with systemic administration. Some synthetic prostaglandins, including the 15-methyl prostaglandin E_2 derivatives, have been introduced recently, and can be used in much lower doses as they are more resistant to metabolism. The ultimate goal is to develop compounds with specific uterine stimulant actions so as to avoid side effects.

The practice of 'accelerating' labour by artificial induction has become widespread and this increasing intervention in a natural process has attracted lively controversy. No doubt both hospital staff and mothers benefit from convenience and the savings in time. However, neither the short- nor the long-term risks of the procedure have been fully evaluated, and it is possible that induced labours are more painful because of the increased forcefulness of the contractions. There is also evidence from controlled clinical studies that induction of labour with oxytocin is associated with higher incidence of fetal distress and low Apgar scores (see section 12.12). However, it must also be remembered that induction is often used when there are medical complications or potential dangers to the fetus, and this may complicate any comparison between drug-treated and control groups. Certainly, there is agreement that the induction of labour or enhancement of sluggish uterine activity by oxytocic drugs has brought considerable benefits to perinatal and maternal health in cases where there is maternal disease or risk to the fetus.

12.11   Therapeutic abortion

Following a section on the induction of labour, it is appropriate here to discuss the induction of abortion for therapeutic reasons. These may be medical (when the health of the mother would be endangered if the pregnancy were allowed to continue, or if there is evidence to suggest that the fetus is abnormal), or social (if abortion is used to terminate an unwanted pregnancy). Attitudes to the social acceptability in Western society of abortion used as a last-ditch contraceptive method have changed greatly in recent years.

Therapeutic abortion is much safer if performed in the first trimester of pregnancy by the curette methods described briefly below. Second trimester abortions may be induced pharmacologically with oxytocic drugs used in the same manner as for the induction of labour. Surgical methods for terminating pregnancy are not usually practised in the second trimester because of the high risks of haemorrhage and trauma. Artificial termination of pregnancy should not be attempted by any method in the third trimester.

The simplest method for first trimester abortion

is suction curettage. After local anaesthesia of the cervix a catheter is passed into the uterus and the contents sucked out by applying a vacuum. This method is safe and rapid. It represents an advance over dilatation and curettage which requires the insertion into the uterus of a larger catheter after mechanical dilatation of the cervix, followed by disruption and removal of the contents. Hysterotomy may be used as a method for abortion, but it has all the problems and hazards of abdominal surgical operative procedures and is rarely performed for this purpose.

Second trimester abortion is usually induced by the administration of oxytocin intravenously or of prostaglandins into the amniotic cavity. Since the uterus is much less sensitive to stimulant drugs during mid-pregnancy, the doses used have to be high, and expulsion is often very prolonged. Side effects are common and may be severe. Recently it has been found that prior administration of prostaglandins often potentiates the actions of oxytocin, so it might be possible to exploit the actions of both substances without having to use high doses that produce side effects. Other methods for the induction of second trimester abortion, such as by injection of hypertonic saline or urea into the amniotic fluid, may soon be completely supplanted by the newer and safer methods using specific drugs.

12.12 Fetal monitoring

In addition to simple time-honoured aids such as the thermometer, sphygmomanometer and stethoscope, there are several recent sophisticated techniques which enable more aspects of fetal welfare to be monitored. These have contributed significantly to the reduction in perinatal mortality observed in recent years, largely because they enable labour to be monitored with a greater degree of precision and allow the earlier recognition of situations of potential danger to the fetus.

The fetal heart rate can be monitored by applying a skin electrode to the presenting scalp or maternal abdomen. The fetal electrocardiogram is obtained as a potential difference between this electrode and a reference maternal electrode, usually applied to the vagina or thigh. The record is often displayed as the fetal heart rate, as in figure 12.11, together with uterine contractions recorded by tokodynamometry (see section 12.5). Figure 12.11 shows a record of fetal heart rate illustrating normal beat-to-beat variations of up to 5 per minute (a), as well as additional records showing substantial slowing of the fetal heart rate, either during (b) or after (c) uterine contractions. The former are probably normal (see section 12.5), but the latter may indicate fetal asphyxia. Whatever the cause, in clinical practice possible fetal hypoxia as suggested by such fetal heart rate signs would be checked by measuring the pH of the fetal blood as described below. Fetal heart activity may also be monitored by ultrasonography (see chapter 10), with the advantage that the method is non-invasive.

Important information concerning fetal welfare may be obtained by measuring fetal blood pH after taking a small sample from the presenting scalp. This is visualised through an amnioscope, but is only possible after the membranes have ruptured. The pH value of fetal capillary blood is usually about 7.30 at the beginning of labour, and reduces to about 7.20 at the end; lower pH values indicate severe hypoxia, which is permanently damaging to the brain if maintained.

The infant's condition at or soon after delivery (for example at 1 or 5 minutes) can be simply and usefully assessed using the Apgar method of scoring. The five clinical signs of heart rate, respiratory effort, muscle tone, reflex irritability and body colour are each scored on a scale 0 to 2. Total scores of 7–10 are achieved by normal vigorous babies; moderately depressed infants score 4–6, and require some measure of resuscitation after birth. Severely depressed babies, for whom there is a poor prognosis and 20 times greater risk of death within a month, score 0–3. More than three-quarters of newborn babies score 7 or more and are healthy; of the low scores, many are premature or small-for-dates because of growth retardation, or have been severely traumatised during a difficult labour. Many of them later show evidence of permanent damage such as neurological disturbance.

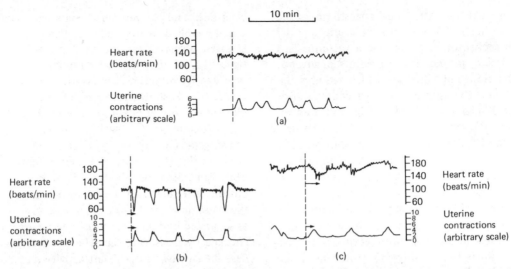

Figure 12.11   Monitoring of fetal heart rate and uterine contractions, showing (a) normal pattern of beat-to-beat variations in heart rate. The other two types of brady cardia illustrated – (b) early cardiac deceleration, (c) late cardiac deceleration – occur after forceful uterine contractions, and may indicate fetal hypoxia which could be investigated by fetal scalp blood sampling unless delivery was instituted without further delay. The late cardiac deceleration pattern is usually ominous and does not augur well for fetal welfare; note the high basal heart rate (Redrawn from Beischer, N. A. and Mackay, E. V. (1976). *Obstetrics and the Newborn*, Saunders, London)

Perinatal mortality increases markedly as birth weight decreases, and is virtually 100 per cent in babies weighing less than 1 kg. Since these babies are extremely premature, a similar relationship could be drawn between perinatal mortality and gestational age at birth. Other factors, such as maternal age, number of previous children, social class and smoking habits, also affect perinatal mortality.

Further reading

Danforth, D. N. (ed.) (1977). *Obstetrics and Gynaecology*, 3rd edn, Harper & Row, New York

Knight, J. and O'Connor, M. (eds.) (1977). *The Fetus and Birth*, Ciba Foundation Symposium, No. 47 (new series), Elsevier, Amsterdam

Liggins, G. C., Forster, C. S., Grieves, S. A. and Schwartz, A. L. (1977). 'Control of parturition in man', *Biology of Reproduction*, **16** 39–56

Llewellyn-Jones, D. (1977). *Fundamentals of Obstetrics and Gynaecology*, vol. 1, Obstetrics, Faber & Faber, London

Adaptations of the Newborn to Extrauterine Life

13.1 Introduction

The word 'neonatal' is used to define the first 28 days of extrauterine life. It is during this period that the majority of infant deaths occur. However, the term has no special physiological significance as many of the changes required for extrauterine life follow a different time course; some occur at birth whereas others are more protracted and take place over a period of weeks or months.

13.2 The effects of birth on the infant

Even normal rapid delivery stresses the infant. Some degree of stress is probably important in activating physiological mechanisms essential for survival after birth. In a normal delivery the fetus is subjected to a degree of asphyxia due to fluctuations in placental blood flow and this may cause respiratory acidosis and a rise in heart rate. Typical changes in the respiratory gas content of scalp capillary blood at the beginning and end of labour are shown in table 13.1. This degree of asphyxia during birth is sufficient both to increase the secretion of catecholamines from the adrenal medulla (thus mobilising glycogen and lipid stores) and also to stimulate the sympathetic nervous system generally. These effects combine to produce an active and alert fetus at birth. Any respiratory acidosis at birth is rapidly corrected when ventilation begins.

Difficult and prolonged labour leads to more marked asphyxia and acidosis. The fetus may show metabolic as well as respiratory acidosis as many tissues adopt lactate-forming anaerobic glycolysis to obtain energy. This sort of severe asphyxia slows the fetal heart rate causing a fall in arterial blood pressure; the newborn baby is limp and depressed and does not make the transition to extrauterine life easily. Severe metabolic acidosis may not be corrected for many hours after birth.

Both fetus and newborn can tolerate degrees of asphyxia or hypoxia that would severely compromise or even kill an adult, but this ability diminishes with age. Both fetus and newborn can divert a considerable proportion of the cardiac output to the central nervous system thus supplying it with oxygen and glucose and protecting it at the cost of hypoxia elsewhere. It has also been suggested that fetal tissue cytochromes have high affinity for oxygen and can extract it from blood at unusually low partial pressures. Nevertheless, the brain is

Table 13.1 Changes in scalp blood values of the fetus during labour

	Onset of labour	End of labour
O_2 saturation (%)	42	30
pO_2 (mmHg)	20	17
pCO_2 (mmHg)	44	51
pH	7.31	7.28

very vulnerable to hypoxia, and severe asphyxia at birth may impair intellectual development. It is estimated that irreversible brain damage occurs within 10 minutes of the onset of total asphyxia at birth compared with about 4 minutes in the adult. Severe asphyxia at birth is associated with micro-haemorrhages in the cerebral circulation and leads to conditions such as spasticity.

13.3   Initiation of ventilation

The preceding discussion shows that the most urgent need of the newborn is to start ventilation. Many factors appear to interact to initiate the first breath. A mild degree of asphyxia and acidosis sensitises the medullary chemoreceptors thus increasing ventilatory drive (see section 11.11). The fetus is delivered from a wet, warm environment into a relatively cold one in which evaporation of amniotic fluid rapidly reduces its skin temperature. It is also transferred from an environment where it is supported in an essentially weightless state by amniotic fluid to one where the full effects of gravity are felt for the first time. Finally the newborn is squeezed and manipulated during birth to an extent that is certainly stressful. No doubt all three factors help to stimulate the first breath.

Experiments have been conducted during caesarean delivery of term fetal lambs to investigate the relative importance of these factors. To avoid respiratory depression, the ewes were given spinal anaesthesia. Lambs delivered with the umbilical circulation intact but allowed to become cool began to breathe when the rectal temperature had dropped by 3–4°C regardless of the time elapsed since delivery. Lambs that were delivered and kept warm with the umbilical cord clamped—thus producing asphyxia without cooling—started to breathe about 1 minute after the cord was clamped and were breathing regularly after 10 minutes. Both cooling and clamping applied together led to very rapid initiation of ventilation. Observations with human babies agree because there is a small but significant reduction in the time elapsing before the first breath if the cord is clamped immediately at birth. Immediate clamping of the cord and incidental cooling is usual in many delivery rooms and most newborn babies make the first gasping ventilatory movements about 6 seconds after cord clamping.

The problems of initiating ventilation are not simply overcome by providing a sufficient stimulus to breathe because at birth the lungs are full of fluid (see section 11.11) and the alveoli are in a relatively collapsed state. Much of the lung fluid from the upper respiratory tract is lost during delivery but the bronchioles and alveoli remain fluid-filled. Surface tension forces at the gas—liquid interfaces oppose filling of the lungs with air. Indeed as air is drawn into the lungs the area of the gas—liquid interface increases and so does the force opposing aeration. The lecithin surfactant produced by the type II alveolar cells (section 11.11) is particularly important as it reduces the surface tension effect. Nevertheless, considerable ventilatory effort has to be applied in order to fill the lungs with air and negative intrathoracic pressures of up to −40 or −60 cm of water have been recorded in human infants during the first inhalation.

Figure 13.1 shows intra-oesophageal pressure in the human neonate plotted against lung volume. During the first breath (a), 33 seconds after birth, a negative pressure of 60 cm of water was needed to inflate the lungs with 40 ml of air. A considerable positive pressure also had to be generated to empty the lungs. Both observations show that the compliance of the lung is very low (i.e. that the resistance to inflation is high). Subsequent breaths are achieved with much smaller changes in oesophageal pressure and need far less mechanical work, showing that lung compliance has increased. The corresponding changes in intra-oesophageal pressure during quiet breathing in an adult are about −3 to −6 cm of water. A minority of babies do not show such a marked drop in intra-oesophageal pressure during the first breath as in the example given. Where a large pressure drop occurs it is thought that the glottis is initially closed as the negative pressure is generated and then suddenly relaxed thus allowing air to enter the lungs rapidly and aiding inflation. Once the infant

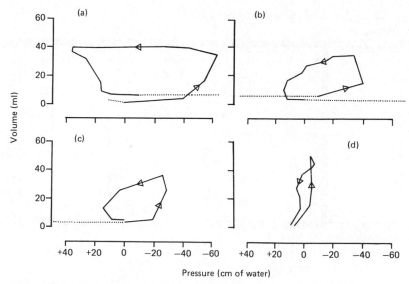

Figure 13.1 Lung pressure–volume relationships during (a) the first breath, (b) the second breath, (c) the third breath, and (d) after establishment of breathing (40 min) (Redrawn from Smith, C. A. (1963). *Scientific American*, 209(4), pages 27–35)

has initially inflated its lungs the lung fluid is reabsorbed rapidly. This is because of its low colloid osmotic pressure of 0.2 mmHg compared with 21 for that of plasma.

Surfactant is also important in maintaining lung stability after inflation because it prevents collapse of the alveoli during exhalation and allows alveoli of differing radii to coexist. The smaller the alveolus the greater is the surfactant-induced reduction in surface tension and hence transmural pressure, thus offsetting the tendency of small alveoli to empty into larger ones.

The mechanical work necessary for the first filling of the lungs with air is performed by strong contractions of the diaphragm. The ribs and sternum of the newborn are extremely flexible and the chest may even become concave during the first few inhalations whilst considerable negative pressures are being generated.

13.4 Cardiovascular changes at birth

A second crucial event at birth is the rearrangement of the fetal circulation to produce the adult circulatory pattern (figure 13.2). The changes that

take place are principally dependent upon the arrest of the umbilical circulation and thus of placental perfusion and upon the rapid increase in pulmonary blood flow which results from lung inflation and expansion. These changes are not as rapid or completed as soon as has often been supposed.

Blood flow in the umbilical vessels persists for several minutes if the cord is not clamped. The walls of the vessels contain smooth muscle which although not innervated is extremely irritable and prone to sustained contracture. The umbilical arteries have thicker muscle layers than the vein and generate higher intraluminal pressures, for example up to 150 mmHg, sufficient to arrest the placental circulation. Such myogenic activity can be provoked by stretching or handling the cord or allowing it to cool as the infant is delivered, and is potentiated by stress-released catecholamines. The vessels are more likely to constrict if the infant has started breathing and less likely to if it has not, since their irritability increases as a function of the oxygen tension. It is possible that vasoactive prostaglandins or thromboxanes may contribute to vasoconstriction as their synthesis is favoured in the presence of oxygen.

At least two mechanisms cooperate to produce

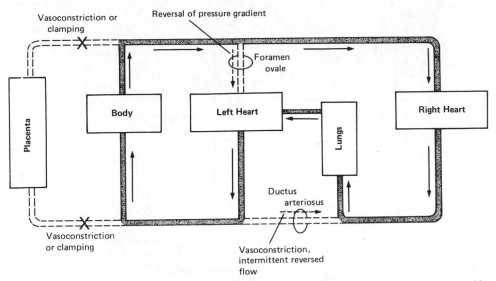

Figure 13.2   Diagram showing the transition from the fetal to adult type circulation. Compare this figure with figure 11.6 and table 13.5

closure of the foramen ovale between the two atria. Arrest of umbilical blood flow reduces venous return in the inferior vena cava and decreases pressure in the right atrium. Secondly the rapid increase in pulmonary blood flow increases venous return and pressure in the left atrium. Thus the fetal to neonatal transition reverses the pressure gradient across the foramen ovale so that the thin septum primum is pushed against the septum secundum. There is a dramatic increase in pulmonary blood flow at birth due to a large reduction in resistance to flow in the newly inflated lung. This is partly because lung expansion reduces the tortuosity of the capillaries but also because of vasodilation of the pulmonary vessels in response to the higher partial pressures of oxygen in the blood. We have noted that the umbilical vessels show exactly the opposite response to oxygen tension, but the reasons for the differing responses are not known.

The reversal of the pressure gradient across the foramen ovale is accentuated by the continued patency of the ductus arteriosus. The pulmonary arterial pressure exceeds that in the aorta in the fetus because the vascular resistance of the lungs is high. At birth the vascular resistance of the lungs decreases dramatically and pulmonary arterial pressure falls by more than half, so reversing flow in the ductus arteriosus. This change of flow augments blood flow through the lungs and the rise in left atrial pressure.

At this stage closure of the foramen ovale is reversible and interruption of ventilation or a fall in alveolar oxygen tension causes vasoconstriction of the lung capillaries. This reverses the pressure changes across the foramen ovale and the circulation reverts to the fetal pattern. In most neonates during the first few days of life the closure of the foramen ovale is probably incomplete and intermittent and occasional cyanotic episodes may be due to its reopening. After a few days of more or less permanent contact the septum primum begins to fuse with the septum secundum permanently effecting closure of the foramen ovale. Patency of the foramen can be demonstrated anatomically in a large number of adults although functional closure is usually completed through the action of the pressure gradient.

In the mature fetus the ductus arteriosus is almost as wide as the aorta. The most important stimulus for ductus closure is the rise in oxygen tension of arterial blood. Since ductus smooth muscle is not innervated, it is possible that humoral factors may participate in the same manner as for umbilical vasoconstriction but in this case prosta-glandins may serve to keep the vessel dilated.

Functional closure of the ductus arteriosus by vascoconstriction occurs within a few hours of birth and is followed by fibrosis and obliteration of the lumen within about 8 days. Intermittent flow in the partly constricted ductus arteriosus can persist for several hours after birth during each cardiac cycle when the aortic pressure is at a maximum.

Less is known about the closure of the ductus venosus and it may occur as an extension of vaso-constriction in the umbilical vein. Its closure is important because blood from the gut, which before birth bypassed the liver, now perfuses its sinusoids. The interpolation of this extra resistance in the venous return further reduces right atrial pressure and so contributes to closure of the foramen ovale.

It was mentioned that the closure of these structures is not immediate or permanent and indeed in some individuals may never be fully completed. Although some measure of anatomical patency may not adversely affect function, gross physiological patency is very serious and surgical correction is usually necessary.

Continued patency of the foramen ovale produces a cyanotic 'blue baby' due to the admixture of venous and arterial blood. Continued patency of the ductus arteriosus is extremely serious because it can lead to heart failure due to overloading of the left ventricle. Closure of the ductus venosus is invariably complete. Figure 13.3 illustrates the timing of closure of these vascular channels as judged from post-mortem material.

13.5 The respiratory system of the newborn

The rate of ventilation in the neonate is high compared with that of the adult and the minute volume is about 50 per cent higher in terms of body weight. Ventilation is often irregular and is interspersed with periods of shallow breathing

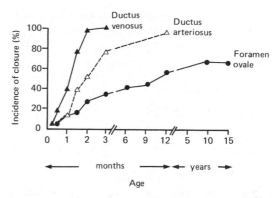

Figure 13.3   Closure of the special vascular channels of the fetus after birth. The data were gathered from post-mortem material so may not reflect the rates of vessel closure in healthy human infants. Note the changes in the time scale

reminiscent of the fetal pattern. The reflexes associated with lung inflation in the newborn appear to be different: the Hering–Breuer reflex increasing expiratory centre activity as the lungs are filled appears to be inoperative and instead the infant exhibits the paradoxical reflex of Head where lung inflation excites the inspiratory centre and produces further inhalation. This reflex may be important in the initial opening of the lungs and in maintaining their expansion. For the first few weeks the infant can only breathe through the nose and this has the advantage that suckling need not be interrupted in order to breathe. However, about 50 per cent of the total airway resistance is in the nasal passages. The oxygen consumption of the newborn is similar to that of the term fetus (about 6 ml/kg min) compared with 4 in the adult), but rises rapidly by 40 per cent in the first few hours after birth and stabilises at about 8 ml/(kg min) at 2 weeks. This high level of oxygen consumption may be due to the relatively larger size of the metabolically active brain and liver but might also be due to poor control over temperature regulation as discussed below.

Table 13.2 shows a number of ventilatory and respiratory values for the newborn compared with the adult. It must be borne in mind that accurate experimental study of lung function in the infant is difficult for obvious reasons. Most of the differences between neonate and adult are self-explanatory but one or two points should be made. The

Table 13.2   Lung function and respiratory values
of the neonate compared to the adult

Function	Newborn	Adult
Body weight (kg)	3.3	70
Ventilatory rate (per min)	25–50	12
Mean minute volume at rest (ml)	500	6500
Tidal volume (ml)	18	500
Vital capacity (ml)	120	4500
Residual volume (ml)	40	1500
Functional dead space (ml/kg)	2.2	2.2
Bronchiole diameter (mm)	0.1	0.2
Compliance $\Delta V/\Delta P$ (ml/(cm H$_2$O))	5	165
Exchange surface area (m^2)	3	60
Oxygen diffusion capacity (ml/(mmHg min))	2.5	20

high airway resistance in the neonate is due both to nasal resistance and to the small bronchiolar diameter and means that the energy cost of breathing is greater in the neonate than in the adult, particularly as lung compliance is low. It is estimated that about 6 per cent of the total oxygen consumption of the neonate is used for ventilation compared with about 2 per cent in the adult. Although the oxygen diffusion capacity of the neonatal lungs is apparently small, calculations show that it is more than adequate.

Control of ventilation by chemoreceptor reflexes in the newborn is functional at birth but differs qualitatively from that of the adult. Exposure to a hypoxic mixture of 15 per cent oxygen in nitrogen causes a rise in minute volume for about 1–2 minutes followed by a fall in the minute volume to below the original value even when the hypoxic gas mixture is still being administered. The initial increase in minute volume is probably due to the stimulation of peripheral chemoreceptors and the decline to hypoxic depression of the medullary respiratory centres in a manner similar to that observed in the fetus (see section 11.11). This response is dependent upon the environmental temperature and the initial rise in minute volume is abolished if the infant is in a cool environment. As in the adult, exposure to 100 per cent oxygen produces a diminution of the minute volume followed by a rise as blood carbon dioxide tension increases.

Ventilatory responses to hypercapnic stimulation are well developed in the newborn who shows a more sensitive response to carbon dioxide than does the adult. The addition of 2 per cent carbon dioxide to inspired air may increase the minute volume by as much as 80 per cent over a 5-minute period.

It is thus apparent that the control of breathing in the neonate has some similarity with that of the fetus, particularly as the central medullary chemoreceptors are dominant. The neonatal pattern represents a transitional state to the adult type of regulation. The sensitivity of the peripheral chemoreceptors to oxygen probably adjusts rapidly at birth to take account of the raised oxygen tension in arterial blood.

13.6   The cardiovascular system of the newborn

Nervous control of the cardiovascular system is well developed at birth and improves rapidly in the first few days of life so that the neonate is soon able to adjust its cardiac output and blood pressure sufficiently to meet changing conditions. The carotid sinus baroreceptors are functional at birth and a fall in blood volume leads to reflex vasoconstriction. This response improves in the first few days of life. Stimulation of the carotid baroreceptors causes reflex bradycardia and this may be the most important mechanism for the control of blood pressure in the first few days of life. At birth peripheral blood vessels constrict readily in response to cold but the capacity for vasodilation in response to a rise in body temperature is not established for

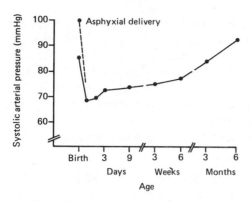

Figure 13.4 Changes in systolic arterial pressure after birth and in early development. Pressure is higher in infants showing asphyxia during delivery (Redrawn from Dawes, G. S. (1968). *Foetal and Neonatal Physiology*, Year Book Medical Publishers, Chicago)

Table 13.3   Cardiovascular parameters of the neonate compared to fetal and adult values

Function	Fetus	Neonate	Adult
Arterial blood pressure (mmHg)	70/45	70/45	120/80
Pulmonary arterial pressure (mmHg)	(higher)*	35/15	30/10
Pulse rate (per min)	140	140	70
Cardiac output (l/min)	0.6	0.6	5
(ml/(kg min))	(similar)*	140	70
(l/(m² min))	(similar)*	2.5–3.0	2.5–3.0
Limb blood flow (ml/(100 g min))	?	4	2
Left atrial pressure (mmHg)	(lower)*	2±1.5	5
Right atrial pressure (mmHg)	(higher)*	0±1.4	0

* With respect to the neonate, but precise values have not been obtained.

a few days. Systemic arterial blood pressure falls for about the first 12 hours post-partum as the effects of birth asphyxia are corrected and then rises gradually during the first few months of life (figure 13.4). The mechanisms for autoregulation of blood flow in brain, heart and lung are well developed at birth.

Table 13.3 compares cardiovascular parameters of the newborn with fetal and adult values. Once the effects of asphyxia have worn off, systemic arterial blood pressure is similar to that of the fetus but is low compared with that of the adult because peripheral resistance is low. Peripheral blood flow is high. The gradual rise in systemic blood pressure seen during the first few weeks of life probably results from changes in peripheral resistance due to increased vascular tone. Pulmonary arterial pressure is high post-partum but declines to adult values within a few days as the pulmonary resistance to flow decreases (figure 13.5). It is not feasible to measure pulmonary arterial pressure in the fetus (hence the estimate in table 13.3), but it must be higher than the systemic arterial pressure to account for the observed direction of flow in the ductus arterious.

The neonatal pulse rate is similar to that of the fetus and falls gradually with age, reaching 90 at 6 years and 70 by about 13 years. The large cardiac output per kilogram body weight of the newborn (table 13.3), is generated by the high pulse rate, and as in the fetus control is largely produced by

variation in heart rate rather than stroke volume. However, when the cardiac output is expressed in terms of body surface area a value very similar to that of the adult is obtained, 2.5–3.0 l/(m² min), and is considered below in relation to the control of body temperature.

The great veins of the newborn have a considerable capacity and can accommodate the widely varying blood volumes which are present in different babies at birth. Variations of up to 30 per

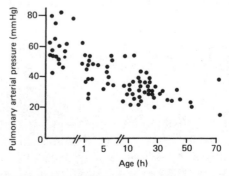

Figure 13.5 Pulmonary arterial pressure as a function of age (Redrawn from Dawes, G. S. (1968). *Foetal and Neonatal Physiology*, Year Book Medical Publishers, Chicago)

Table 13.4   The effects of early and late cord clamping on blood values in the neonate

	Age post-partum	*Time of cord clamping*	
		early (10–22 s)	late (5 min)
Blood volume (ml/kg)	30 min	78	99
	24 h	86	96
Haematocrit (%)	30 min	47	59
	24 h	44	62
Mean arterial BP (mmHg)	5–10 min	44	69
	4 h	52	71
Capillary blood pH (heel)	30 min	7.24	7.30
Capillary blood pCO_2 (heel)	30 min	55	45

cent in blood volume occur depending on how much of the placental blood content reaches the neonate before the cord is clamped (table 13.4). If the cord is clamped early the initial blood volume is low and rises with time; the opposite obtains if the cord is clamped late.

The fact that the foramen ovale and ductus arteriosus retain a degree of patency is demonstrated by the figures in table 13.5 since left ventricular output is higher than the right and pulmonary blood flow is higher than right ventricular output. This situation must arise from recirculation of blood from aorta to pulmonary artery through the ductus arteriosus. The left to right heart shunt through the ductus arteriosus has been calculated

Table 13.5   Cardiac output in the newborn

Age (h)	10	(range 2–28)
Weight (kg)	3.2	
LV output (ml/(kg min))	348	
RV output (ml/(kg min)	233	
Pulmonary flow (ml/(kg min))	305	
L to R shunt (% LV output)	38	
R to L shunt (% RV output)	20	

LV, left ventricle; RV, right ventricle; L, left; R, right.

at approximately 38 per cent of the left ventricular output, and the right to left shunt through the foramen ovale is estimated at 20 per cent. At birth the right ventricular wall is thicker than the left demonstrating the greater work load in fetal life on the right heart. This position is rapidly reversed by left ventricular hypertrophy induced by the load associated with the postnatal circulatory pattern.

13.7   Metabolism in the newborn

The considerable store of glycogen which is built up in skeletal muscle and to a lesser extent in the liver during fetal life is sufficient to provide energy for metabolism during delivery and the first hours of postnatal life. Glycogen is mobilised in response to circulating catecholamines but is rapidly replaced when feeding starts. At birth the respiratory quotient is 1.0 indicating that glucose is the principal metabolic substrate but it falls during the first few days of life to about 0.7 (a similar value to that in an adult diabetic), because fat stores and protein are mobilised and milk is utilised. A newborn baby commonly loses about 10 per cent of its birth weight in the first 2–3 days of life, but most of this is due to a reduction in extracellular water rather than to extensive tissue catabolism.

The neonate cannot efficiently regulate its blood glucose and is usually hypoglycaemic for the first few days—figure 13.6(b). There are several reasons for this. Compared to the adult the neonatal liver is immature and the enzymes concerned with glucose metabolism (especially hexokinase, phosphorylase and glucose-6-phosphatase) do not reach adult levels for 2–3 weeks. Glycogenolysis and gluconeogenesis are relatively slow processes in the newborn and a fall in blood glucose cannot rapidly be corrected. The glycogen stores of the liver and muscle of babies whose delivery has been protracted are severely depleted and any subsequent hypoglycaemia may be greater. Another aspect of glucose metabolism in the newborn concerns insulin; for some time after birth secretion in response to a glucose load is small and sluggish (as in the fetus), despite there being adequate insulin in the beta islet cells. It appears that these cells still lack

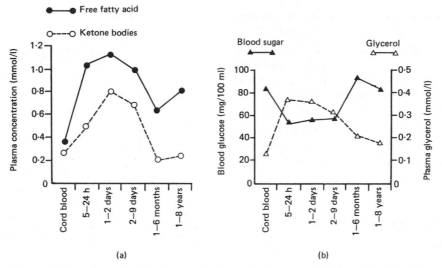

Figure 13.6   Changes in blood concentrations of glucose and other metabolites. (Redrawn from Dawes, G.S. *Foetal and Neonatal Physiology,* **Year Book Medical Publishers, Chicago)**

sensitivity to glucose but respond better to amino acids as in the fetal period (see section 11.13).

Thus blood glucose levels in neonates may fluctuate considerably and values as low as 20 mg/100 ml of blood have been recorded. In an older child or an adult such falls in blood glucose levels would produce convulsions and hypoglycaemic coma and probable neurological damage, but in the newborn may provoke an apnoeic attack but nothing worse. It appears that the central nervous system of the neonate is partially protected against hypoglycaemia. It is probable that the neonatal brain is able to utilise other metabolic substrates such as free fatty acids, glycerol and ketone bodies, all of which are present in high concentrations in plasma at this time (figure 13.6).

High levels of free fatty acid and glycerol in neonatal plasma occur because of the lipolytic effects of the high levels of growth hormone which are present at and following birth and as a result of the stimulation of lipolysis in brown fat by noradrenaline. The oxidation of fatty acids and glycerol produces ketone bodies which accounts for their high plasma levels at this time (figure 13.6).

Since blood glucose levels in the newborn are dependent on its immediate nutritional state, glucose homeostasis is best maintained by allowing it to feed on demand.

The relative immaturity of the neonatal liver has a number of important consequences. For example, the rate of synthesis of plasma proteins is low and there may be a transient decline in their plasma concentrations. The neonatal liver also has a poor ability to metabolise foreign substances such as drugs by either oxidative or conjugation routes. The ability to conjugate bilirubin with glucuronic acid to form water-soluble bile pigments which can be excreted in the urine is deficient, and underlies the jaundice which is common in the first few days of life. Jaundice is due to the accumulation of bilirubin in the skin and may be particularly severe in cases of rhesus isoimmunisation where there is considerable haemolysis and release of blood pigments (see section 10.6). Since the blood–brain barrier of the neonate is more permeable than that of the adult, bilirubin may reach the brain and cause kernicterus and permanent neurological damage by deposition in the basal ganglia.

In some babies blood clotting may be defective because of low plasma prothrombin activity due to a relative lack of the vitamin K prosthetic group. Most vitamin K is derived from the gut microflora but because the gut at birth is microbiologically sterile formation of prothrombin is limited.

The relative immaturity of the liver in the newborn means that the half-lives of many drugs in the body are greatly extended and the detoxification of many substances is slow. Thus drugs have to be administered with great caution.

13.8   Temperature regulation in the newborn

The newborn baby has considerable difficulty in regulating its body temperature. The ratio of surface area of skin to body weight is more than twice that of the adult whereas the ratio of cardiac output to body surface area is the same. Furthermore, the subcutaneous layer of insulating fat is relatively thin and therefore makes potential heat loss even greater. At birth the neonate must adjust from conditions where there is no need for temperature control or conservation of heat to those of a comparatively unfavourable environment in which heat is easily dissipated. The large increase in oxygen consumption shortly after birth is accompanied by a surge of thyroid stimulating hormone release from the pituitary gland and this probably serves to increase the basal metabolic rate by increasing thyroid hormone secretion.

The core body temperature of the neonate drops considerably during the first few hours after birth but then begins to rise as oxygen consumption increases and thermogenesis begins (figure 13.7). The peripheral vasoconstrictor mechanisms present at birth are insufficient to prevent this initial fall in temperature. Normal body temperature is not regained until about 12 hours post partum and for the first few weeks of life may still fluctuate greatly. Table 13.6 shows a comparison of heat production in the neonate and adult and illustrates that although heat production per kilogram of tissue in the newborn is about 1½ times that of the adult it is much less in terms of body surface area.

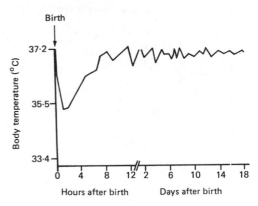

Figure 13.7   Body temperature at birth and in the neonatal period (Redrawn from Guyton, A.C. (1971). *Textbook of Medical Physiology*, Saunders, Philadelphia)

It is thus evident that babies must be kept well wrapped and in a warm environment to prevent heat loss. Thermogenesis begins when a critical temperature difference of 1.5°C between the skin and the environment is exceeded and thereafter oxygen consumption increases by 0.6 ml/min for every 1°C difference. Oxygen consumptions of 15 ml/(kg min) have been recorded in cold-stressed infants, indicating a considerable capacity for thermogenesis.

The newborn baby is unable to shiver and thus this mechanism of heat generation is unavailable. However, a special mechanism for the rapid production of heat exists; at birth there are

Table 13.6   Metabolic rate in the newborn and adult

	Newborn	Adult
Surface area of body (m^2)	0.21	1.73
Body weight (kg)	3.3	70
Basal metabolic rate:		
(i) absolute (kcal/24 h)	115	1610
(ii) in terms of body surface area (kcal/(m^2 h))	22.8	38.7
(iii) in terms of mass (kcal/(kg·h))	1.50	0.96

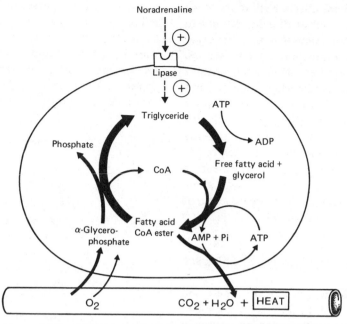

Figure 13.8 **Breakdown of triglyceride to yield useful heat in the brown fat cell of the neonate. About 160 kcal/mol of triglyceride are produced during each turn of the cycle** (Redrawn from Swan, H. (1974), *Thermoregulation and Bioenergetics*, Elsevier, New York)

large deposits of *brown fat* which are located around the nape of the neck and shoulders, between the scapulae and around the kidneys. Thermogenesis is accomplished by means of stimulation of brown fat cells by catecholamines released by nervous stimulation or secreted into the circulation from the adrenal medulla. Activation of a lipase results in the release of free fatty acids and glycerol from the triglyceride stores, but instead of being completely oxidised most free fatty acid is resynthesised into triglyceride by incorporation of α-glycerophosphate (figure 13.8). There is consequently only a modest depletion of the triglyceride stores, and heat is released from the ATP and α-glycerophosphate consumed during each cycle. The nervous control of this efficient source of heat production means that it can be activated rapidly. In cold-stressed infants the plasma levels of free fatty acids and glycerol are elevated as the result of lipolysis and these compounds can then be oxidised to yield heat by conventional routes.

13.9 The neonatal kidney

The fetus produces large volumes of dilute urine but there is no risk that its plasma composition will change markedly because any osmotic imbalance is rapidly corrected across the placenta or by fetal swallowing (see sections 11.7, 11.9 and 7.8). Mature kidney function develops by 1 month of age but up to this time urine production resembles the fetal pattern. The neonatal kidney is unable to conserve or eliminate solutes efficiently and urine can only be concentrated to about 1.5 times the plasma osmolarity, compared with 3–5 times in the adult. Thus alterations in fluid intake can easily produce an osmotic imbalance and dehydration can occur very easily. It is therefore important to dilute formula feeds and cow's milk correctly so that sodium chloride and other ingredients are not present in too high a concentration. The neonatal kidney is also unable to compensate acid-base imbalances rapidly and this is why any metabolic acidosis that occurs at birth takes a long while to correct. The dangers of dehydration and acidosis are obviously minimised in the infant that is allowed to take human milk whenever it wishes.

The glomerular filtration rate in the neonate is low, about two-thirds of the adult value in terms of total body water. Although antidiuretic hormone is present in the posterior pituitary at birth, the distal nephrons of the kidney appear to be insensitive to its action for at least the first week of life and hence water retention is poor. The neonate responds to a water load by an increase in glomerular filtration rate rather than by a reduction of antidiuretic hormone secretion.

13.10   The neonatal gastrointestinal tract

The gastrointestinal tract is able to digest and absorb milk at birth. The first feed is often distilled water to correct any dehydration and is usually given within the first 6 hours after birth. This is then followed by breast or bottle feeding. Milk is a perfectly adequate food until the infant is old enough to supplement it with homogenised or solid food and indeed in some cultures babies are not weaned for 2 years or more.

The ability to absorb fat in early life is limited because the liver is unable to produce the large quantities of bile salts necessary for its complete emulsification. This is why fat-rich cow's milk that has not been diluted leads to the production of fatty faeces (steatorrhoea).

The first stools consisting of meconium are passed during the first day of life, but meconium usually disappears from the stools within about 4 days.

13.11 The central nervous system

In the newborn human baby cortical function is relatively immature compared with some species, but its development accelerates rapidly after birth as sensory input is greatly enhanced. Reflexes are usually depressed for the first 24 hours of life as a result of the mild asphyxia of birth and the infant is relatively quiescent. After this time several reflexes can normally be elicited readily as listed below. In severely asphyxiated or unhealthy babies with low Apgar scores (see chapter 12), these reflexes are greatly depressed and take longer to appear. There is also a higher incidence of neurological damage in these babies.

Principal reflexes in the newborn

(1)   The grasping reflex. If a finger or a pencil is placed in the infant's palm the hand will close to grasp it firmly.

(2)   Moro embrace reflex. If the baby is held to the chest it will extend its arms to grasp the holder.

(3)   Blinking of the eye if the lid is touched.

(4)   Withdrawal of a limb from a painful stimulus.

(5)   Turning the head to free the nostrils. This enables the baby to breathe without having to remove its face from the breast.

(6)   Rooting for the breast. The baby makes vigorous movements with its head to locate the nipple if it is held to the breast.

(7)   Walking reflex. If the infant is held under the armpits so that its feet just touch a firm surface it will make walking movements. This reflex is less readily elicited as the infant gets older.

(8)   Falling reflex. If the head is raised and allowed to fall back on the cot the infant will throw its arms out sideways in an attempt to break the fall.

The grasping and Moro reflexes are commonly used to assess the reflex ability of the newborn. The functions of these reflexes is obscure, but they may be ancestral relics related to vital reflexes in those primate species in which the infant is carried grasping on to the mother's fur.

The newborn baby also shows a general awareness of its surroundings and reacts to changes in sound and light by movements of the limbs, eyes and head and by changes in ventilatory rate and vocalisation.

The newborn baby sleeps for periods of about 3

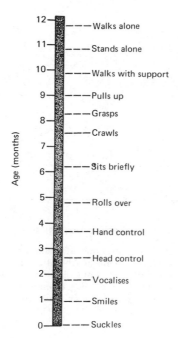

Figure 13.9 indicators on vertical age scale (months):

12 — Walks alone
11 — Stands alone
10 — Walks with support
9 — Pulls up
8 — Grasps
 — Crawls
7 —
6 — Sits briefly
5 — Rolls over
4 — Hand control
3 — Head control
2 — Vocalises
1 — Smiles
0 — Suckles

Age (months)

Figure 13.9   Some of the principal stages in the behavioural development of the infant during the first year of life. Individual variations for these milestones between normal infants is very wide (Redrawn from Guyton, A. C. (1971). *Textbook of Medical Physiology,* **Saunders, Philadelphia)**

hours interspersed with short periods of wakefulness. Rapid eye movement (REM) sleep occupies about 40 per cent of the sleeping time compared with about 20 per cent in the adult; this type of sleep is associated with typical slow wave patterns on the electroencephalogram and with dreaming in the adult.

Figure 13.9 illustrates some of the major behavioural milestones during the first year of life.

13.12   The problems of prematurity

A premature baby may be defined as one whose development and homeostatic mechanisms are insufficiently advanced to enable it to make the transition to an independent life without a considerable risk of death. This definition includes all babies whose development would have proceeded normally to term had they not been born early,

but excludes those babies with specific malformations or defects. However, there is no clear-cut definition of prematurity in terms of menstrual age or size at birth and the term premature should only be used in a general sense. Because of this difficulty other more exact but arbitrary distinctions are made. Some authorities simply regard a baby of less than 37 weeks of gestation (*pre-term*) or less than 2.5 kg (*low birth weight*) as premature.

The two major problems faced by the premature baby are temperature regulation and ventilation. The smaller size of the premature baby means that its surface area to volume ratio is even greater than usual and thus affords a huge area for heat loss. Furthermore, since fat is only formed late in gestation (see chapter 11), the layer of subcutaneous insulating fat is thinner. Lack of subcutaneous fat also occurs in babies whose growth *in utero* is retarded because of poor nutrition. Stores of brown fat and glycogen in muscle and liver are also reduced in premature babies. Additionally the vasomotor responses are less well developed in premature babies and the ability to reduce heat loss by peripheral vasoconstriction is more limited. Since the premature baby can do little to limit heat loss and lacks adequate metabolite reserves to generate extra heat it must be maintained in a warm incubator.

There may be severe difficulties with ventilation in the premature baby and this is the major cause of mortality. It was noted previously (see figure 11.13) that there is an association between plasma cortisol and the formation of lecithin lung surfactant. The plasma cortisol levels and surfactant production are very low in premature babies and thus their lungs are very difficult to expand. They also tend to collapse again after each exhalation. This lowers the diffusion capacity of the lungs and considerably increases the work needed for ventilation. The premature baby often grunts as it breathes because it tries to prevent alveolar collapse by expiring through a closed glottis; the sternum bows inwards at each inhalation. This condition is called the *respiratory distress syndrome* and is common in pre-term babies weighing less than 2 kg. The baby rapidly becomes exhausted, hypoxic, hypercapnic and acidotic.

Respiratory distress syndrome is also called hyaline membrane disease because *post mortem* the alveoli are seen to be filled with concentric accumulations of lipid material when examined under the microscope. This material impedes gaseous exchange and contributes to the lowering of the diffusion capacity. Respiratory distress syndrome can be treated by ventilating the infant artificially at a positive airway pressure with gas mixtures enriched with oxygen. The ventilator is designed so that the pressure in the lungs always exceeds atmospheric pressure thus maintaining expansion of the alveoli. The use of gas mixtures containing more than 80 per cent oxygen has to be avoided because this frequently leads to invasion of the vitreous humour of the eye with blood vessels and subsequent blindness. A premature baby which is not ventilated artificially usually shows breathing movements of fetal type characterised by periods of very shallow breathing or apnoea, and its circulation is often on the brink of reversion to the fetal pattern. Respiratory distress syndrome is common in the babies of untreated diabetics and here the development of the lungs appears to be specifically retarded in relation to other systems.

If lung immaturity is suspected, for example when spontaneous labour begins pre-term or if induction before term is planned, fetal lung development can be assessed by measuring the amount of surfactant in amniotic fluid. If the concentration of lecithin is below 4 mg/100 ml of amniotic fluid (figure 13.10), or the ratio of lecithin to sphingomyelin is less than 2:1, then the lungs are likely to be immature. In many cases the maturation of the fetal lungs can be accelerated by the administration to the mother of a synthetic corticosteriod.

The feeding of premature babies usually presents little problem as the development of the gut is well advanced in the third trimester. Sometimes the reflexes of deglutition are poorly developed and the baby has to be fed by intragastric tube.

13.13   Mortality in early life

There are three useful indices relating to mortality in the neonatal period and in early life —

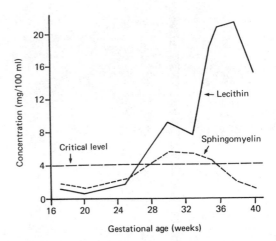

Figure 13.10 Concentrations of pulmonary surfactants lecithin and sphingomyelin in amniotic fluid. The dashed line shows the critical level of lecithin, below which there is a high probability of ensuing respiratory distress syndrome in the newborn (Redrawn from Avery, M. E. *et al.* (1973). *Scientific American*, **228(4)**, pages 75–85)

infant mortality, neonatal mortality and *perinatal mortality* — and their definitions are given in table 13.7 together with data for England and Wales in 1976. Whilst infant and neonatal mortality refer only to deaths after live birth (within a year and 28 days respectively), the figure for perinatal mortality includes deaths during the first week and stillbirths occurring after 28 weeks of gestation. Spontaneous labour resulting in a birth before 28 weeks, whether alive or dead, is referred to as a spontaneous abortion (see chapter

Table 13.7   Mortality in early life

		Incidence per thousand (England & Wales, 1976)
Infant mortality	Deaths in the first year of life after live birth	14.3
Neonatal mortality	Deaths in first 28 days after live birth	9.7
Perinatal mortality	Number of stillbirths plus deaths in first 7 days of life after live birth	17.7

10). An important contribution to the mortality figures is made by deaths due to abnormalities such as congenital malformations and to a lesser extent inborn errors of metabolism; in fact as other causes for mortality such as infection or prematurity decline in importance, the proportion of deaths due to congenital abnormalities increases, even though there is no increase in their absolute incidence.

It is important to reflect that the frequency of mortality in early life has decreased markedly in the last 150 years, due largely to improvements in hygiene, education and perinatal care, as well as because of the introduction of antibiotics and vaccinations for the control or prevention of infections. About 100 years ago in Britain, the infant mortality rate was of the order of 150 per thousand (cf. 14.3 in 1976), and more than one-half of the deaths were directly attributable to infection. The rates of mortality in countries with poorly developed medical and antenatal facilities still remain high, particularly in the tropics, and it is hoped that simple preventive and educational measures may reduce many of these early deaths. By contrast, in the developed countries most early deaths occur because of abnormalities or because of inadequate intrauterine development or prematurity, and the recent continued reduction in these deaths is attributable in part to the provision of facilities for fetal monitoring and improvements in the care of premature babies. Nevertheless, the likelihood of death in the neonatal period or in the first year of life is greater than at any time between birth and old age.

Further reading

Comline, R. S., Cross, K. W., Dawes, G. S. and Nathanielsz, P. W. (eds.) (1973). *Fetal and Neonatal Physiology* (Barcroft Centenary Symposium), Cambridge University Press

Dawes, G. S. (1968). *Fetal and Neonatal Physiology*, Year Book Medical Publishers, Chicago

Young, M. (1976). 'On being born', in *Companion to Medical Studies*, vol. 1, Blackwell, Oxford

The Breast and Lactation

14.1 Introduction

The breast or *mammary gland* provides milk for the nourishment of the newborn mammal. This system of postnatal nutrition is considered to be of such evolutionary importance as to justify its taxonomic use for an entire class of animals. The structural and behavioural complexity of the mammal requires a considerable degree of post-natal development and growth, and the phenomenon of suckling enables the mother to provide extrauterine nutrition while the young are maturing sufficiently to feed themselves. This places a great burden on the mother who devotes much energy to the nurture of her young. One obvious consequence is that reproductive rates of mammals are low in comparison to other types, but the success rate is higher because parental care and feeding of the young are so well developed.

The growth of the breast, its structure and the mechanisms responsible for the formation and release of milk will be discussed in this chapter. The breast is essentially an alveolar gland derived from skin, in which milk is synthesised (*lactogenesis*) and released (*lactation*) after appropriate hormonal and neural stimuli. Breast growth falls into four phases in the human. From birth to puberty the breast is quiescent and grows at the same rate as the rest of the body; at puberty there is a phase of accelerated development under hormonal stimulation; during pregnancy and lactation there is a further phase of growth during which alveolar milk synthesis occurs; finally, after lactation, and especially after the menopause, the mammary gland regresses. In the male the mammary gland remains rudimentary throughout life, approximating in form and structure to that of the prepubertal female.

14.2 Structure and function of the adult mammary gland

The variations in structure and function of the mature mammary gland are complex, so it is preferable to describe the detailed structural features of the lactating gland before considering its embryological origins and its growth and development through the different phases of life.

The mammary glands are paired, and lie in the superficial fascia over the pectoralis major muscle. They are connected to the skin and supported by fibrous sheets and, although essentially circular in frontal view, contain several tail-like processes, the principal of which runs upwards and laterally towards the axilla. Thus the mature mammary gland has the shape of an inverted comma when viewed from the front.

Each gland is a compound tubuloalveolar gland consisting of 15–25 irregular lobes of glandular tissue radiating out from the nipple (figure 14.1). Both the nipple and the surrounding circular area of skin, the *areola,* are firmer than the surrounding breast tissue, do not contain much fat, and are pigmented, especially in pregnancy. Each lobe is drained by a *lactiferous duct*

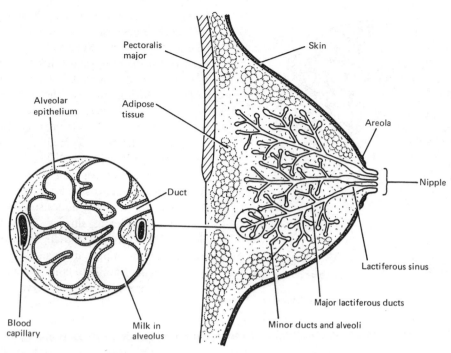

Figure 14.1   Vertical section of lactating breast

lined with stratified squamous epithelium, into which the primary terminal ducts of the lobules empty. However, the lactiferous duct from each lobe passes to the apex of the nipple and opens to the surface independently, although each has a dilation in the region beneath the areola, the *lactiferous sinus.*

Each lobe is subdivided into many lobules, each of which comprises elongated tubules, the *alveolar ducts,* covered with sac-like *alveoli.* The lobules are separated by thin connective tissue septa, and the stroma also contains adipose tissue. The proportions of connective tissue and fat vary between individuals and also according to physiological state. The considerable differences in size of the breasts between women are largely due to variations in the amounts of adipose tissue. In the non-pregnant woman the alveili are hardly developed at all and the ducts end in a fine array of smaller, branching ducts.

During pregnancy there is considerable growth of the breast in cellular terms, although its size sometimes does not increase markedly. In the first half of gestation the duct system grows and extensive branching of its terminal parts takes place to form alveoli, mainly at the expense of the interlobular adipose tissue. The fat lost may provide some of the metabolic energy necessary for growth. Each alveolus is lined with secretory epithelial cells, the shape of which depends on the state of distension of the alveolus. Thus they are flattened when the sac is engorged with milk, but tall and columnar when nearly empty. Underneath the alveolar cells lies a basket-like network of myoepithelial cells (figure 14.2) supported by a basal lamella in contact with the numerous adjacent capillaries. The contractile function of the myoepithelial cells surrounding the alveoli was correctly postulated as long ago as 1894, but it should be noted that they are not homologous with smooth muscle cells since they derive from epithelium rather than from connective tissue. Myoepithelial cells also surround the ducts and can be identified even in the fetal mammary gland.

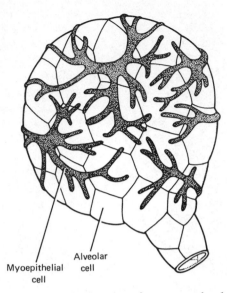

Myoepithelial cell   Alveolar cell

Figure 14.2   Surface view of mammary alveolus

In the latter part of pregnancy the rate of cellular proliferation slows and subsequent enlargement of the breast is largely due to distension by the products of secretion. At this stage colostrum is produced rather than milk: this is watery and rich in proteins, but does not contain much fat (see section 14.11). However, not all alveoli secrete at the same time and so the histological appearance of the gland varies from one area to another. The secretory function and ultrastructure of the alveolar epithelial cell is discussed separately below.

These structural changes in the breast during pregnancy and lactation are principally under endocrine control. Breast growth at puberty involves proliferation of the duct system and accumulation of adipose tissue, and is initiated by circulating oestrogens and completed by the synergistic actions of progesterone and oestradiol. Growth hormone, insulin and glucocorticoids may play subordinate or permissive roles, but prolactin is probably not critical. These hormones plus prolactin (and perhaps placental lactogen) are vital for further breast development during pregnancy. The fall in placental steroids after parturition enables prolactin to exert its important actions on lactogenesis and lactation, and the other hormones continue to have permissive or synergistic actions. Finally, oxytocin release is essential for the removal of milk and for continued milk secretion during suckling *(galactopoiesis)*.

The characteristics of the nipple have been mentioned. The lactiferous ducts open at its surface (see figure 14.1) but in the resting gland are plugged by keratin formed by the stratified squamous epithelial cells. The dense connective tissue of the nipple contains a network of smooth muscle fibres which pass circumferentially around the nipple and its base, and also lie longitudinally along the lactiferous sinuses. They have attachments to the skin, and their function is for the erection of the nipple during suckling and sexual arousal and in response to cold. The nipple contains a profuse supply of sensory nerve endings, and it is stimulation of these afferent pathways which activates the neuroendocrine reflex concerned with milk ejection (see section 14.10).

The intercostal nerves contain these somatic afferent nerves and also sympathetic fibres which supply the smooth muscle of the blood vessels and of the nipple. There is no parasympathetic innervation, and autonomic nervous control over mammary gland function appears to be minimal. Blood is supplied from branches of the intercostal, internal thoracic and lateral thoracic arteries, and is drained by the corresponding veins. Blood flow is much increased during lactation as there is a high demand for metabolic substrates. The lymphatic drainage is also well developed, and passes mainly to the parasternal, interpectoral and apical axillary nodes.

14.3   Embryological development of the mammary gland

The mammary glands originate from the skin as specialised ectodermal structures, probably derived from sweat glands. They differentiate as bilateral linear thickenings of the epidermis of the ventro-lateral aspect of the body; the first raised band of ectoderm (the mammary band) appears by the fourth week of gestation but disappears, whilst a second narrower ridge of ectoderm develops on either side of the midline. This is the *mammary crest.* In the human, the cranial end proliferates to form a mammary bud which sinks into the differentiating mesenchyme, figure 14.3(a), and the rest of the mammary crest regresses. The position and number of future mammary glands characteristic of a given species is determined at this stage by the manner in which the mammary crest becomes divided into mammary buds. In man, accessory nipples may develop at other points along the mammary crest, caudal to the mammary glands proper.

The mammary bud is originally lenticular in shape, but then becomes conical as it grows downwards from its base to form a cord-like structure (primary mammary cord) attached to the epidermis – figure 14.3(b). Its distal part extends into the mesenchyme and a number of solid cellular sprouts develop from it as it pushes inwards. Only after this cellular proliferation at the third or fourth month of gestation is there any visible elevation of the epidermis to show the location of the mammary glands – figure 14.3(c). The cellular sprouts later develop lumina to become ducts lined with two layers of cuboidal cells, but alveoli are absent at this stage.

The epithelial arborisation occurs within a matrix of differentiating mesenchyme. Two types of mesenchymal differentiation occur, forming the smooth muscle and the connective tissue of the nipple, lobules and interlobular septa.

Towards birth, the superficial ectoderm of the bud desquamates and keratinises to leave an inverted nipple; when the underlying dermis thickens the nipple is pushed upwards and everts – figure 14.3(d). The duct system corresponds to the adult pattern in that the primary cellular sprouts are completely canalised to form the *lactiferous ducts,* and the secondary outbuddings open their lumina to form the ducts of the gland.

This complex series of cellular changes appears to be under hormonal control, principally mediated by oestrogens, progesterone, growth hormone, prolactin and insulin. Development of the mammary gland in the male rat is much attenuated, apparently because the normal pattern of growth (which is female) is diverted by the actions of androgens released from the fetal testis. There is little evidence of this in man, however, and there are no obvious differences in mammary gland structure between male and female fetuses, but it is thought that the administration of steroids to

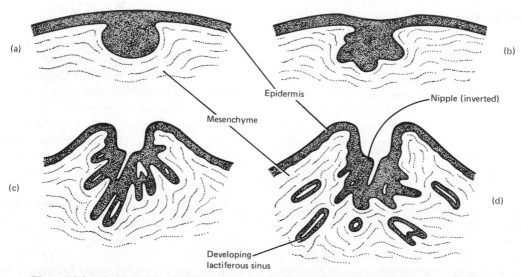

Figure 14.3   **Development of the mammary gland. (a)–(d) show transverse sections of the mammary crest at stages from the 10th week of development until near term. Progressive downgrowth, arborisation and canalisation of the epithelial rudiment are seen. Shortly after the stage shown in (d) the nipple everts**

pregnant women during the first trimester of pregnancy may induce congenital malformations of the fetal mammary gland.

14.4   Growth of the breast from birth through puberty and until pregnancy

There is very little growth of the mammary gland between birth and puberty. This is a quiescent phase, during which the breast grows at the same rate as the rest of the body.

However, there is sometimes mammary activity in both sexes at birth during which a clear fluid ('witch's milk') composed of water, fat and cellular debris may be secreted. This occurs because of transient proliferation, growth and dilation of the ducts and lobules, and is probably caused by the high levels of steroids to which the fetus is exposed in late gestation. This secretion may persist for up to 3 weeks, after which the lobules and ducts regress.

In all mammalian species there is marked acceleration in the growth of the female mammary gland at the time when adult ovarian activity is established. Thus the structural development of the breast coincides with the acquisition of fertility. In the human female, breast development occurs during puberty, but starts before the first menstrual period and well before the ovary is fully functional; thus the growth of the breast is usually the first sign of the onset of puberty, and precedes ovulation and secretion of progesterone from the corpus luteum by several years. This implies that the breast growth and development in early puberty is due to the effects of circulating oestrogens rather than to progesterone, because this latter hormone is released only in the luteal phase of a fully established menstrual cycle. In Britain and the USA, the mean age at which the first signs of breast development are evident is about 11 years, and full growth of the duct and stromal tissue to give the adult form is achieved by about 15½ years. Interestingly, man is the only primate in which significant breast growth occurs at puberty; in other species, including the great apes, it occurs only during the first pregnancy.

The principal features of development of the external breast during puberty are that the breast grows greatly in size and changes in contour from conical to hemispherical, and that the areola and nipple acquire pigmentation and enlarge.

At puberty there is extensive growth and branching of the duct system, proliferation and canalisation of tubuloalveolar units at the tips of the branching ducts and differentiation of the connective tissue to form interlobular septa and adipose tissue. The epithelial structures are formed by a double layer of cells: the epithelial cells which line the ducts are covered with a meshwork of myoepithelial cells. Further growth and enlargement of the breast may occur after puberty, but this generally reflects the accumulation of more periglandular adipose tissue. Indeed, in the non-lactating woman, the external size of the mammary gland is not a reliable indicator of the amount of secretory tissue within, because the proportion of adipose tissue is so variable. Although the breast grows considerably at puberty it does not yet acquire the true alveolar milk-secreting cells and hence is not capable of lactogenesis.

It is probable that there is a degree of structural change in the breast during the menstrual cycle, but accurate generalisations are hard to make. There is evidence that duct growth occurs during the oestrogen-dominated follicular phase and that progesterone secreted in the luteal phase promotes further extension of the duct system and the laying down of some alveoli. Progesterone may also cause fluid retention, and this contributes to the engorgement or fullness of the breasts experienced by some women in the luteal phase of the menstrual cycle. High dosage oral contraceptives often have a similar effect.

14.5   Prolactin and the endocrinology of lactogenesis

Prolactin has a central role in the physiology of the breast. It is a polypeptide hormone released from the anterior pituitary gland which stimulates the growth of the mammary gland and the formation of milk. Prolactin has diverse actions unparalleled by any other hormone, and its effects vary considerably between species, but in all mammalian species it is mammotropic and lactogenic. A common denominator in its other actions seems to be an involvement with reproduction, albeit indirectly, and it may arguably be regarded as the least specialised but most intriguing of the adenohypophyseal hormones.

Prolactin is very closely related to growth hormone and placental lactogen. All three hormones contain 190 amino acids, with many identical sequences, and it is probable that they have all arisen from a common ancestral peptide by a series of gene duplications preserved by evolution. In some species there is considerable overlap in properties; in man, growth hormone and prolactin have weak lactogenic and growth-promoting actions respectively, and human placental lactogen has both actions, although admittedly it has low potency. The structure of human placental lactogen is closer to growth hormone than to prolactin and this is used as a justification by those who prefer the name human chorionic somatomammotropin for this hormone.

It proved very difficult to establish that human prolactin and growth hormone are indeed different substances, because of the overlap in properties and the minute amounts of prolactin normally to be found. Histological examination of pituitaries taken at necropsy from pregnant women reveal 'pregnancy cells' which stain in a manner similar to prolactin-containing cells in the pituitaries of animals in which the hormone is unambiguously differentiated from growth hormone. These cells are more abundant during late pregnancy and lactation, and can be distinguished histologically from the acidophil cells which contain growth hormone. In addition they do not stain when treated with fluorescent anti-human growth hormone sera. Human prolactin has now been purified and anti-human prolactin antibodies prepared, thus permitting the development of a specific prolactin radioimmunoassay and determination of the complete amino acid sequence.

Secretion of prolactin increases throughout pregnancy until term, during which time further breast development takes place together with the formation of milk in the alveoli. Oestrogens, progesterone and prolactin are all vital for this and placental lactogen may also contribute, with glucocorticoids and insulin again exerting permissive roles.

After parturition, steroid hormone levels fall rapidly, but pituitary prolactin secretion increases, especially in response to suckling. The change in relative hormone dominance precipitates the secretion of milk: during pregnancy breast development and some lactogenesis occur but lactation itself is inhibited, possibly because the steroid hormones inhibit the lactational actions of prolactin and its release. Oestrogens are often administered therapeutically to inhibit unwanted post-partum lactation. The precise mechanisms underlying these complex hormonal actions are not known. Lactation stops if prolactin levels are suddenly reduced during nursing by experimental hypophysectomy in animals, or clinically in women by the administration of drugs which inhibit prolactin release.

14.6   Control of prolactin secretion

Secretion of prolactin differs from that of all other anterior pituitary hormones because it is under inhibitory rather than stimulatory control from the hypothalamus. The 'prolactin inhibitory factor' which was sought for a decade or more appears to be dopamine rather than a peptide as anticipated. Drugs known to stimulate central nervous system dopamine receptors, such as apomorphine and bromocriptine, inhibit prolactin release and can be used for the treatment of galactorrhoea associated with hyperprolactinaemia or to suppress puerperal lactation when it is not required. By contrast, elevation of plasma prolactin levels may be a side effect of therapy with dopamine receptor antagonists such as the phenothiazine and butyrophenone tranquillisers. Morphine and the naturally occurring opioids, β-endorphin and the enkephalins, also stimulate prolactin release, but this may be mediated indirectly by altering hypothalamic release of prolactin inhibitory factor.

Prolactin is often released physiologically at the

same time as growth hormone although, paradoxically, the pharmacological effects on the release of the two hormones of the drugs just mentioned are opposite. Prolactin levels are increased during sleep and stress, in both women and men, and rise very markedly during late pregnancy and suckling, as described above. Levels rise after sexual intercourse (in women) and after strenuous exercise, hypoglycaemia, and in hypothyroidism, but decrease when plasma glucose levels rise. Mean plasma prolactin levels in women are slightly higher than in men. There is about 100 times more growth hormone than prolactin in the normal non-pregnant human pituitary.

There is also some evidence for a prolactin releasing factor, although it is much less substantial than that obtained for dopamine as prolactin inhibitory factor. For example, it is known that the tripeptide thyrotropin releasing hormone (TRH) stimulates prolactin release as well as diminishing the secretion of growth hormone, although it is doubtful whether TRH regulates prolactin secretion physiologically. In the rat pituitary, TRH does this by increasing the messenger RNA-dependent synthesis of prolactin. It is of interest that both prolactin and growth hormone are synthesised intracellularly in the forms of 'pro-hormones' containing 20–30 extra hydrophobic amino acids which are cleaved before release of the hormone from the secretory cell. Very recent work suggests that many polypeptide hormones are made in this way, and that the extra peptides are vital for the passage of the hormone across the plasma membrane.

14.7   The alveolar cell

Some comments on the general features of the milk-secreting alveolar cell are appropriate before discussing milk itself. The cells of the alveolar epithelium have an exceptionally high capacity for the biosynthesis of lipid, carbohydrate and protein. The lactogenic cell is indeed remarkable and offers much scope for investigating the relation between cell structure and synthetic function.

Figure 14.4 shows a diagram of a fully developed lactating alveolar cell. It contains numerous mitochondria, abundant rough endoplasmic reticulum, mainly in the basal part of the cell, and a well-developed supranuclear Golgi complex containing flattened cisternae and associated vacuoles and microvesicles. These cytoplasmic organelles increase in number during late pregnancy and after the onset of lactation, reflecting the conversion of the alveolar cell from a resting to a fully secretory state. Morphometric studies have shown that proliferation of mitochondria precedes growth of the endoplasmic reticulum and Golgi complex, and reaches a plateau before parturition. Thus the cell increases its capacity for energy transduction before proliferation of the synthetic machinery. By contrast, the increase in number of the other organelles continues until lactation is well established.

The alveolar cells are firmly joined to one another near the apical surface by tight junctions. The apical plasma membrane has an essentially smooth surface apart from a few projecting microvilli, whereas the basolateral membranes are highly folded. This may reflect the high capacity of the alveolar cell for the uptake and transport from the extracellular space of substances originating from the perfusing blood. Substances actively taken up by the alveolar cell include amino acids, glucose, acetate and free fatty acids.

The most characteristic features of the lactating cell are the presence in the cytoplasm of abundant protein granules (0.04–0.12 μm diameter) and lipid droplets (1.0–4.0 μm diameter) which are most numerous towards the apical surface. It is now known that the specific milk proteins are synthesised in the rough endoplasmic reticulum and are then transported in microvesicles to the Golgi complex where, in the presence of calcium, they are packaged and condensed into secretory granules prior to secretion. The vesicles containing protein are secreted by exocytosis, the vesicle membrane becoming incorporated into the plasma membrane. Protein granules are not found in the developing alveolar cell before lactation.

The lipid droplets are much larger than the protein granules and increase in size towards the apex of the cell. They are found from late pregnancy

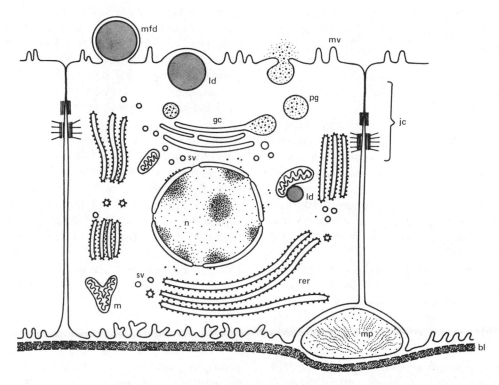

Figure 14.4 Active mammary alveolar cell. Milk proteins synthesised at the rough endoplasmic reticulum (rer) are carried in small vesicles (sv) to the Golgi complex (gc) where they are modified and concentrated. They are released as protein granules (pg) which fuse with the apical plasma membrane and release their contents by exocytosis. Lipid droplets (ld) formed in the cytoplasm migrate to the apex and are released packaged in an envelope of plasma membrane as milk fat droplets (mfd). (m, mitochondrion; n, nucleus; mv, microvilli; jc, junctional complex; mp, myo-epithelial cell process; bl, basal lamella)

onwards and become larger and more numerous as parturition approaches. It is believed that the fats are synthesised in the basal parts of the cell and coalesce in the cytoplasm into large droplets which are then secreted whole by pinching off from the apical plasma membrane. This mode of secretion (figure 14.4) explains why the secreted lipid globules are surrounded by a single layer of membrane as revealed by microscopic studies and biochemical analysis.

The biosynthesis of lactose is described in section 14.8. There is uncertainty about its mode of secretion: it appears to be synthesised at the Golgi complex and is probably released in the same vesicles as the milk protein. Alternatively, it may be secreted by a direct membrane transport mechanism, but no evidence of such a system has yet been produced. The apical plasma membrane is impermeable to lactose.

The high metabolic and synthetic activity of the fully developed lactating alveolar cell is discussed below in relation to the formation of lipid, proteins and lactose. It is worth noting here that studies of mammary gland nucleic acids have shown that there is a large increase in RNA relative to DNA during the latter part of pregnancy and after parturition. Prolactin administration also causes similar changes in suitably primed mammary tissue, but both insulin and glucocorticoids are necessary for the maturation of the gland and translation of messenger RNA.

14.8   Milk

Since the only food of most newborn mammals is the mother's milk, it is hardly surprising that milk is an almost complete food. It contains proteins, lipids, carbohydrates, minerals and vitamins, and its special nutritive value derives from an ideal combination of energy-rich fuel and metabolic substrates. The energy content of human milk is roughly 700 kcal/l and the infant derives about 60 per cent of its required calories from the oxidation of proteins which are thus utilised for growth. The composition of milk for any given species has evolved to suit the needs of the newborn, so that substitution with milk from another species may not be satisfactory and can result in intolerance or failure of normal growth.

The compositions of human and bovine milk are given in table 14.1. Cow's milk is richer in protein but contains less carbohydrate, and is therefore not an exact substitute for human milk. Human babies fed by bottle are usually given preparations of cow's milk which have been diluted to reduce the protein concentration and enriched in carbohydrate by addition of lactose or sucrose.

The components of milk will be discussed in terms of their biosynthesis and their nutritive value and utilisation by the newborn.

Carbohydrate

Lactose is the principal carbohydrate present in mammalian milk, and is the sole disaccharide found in mammals. It occurs only in milk, and is formed by the energy-dependent condensation of glucose with galactose. The uniqueness of this biosynthetic pathway to the mammary gland derives from the presence in the alveolar cells of the 'lactose synthesising enzyme'.

The main precursor of both of the monosaccharides used in lactose synthesis is glucose which is taken up from blood perfusing the breast. The steps by which glucose is phosphorylated and converted to UDP-galactose are summarised in figure 14.5. The final step in lactose synthesis is conjugation of UDP-galactose with glucose by the formation of a $\beta(1-4)$-glycosidic bond similar to that formed in plants during sucrose synthesis.

The lactose synthesising enzyme is of considerable interest. The partially purified 'enzyme' has been resolved into two components, a high molecular weight A protein and a second much smaller B protein. It is now known that the larger component, which is found mainly in the microsomal fraction, is the familiar enzyme galactosyl transferase and that the B protein is the whey protein α-lactalbumin, long recognised as an important characteristic protein found in milk. Galactosyl transferases are found in many tissues and are involved in diverse synthetic pathways, including glycoprotein and polysaccharide synthesis; they transfer N-acetyl glycosamine to an appropriate acceptor. In mammary lactose synthesis, interaction of galactosyl transferase with a α-lactalbumin increases the affinity of the enzyme for the substrates UDP-galactose and glucose. It is believed that α-lactalbumin causes a conformational change in the enzyme, thus altering the geometry of the active site, and it is therefore called a *specifier* since it effectively specifies the substrate of the enzyme.

By itself α-lactalbumin is inactive but is found in relatively high concentrations in milk, accounting for 2 per cent of the total milk protein. It is made on the rough endoplasmic reticulum and migrates to the Golgi complex where it binds to galactosyl transferase and initiates lactose synthesis. After catalysis, α-lactalbumin is released as well as lactose and is subsequently secreted, so that overall control of the rate of lactose synthesis may depend upon the concentration and rate at which the α-lactalbumin passes through the Golgi complex. It is believed that lactose is secreted from the alveolar cell in the small dense granules, packaged with the milk proteins (see section 14.7).

During pregnancy the levels of galactosyl transferase in the mammary gland increase but this

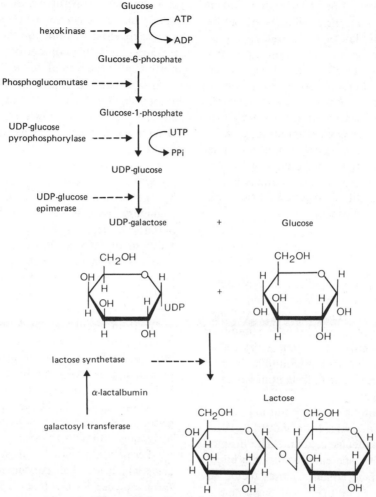

Figure 14.5   Biosynthesis of lactose

is not accompanied by any alteration in α-lactalbumin concentration because its formation is inhibited by progesterone. At parturition there is a large increase in the formation of the specifier protein and this initiates lactose synthesis.

The specific evolutionary advantage of lactose as the principal source of carbohydrate in milk remains obscure although a number of interesting explanations have been offered. Two comments concerning the properties of lactose are relevant. The first concerns the osmotic pressure of milk; clearly it is desirable that milk should have the same osmolarity as plasma so that further energy

does not have to be expended in keeping its fluid composition constant. The principal osmotically active component of milk is lactose, but if the carbohydrate were present in the form of monosaccharides like glucose only about one-half of the calorific value could be accommodated at the same osmolarity. Secondly, the alveolar cell membrane is impermeable to lactose but highly permeable to glucose so that, in contrast to lactose, retention of glucose would require energy expenditure.

Lactose is digested by hydrolysis to galactose and glucose by the enzyme lactase. The galactose is then converted to utilisable glucose by phosphorylation and epimerase action. Lactase is found in the epithelial cells lining the small intestine but its activity is relatively low even in the newborn. After weaning it declines to very low levels, and large amounts of lactose often cannot be properly digested by adults. Certain people are upset by large amounts of lactose in the diet due to a genetic deficiency in lactase (lactose intolerance). Another much rarer lactose intolerance condition, *galactosaemia*, is caused by the genetic deficiency of an enzyme required for the breakdown of galactose. Digestion of lactose leads to an accumulation of galactose which cannot be digested further, and which has several toxic effects.

Fats

Lipids are present in human milk in concentrations of about 3–4 per cent by weight, and are an important source of metabolic energy. Although human and cow's milk contain similar amounts of fat (see table 14.1) milk fat content varies widely between species: only traces are found in the milk of the horse, whereas seal milk contains over 50 per cent fat by weight.

Milk fat is present as a stable emulsion of small globules ranging in diameter from about 1 to 10 μm suspended in an aqueous medium. The droplets are prevented from coalescing by the thin bimolecular lipid membrane which encloses them; this membrane derives from the apical membrane of the alveolar cell during the secretion of the milk droplet (see above) and contains proteins and

phospholipids, together with small amounts of sterols and of glycolipids. These latter lipid substances together account for about 15 per cent of the total milk fat content of human milk, but a much smaller fraction of bovine milk.

Most of the lipid in milk is present as triglyceride, accounting for 85 per cent of human milk lipid and 97 per cent in cow's milk. The mammary gland is one of the most active lipid forming tissues of the body.

It was originally thought that most of the triglyceride in milk derives from fatty acids taken up by the mammary gland. It is now known that mammary tissue is itself capable of the synthesis of fatty acids, and it is probable that *de novo* synthesis of fatty acids from two-carbon sources accounts for as much as 60 per cent of the total milk triglyceride. None the less, there is good evidence from perfusion studies that the mammary gland can take up blood-borne triglycerides efficiently from circulating chylomicra and very low-density lipoproteins after hydrolysing them to free fatty acids. This is achieved by the action of lipoprotein lipases which are present in large concentrations in the actively secreting mammary gland. The resulting fatty acids are transported into the alveolar cells and resynthesised into triglycerides by conjugation with glycerol.

The principal route for the synthesis of the fatty acids which are then condensed with glycerol to form triglycerides involves the formation of acetyl coenzyme A (acetyl-CoA) and NADPH in the cytoplasm of the alveolar cell and the conversion of acetyl-CoA to malonyl-CoA, followed by the orderly addition of malonyl-CoA to a 'primer' or 'template' of either acetyl-CoA or butyryl-CoA until the newly synthesised fatty acid is released from the fatty acid synthetase complex. In nonruminants such as man, glucose serves as the prime carbon source for this process, but in ruminants such as the cow the major source of carbon for fat synthesis is acetate derived from microbial carbohydrate fermentation in the rumen rather than from glucose. This accounts for the high proportion of short chain saturated fatty acids found in their milk fat. These fatty acids are responsible for the characteristic flavours of butter and cheese.

Table 14.1   Composition of human and bovine milk

	Per cent by weight	
	human	cow
Water	87.5	87
Total solids	12.5	13
Protein	1.0–1.5	3.0–4.0
Fat	3.0–4.0	3.5–5.0
Carbohydrate	7.0–7.5	4.5–5.0

The key enzyme in the synthesis of fatty acids in the mammary gland is acetyl-CoA carboxylase from which malonyl-CoA is formed. It is probably the rate limiting step and its level increases markedly at the initiation of lactation. A large amount of energy is built up into the fatty acid: for example synthesis of 1 mol of palmitic acid requires 14 mol of NADPH, underlining the huge energy investment by the mammary gland in fat synthesis.

A very diverse pattern of fatty acids is formed in the mammary gland. Although more than 150 different fatty acid chains have been described in cow's milk, only 15 of them comprise 1 per cent or more of the total. In human milk, palmitate, oleate and linoleate account for more than three-quarters of the total milk fatty acid content. Of these, linoleic acid is derived from dietary sources, since mammalian cells are not capable of the synthesis of this polyunsaturated fatty acid.

Triglycerides are formed by the esterification of the fatty acids with glycerol in the particulate fraction of the alveolar cell, most probably on the rough endoplasmic reticulum.

Proteins

The protein content of milk in various species ranges from 1 to 20 per cent, and these proteins are generally classified into four principal types: casein, α-lactalbumin, β-lactoglobulin and immunoglobulins. Casein is found in the largest amounts, and accounts for about 80 per cent of the protein in cow's milk and 40 per cent in the human. It provides the principal source of amino acids for the suckling young. Casein is stabilised in milk in the form of complex micelles to prevent precipitation. Caseins are extremely hydrophobic and will precipitate readily in acid conditions forming curds, leaving the other milk proteins in solution as whey. Casein is thus easy to prepare and purify, and several distinct proteins have been demonstrated. The principal casein proteins are designated as α, β and κ; of these both α and β contain a high proportion of proline residues which prevent the formation of secondary structures such as α-helices. κ-Casein contains carbohydrate groups and di-sulphide cross-links and it is this component of the casein micelle which is critical for the maintenance of its stability. Calcium is required for the formation of these micelles. Caseins are readily attacked by proteases, thus serving as a ready source of amino acids, and in the non-ruminant stomach are digested by pepsin. Caseins also contain numerous phosphate groups; together with the high calcium content, this adds to their nutritional value. In cows and goats there is a specific casein-digesting enzyme, rennin, which precipitates casein by removing a glycopeptide fragment, including the carbohydrate, from κ-casein prior to its digestion.

The other proteins in milk are designated as whey proteins and do not precipitate with casein. Human milk contains α-lactalbumin, comprising about one-quarter of the total protein content; its role in lactose biosynthesis has been discussed above. β-Lactoglobulin is found in small amounts in human milk but in much larger concentrations in the milk of ruminants. Its specific function is not known.

Other proteins not manufactured in the mammary gland may also be found in milk. Serum albumins and several enzymes may be found in milk, albeit in low concentrations, and some of these may get into milk from the plasma by passive transfer across the alveolar cell. Of more importance is the presence in milk of relatively high concentrations of immunoglobulins, particularly immunoglobulins A and G (IgA and IgG). In the human, IgA accounts for 90 per cent of the immunoglobulin found in milk and colostrum, whereas in the cow the principal immunoglobulin in both is IgG with only 20 per cent of IgA. The importance of these immunoglobulins for the acquisition of passive immunity by the newborn will be discussed in section 14.11. It appears that IgA in milk is synthesised by plasma cells within the mammary gland, whereas IgG is obtained by selective uptake from the plasma.

Ions, vitamins and other components of milk

The ionic composition of milk is very different from that of plasma, and is maintained by active pumping of ions. The most likely site of this pump is in the basolateral membrane separating the alveolar cell from the extracellular space, and it is probable that the alveolar cell is in partial ionic equilibrium with milk due to the relative permeability to ions of the apical cell membrane. The most important features of the ionic composition of milk are the high levels of calcium ($\times 14$), phosphate ($\times 7$), potassium ($\times 7$) and magnesium ($\times 4$), and low levels of sodium ($\times \frac{1}{8}$) and chloride ($\times \frac{1}{4}$). The figures in parentheses indicate the approximate ratio of the concentrations of the ions in milk compared to plasma. There is ample evidence from these figures that alveolar epithelial cells are highly specialised for active ion transport.

The calcium and phosphate in milk are important for the growth and development of bone; in cow's milk most of the calcium and magnesium ions are complexed with the phosphate groups of the casein micelles or with citrate ions. This prevents the precipitation of calcium as the phosphate, and augments the calcium carrying capacity of milk. The large amounts of calcium secreted in milk imply considerable modification of normal calcium metabolism in the mother which sometimes causes enlargement of the parathyroid glands.

It was stated earlier that milk is an 'almost complete' food. Iron and copper are both present in trace quantities but may sometimes be insufficient if milk is the only source of food for the newborn. For this reason small amounts of iron may be added to cow's milk preparations as a supplement so that iron deficiency anaemia does not develop.

All the water-soluble vitamins are present in milk, most of them in concentrations sufficient for adequate growth and nutrition. However, vitamin C (ascorbic acid) is destroyed during boiling or pasteurisation, and should be added as a supplement to prevent scurvy. Vitamin D levels are also relatively low and rickets due to deficiency of this vitamin may result, particularly if the infant is not adequately exposed to sunlight.

Milk also contains amino acids at a total concentration of about 0.5 per cent which are taken up from blood perfusing the breast. There is a high proportion of proline in milk and this may be related to its important role in the synthesis of collagen.

Certain drugs, for example nicotine or steroid

contraceptives, may also be secreted into milk. This suggests that nursing mothers should use drugs with caution in order to avoid passing them to their babies through the milk.

14.9   Energy inputs in lactation

Lactation places heavy demands upon maternal metabolism because the energy investment in milk synthesis is very large. Thus it is remarkable that the protein and carbohydrate content of milk should remain virtually unaltered even in adverse maternal circumstances. Under conditions of malnutrition or actual starvation the lipid content and total volume may start to fall and maternal vitamin deficiencies are often reflected in the milk.

We can calculate approximate figures for the extra nutritional requirements of a lactating woman. The rate of milk secretion averages about 850 ml per day, although amounts as high as 3 l have been recorded, and about 50 g of fat, 18 g of protein and 100 g of lactose are synthesised. One litre of milk has a calorific value of about 700 kcal. Since it has been estimated that the synthesis of milk is about 80—90 per cent efficient it is apparent that an extra 1000 kcal per day should be allowed for a lactating mother as well as appropriate quantities of water and minerals.

14.10   Milk release

Milk is secreted from the alveolar cells into the alveoli and some passes into the larger ducts and lactiferous sinuses. Only the milk released into the sinuses can be removed by the negative pressure exerted by the infant sucking at the nipple or drained passively by cannulation. In goats and cows which have large cistern-like sinuses the proportion of milk that can be withdrawn is large, but in the human most milk is retained within the alveoli. The remainder can be released or 'let-down' only by active contraction of the myoepithelial cells surrounding the alveoli and ducts. There is abundant evidence that this process of milk ejection is mediated by a neuroendocrine reflex mechanism.

The nipple and areola contain abundant sensory nerve endings which respond to mechanical stimulation, especially to suction and pressure. Most of the fibres are present as free nerve endings and do not terminate in specialised structures. There are both myelinated and unmyelinated fibres and fast and slow adapting responses have been demonstrated. There is some sensory innervation of the connective tissue but not of the alveoli.

Afferent impulses in the intercostal nerves enter the spinal cord by the dorsal roots, pass via synapses in the dorsal grey matter to the dorsal and lateral ascending tracts of the same side, and reach the hypothalamus through several different routes in the brain-stem. They terminate mainly on the neurones of the hypothalamic supraoptic and paraventricular nuclei, thus stimulating release of oxytocin from the axon terminals of these neurones in the neurohypophysis. Circulating oxytocin acts on specific receptors in the myoepithelial cells to trigger their contraction. Suckling also causes release of prolactin from the anterior pituitary and this is important for the maintenance of milk synthesis and secretion.

Striking evidence for the neuroendocrine reflex mediating milk ejection is that ejection does not occur after hypophysectomy but proceeds normally if the efferent nerves to the breast are sectioned. The hormonal nature of the efferent stimulus explains why milk may sometimes be forcefully expressed from one breast during suckling of the other. Oxytocin can be detected in the blood during suckling or milking.

Synthesis of milk slows down and stops when the alveoli are engorged if milk ejection and removal does not occur. It is thought that the pressure exerted on the apical surface of the alveolar cell inhibits the fat droplet and protein granule secretory mechanisms. One consequence of this is that contents of the granules containing protein disrupt and are digested by lysosomes.

Suitable tactile stimulation of the nipple may also activate the milk ejection reflex in the same manner as suckling. Other stimuli which may sometimes cause oxytocin release include events which evoke conditioned auditory and visual reflexes, such as the anticipation of nursing as well as mechanical stimulation of the vagina and reproductive tract. Although the afferent pathways for these reflexes differ from those involved in the milk ejection reflex, they all result in the secretion of oxytocin consequent to stimulation of hypothalamic nuclei. Some of these stimuli may also cause prolactin release, presumably by diminishing hypothalamic release of prolactin inhibitory factor.

Oxytocin is a nonapeptide elaborated in the cell bodies of the supraoptic and paraventricular nuclei of the hypothalamus, and is passed in granules along the axons of the cells into the posterior lobe of the pituitary. Stimulation of the supraoptic and paraventricular nuclei causes oxytocin release, as does microinjection of acetylcholine into the hypothalamus. Oxytocin differs from vasopressin (antidiuretic hormone) by only two amino acids (figure 14.6) and both hormones are specific to the hypothalamus and posterior pituitary. However, certain stimuli are known to effect selective release of one hormone but not the other, and the two hormones have markedly different actions. Thus oxytocin powerfully stimulates contractions of myoepithelial cells of the breast and uterine smooth muscle (see chapter 12) but has no antidiuretic action on the kidney collecting ducts and is a weak vasodilator rather than a powerful vasoconstrictor. These striking differences illustrate how biological activities can be greatly modified by small changes in chemical structure. Injection of oxytocin or inhalation from a nasal spray causes milk ejection in the fully lactating breast but as it is a peptide it cannot be administered orally. The possible role of oxytocin in parturition was discussed in chapter 12.

Milk ejection may be easily interrupted by somatic or psychological stress. Inhibition may occur at the level of the hypothalamus, for example during anaesthesia, to decrease the responsiveness of the neuroendocrine reflex just described and thereby reduce oxytocin release, or at the breast due to the effects of sympathetic nerve stimulation. Stimulation of adrenergic receptors on myoepithelial cells inhibits their contraction and in the mammary blood vessels causes constriction. These peripheral effects tend to suppress lactogenesis and milk ejection.

Contraction of the smooth muscle within the

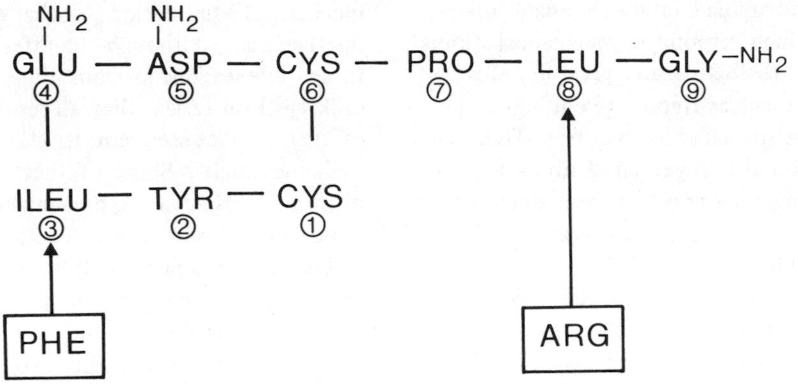

Figure 14.6   Structure of oxytocin. Vasopressin (antidiuretic hormone) has the same structure as oxytocin except for the two amino acids indicated in the boxes

nipple and areola in response to suckling, cold, touch or sexual arousal causes the erection and hardening of the nipple but the mechanisms for this effect are not fully understood. It serves to make the nipple easier to grasp during suckling.

14.11   Colostrum

The first milk secreted at the time of parturition is called *colostrum*, but its composition is very different from normal milk. Colostrum is a clear yellowish liquid which contains more sodium and chloride and much less potassium and lactose than milk. Its ionic composition resembles that of plasma. However unlike milk it coagulates on boiling because it has a much higher protein content, particularly of the immunoglobulins.

In the cow, pig and sheep, colostrum contains very large quantities of immunoglobulins G and M. Passive transfer of these antibodies to the offspring occurs during the first few days of life rather than *in utero*, and placental permeability to immunoglobulins is very low in these species. By contrast in man, immunity to certain antigens is gained passively before birth by passage of IgG across the placenta. However, human colostrum does contain IgA antibodies but in smaller amounts than for the species mentioned above. The antibodies in human milk are not absorbed in the gut and may serve to

neutralise pathogens in the intestine of the new born.

Human colostrum is secreted for the first few days after parturition after which milk production proper takes over as fat and lactose synthesis by the mammary gland get into full swing.

14.12   Lactational amenorrhoea

It is well known that conception does not usually occur during lactation and nursing of an infant at the breast. This is because lactation inhibits the return of regular menstrual cycles by preventing cyclic gonadotropin release from the anterior pituitary, producing a state of *lactational amenorrhoea*. This has been confirmed by comparing plasma hormone levels in post partum lactating women with those from mothers who choose to bottle feed their babies. At present there is speculation concerning the mechanism for lactational amenorrhoea but it is probable that it is due to inhibition of hypothalamo–hypophyseal pathways by the reflexes following breast stimulation during suckling. This suggestion has been offered to explain the suckling-induced secretion of prolactin, which is said to result from hypothalamic inhibition of prolactin inhibitory factor release (see section 14.6), and it is proposed that this same hypothalamic inhibition reduces gonadotropin releasing hormone (GnRH) secretion from the hypothalamus. This would therefore prevent the re-establishment of normal menstrual cycles. It has also been observed that responses to GnRH in women who are breast feeding are much reduced, implying that prolactin may itself inhibit pituitary gonadotropin release by a direct action during lactational amenorrhoea.

Lactational amenorrhoea is a natural mechanism for the adequate spacing of pregnancies so that one infant can be satisfactorily weaned before heavy metabolic demands are once again placed on the mother during her next pregnancy. It has been suggested that lactational amenorrhoea is the single most important mechanism at present limiting population growth because the majority of women in less highly developed countries still practise prolonged breast feeding. For this reason alone breast feeding is to be encouraged, quite apart from the consideration that human breast milk is probably preferable to cow's milk on nutritional grounds. However, lactational amenorrhoea is a very unreliable 'contraceptive', particularly if compared to the methods considered in chapter 6.

14.13 Mammary gland regression after pregnancy and in the menopause

The return of the breast to the non-lactating state involves gradual regression of its complex alveolar structure to a simpler form. This occurs after pregnancy when the infant is weaned from the breast to an independent diet and is marked by replacement of the numerous secretory lobules with connective tissue and fat. There is also a reduction in pigmentation of the nipple and areola as well as a decrease in the overall size of the gland. The breast often does not return to its previous firmness but remains somewhat looser and more pendulous than before pregnancy, due largely to stretching of its ligaments. Milk secretion declines before weaning is complete; the precise reasons underlying the timing of the reduction are not known.

Microscopic examination of alveolar cells undergoing regression shows that there is a decrease in the quantity and organisation of the rough endoplasmic reticulum, mitochondria, Golgi complexes and associated organelles, as well as in the number of protein granules and fat droplets. Lysosomal autophagocytosis is responsible for the removal of all these structures. The lysosomal enzymes are the only enzymes which do not decrease in amount during mammary regression. The nucleus reverts from a smooth round shape to a more irregular and folded form. These changes in the mammary gland are reversible and further hormonal stimulation from the next pregnancy causes development once more to the fully competent lactating state. There is some evidence that capacity for milk production declines after a large number of pregnancies and with advancing maternal age.

Regression of the breast during the menopause is irreversible and proceeds beyond the stages described above. There is a gradual loss of the adipose and connective tissue and shrinkage in overall size. The breast loses its elasticity. In old age it atrophies to a modest fraction of its original adult size and its surface becomes wrinkled. These changes reflect both the withdrawal of steroid hormonal support and the natural ageing processes in the tissue.

Further reading

Cowie, A. T. and Tyndal, J. S. (1971). *The Physiology of Lactation*, Edward Arnold, London

Frantz, A. G. (1978). 'Prolactin', *New England Journal of Medicine*, **298**, 201

Larson, B. L. and Smith V. R. (eds.) (1974). *Lactation: A Comprehensive Treatise*, vols I–III, Academic Press, London

Linzell, J. L. and Peaker, M. (1971). 'Mechanism of milk secretion', *Physiological Reviews*, **51**, 564

Mepham, B. (1976). *The Secretion of Milk*, Edward Arnold, London

Patton, S. (1969). 'Milk', *Scientific American*, **221**, 58

15

Growth, Puberty and Ageing

15.1 Growth

The meaning of the word 'growth' as used by biologists contains some elements that are not immediately obvious from its common use. Growth usually implies an increase in physical dimensions such as length or mass. This can be measured throughout both prenatal and postnatal development and provides a first approach to the detailed biological analysis of growth. In this sense, growth is usually taken to exclude temporary fluctuations in otherwise stable dimensions due to accumulation of fat or water.

More subtle than simple increase in dimensions is growth by increase in complexity, especially that due to the construction of new hierarchies of order in a system. This concept of growth also occurs in non-technical speech in such examples as 'the growth of an idea'. A simple example taken from chapter 8 is afforded by the development of a zygote into a morula which was interpreted in terms of growth or enrichment of the positional information of the cells on which further development is dependent, but which occurs without any increase in size.

A use of the word which is not encountered in everyday speech is *negative growth*. This may imply a reduction in either dimensions or complexity. For example, at the end of lactation the absolute size of the breast decreases and the complexity of organised units in the secretory tree diminishes as described in chapter 14.

The measurement of changes in complexity and organisation is more difficult than measurement of physical dimensions, but is performed routinely whenever the functional competence of a system is examined. Testing of reflex activity in neonates and intelligence testing of children are examples. Such tests are largely empirical because we generally do not understand the functioning of the system well enough to make mechanistic interpretations. Therefore much of the discussion here will be confined to dimensional growth, although the beginnings of a systems approach can be seen in the discussion of the control of the onset of puberty.

The dimensional growth of humans continues up to about 20–21 years of age, but occurs at varying rates during this period. Figure 15.1 shows curves for height and weight for both sexes plotted as a function of age, as well as the rates of increase of the parameters. The rate curves are perhaps the more interesting, since they illustrate very clearly the two periods in childhood when growth accelerates. A small height and weight spurt is sometimes detectable during childhood (5–8 years of age) and is earlier and more marked in boys. The major acceleration of growth occurs during adolescence at puberty (see later). Girls enter this phase before boys, so for a few years they are taller and heavier; however, the boys pass them by about 14½–15 years, and remain taller and heavier (figure 15.1).

Growth curves for different species vary (figure 15.2), depending on the proportion of the life span over which growth is spread. For example,

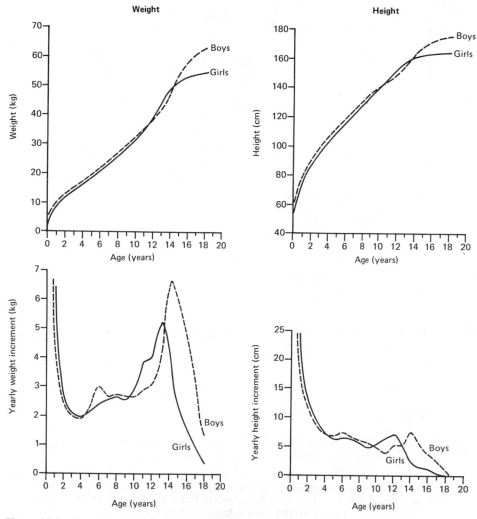

Figure 15.1   Growth curves for boys and girls. The upper curves show the absolute heights and weights and the lower curves illustrate the changes in rates of growth during the various developmental periods (Redrawn from Rhodes, P. (1969). *Reproductive Physiology for Medical Students*, J. & A. Churchill, London)

lower vertebrates such as fish generally tend to increase in length and weight throughout life until senescence sets in, although the rate falls steadily after a juvenile period of rapid growth. A similar general pattern is seen in many mammals, except that the period of fastest growth is confined to the juvenile period and growth in the mature animal is limited to an increase in bulk and muscular development rather than of length or height. The growth curves of primates and man, with two spurts of growth in childhood followed by cessation of growth at adulthood, are thus rather unusual.

However, in general terms the growth curves of an individual organism or of a population under optimal conditions can all be described by sigmoid curves as illustrated in figure 15.2. The only apparent exception is in arthropods in which all dimensional growth has to occur at *ecdysis* (moulting), because at other times the body size is con-

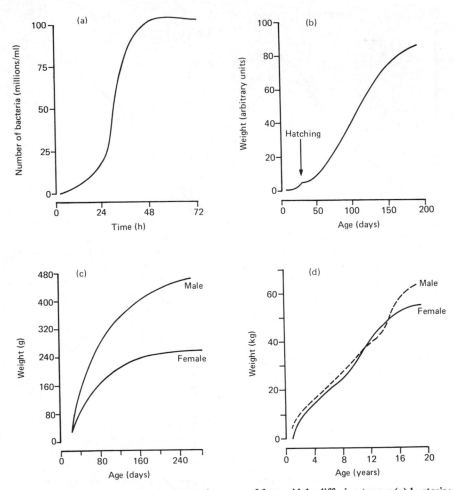

Figure 15.2   **Sketches of typical growth curves of four widely differing types: (a) bacteria; (b) chicken; (c) rat; (d) human (Modified from Timiras, P. S. (1972).** *Developmental Physiology and Aging*, **Macmillan, New York)**

fined by a rigid exoskeleton. Their growth curves show a series of discontinuous steps, but even these yield a sigmoid curve if smoothed out.

We should note that the growth of different organs in man does not occur at the same time or rate. Consider as an example the relatively large size of the human head at birth; after birth there is proportionally much greater growth of the limbs and trunk relative to the head. The change in relative proportions is even more obvious if we compare the fetus with the adult (figure 15.3). There are other striking differences in organ growth in the postnatal period, some of which are

illustrated in figure 15.4 in terms of weight. The brain grows rapidly and exponentially, and completes its growth much sooner than the majority of organs. By contrast, most of the growth of the reproductive organs is delayed until puberty. The adrenal growth curve is interesting: at birth the fetal cortex is present, but this rapidly atrophies during infancy, after which the organ grows towards its adult size.

Although human growth patterns have been well documented in quantitative terms, there is still considerable uncertainty about the ways in which growth is regulated. It is clear that several

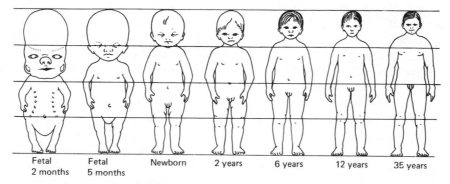

Figure 15.3 Changes in relative proportions of the human body during growth from the fetal period to adult (Redrawn from Scammon, R.E. (1927). *American Journal of Physical Anthropology*, **10, pages 329–336)**

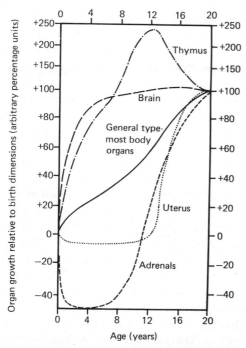

Figure 15.4 Growth curves of different organs of the human plotted so as to show the manner in which growth to the adult size is achieved. The size at birth is taken as 0 and that of the fully grown adult as 100. The graph shows how the brain grows relatively early, whereas uterine growth is delayed until puberty. The adrenal glands regress after birth (see chapter 11) before growing to adult size. Other lymphoid and reproductive organs follow the pattern represented here by thymus and uterus respectively (Redrawn from Timiras, P. S. (1972). *Developmental Physiology and Aging*, **Macmillan, New York)**

hormones play a crucial role in determining the onset, extent and patterns of growth, but their precise functional interrelationships and control remain to be established. The three principal endocrine growth regulators are growth hormone, the thyroid hormones and the sex steroids, although other hormones such as insulin and the glucocorticoids are known to exert permissive or modifying effects.

Hormones of the three principal groups mentioned above stimulate protein anabolism and increase the retention of nitrogen, potassium, phosphorus and calcium which are needed for synthesis of both cellular and extracellular materials. In addition, they all have their own characteristic effects. Growth hormone promotes the growth of many tissues by increasing protein synthesis, probably by stimulating messenger and ribosomal RNA production. It also promotes cellular uptake of certain amino acids, and mobilises fats and carbohydrates so as to make available extra substrates for metabolism. Children with severe hypopituitarism hardly grow at all, principally because of the absence of growth hormone. Their growth can be stimulated by the administration of human growth hormone provided that thyroid hormone replacement is also given. Growth hormone stimulates linear growth and skeletal enlargement, but can only do this before the epiphyses have fused. If growth hormone secretion occurs to excess in the adult, linear growth cannot occur as the epiphyses have closed and a characteristic pattern of bone and soft tissue deformities called *acromegaly* may result.

Thyroid hormone deficiency causes a dramatic reduction in the rate of growth in early childhood. It is known that thyroxine has direct anabolic actions on many cells, causing protein synthesis and cellular growth. Thyroxine and growth hormone act synergistically and both are required for proper growth.

Testosterone has powerful anabolic and growth promoting actions and is largely responsible for the surge of growth during puberty in the male; the smaller amounts of androgens secreted by the ovaries and adrenals in the female also contribute to her pubertal growth spurt. Oestrogen stimulates the growth of certain tissues, most notably those of the female reproductive system and the breasts, but has less powerful anabolic actions than testosterone. Both sex steroids promote epiphyseal closure; thus precocious puberty, although associated with an unusually early spurt of growth, often results in short stature since linear growth of the skeleton is arrested at a relatively earlier stage.

Insulin deficiency results in reduced protein synthesis and reduced growth. Thus adequate insulin levels and pancreatic islet function are required for the full expression of the growth-promoting actions of the hormones mentioned above. Glucocorticoids may also influence growth, since in excess they direct the utilisation of amino acids away from protein synthesis towards gluconeogenesis.

The preceding paragraphs are intended as a brief survey of the hormonal regulation of growth. It is also pertinent to recall that normal growth depends upon adequate supplies of nutrients and oxygen. Deficiencies of these may well prevent adequate growth, as illustrated by the characteristic malnutrition syndromes such as kwashiorkor (protein deficiency), rickets (insufficient vitamin D or sunlight), the reduced rates of growth observed when animals are transferred to high altitude and certain genetically based inborn errors of metabolism which prevent the proper intestinal absorption or utilisation of vital metabolic intermediates. There are many other ways in which growth may

be modified. For example, short stature may result from a variety of genetic disorders, from several types of endocrine malfunction (some of which were mentioned above), or from certain diseases which impair gastrointestinal, renal, pulmonary or cardiovascular function.

Excessive growth (gigantism) is much rarer than dwarfism or stunted growth. Extreme height is often familial, reflecting above-average height of the parents. Some endocrine disturbances, such as overproduction of growth hormone or of thyroxine in childhood, may also cause excessive growth.

Factors which influence the rate of fetal growth have been mentioned in previous chapters. For example, babies born to heavy smokers are generally smaller than average, whereas those of diabetic mothers are frequently considerably overweight. Some heavy fetuses appear to be 'constitutionally large' and exhibit much more rapid growth in infancy than is usual; they often become obese and mentally retarded. It is noteworthy, too, that larger children tend to mature earlier and to reach puberty sooner. This last observation is of interest with regard to the critical body weight theory of the onset of puberty which is discussed later in this chapter.

The preceding discussion, although simplified, has been concerned with established facts about human growth. It is relevant to mention briefly some of the important gaps in our understanding of the subject. For example, how is growth limited? Each species appears to follow a self-limiting pattern of growth, as illustrated by the slowing of the growth curves presented earlier. Does the slowing of growth depend upon genetically programmed instructions in which an active self-inhibitory system swings into action, or does growth decline passively, due perhaps to lack of nutrients or accumulation of inhibitory metabolites? Maybe growth simply slows down because of the ageing of the tissues; if so, what determines ageing?

Another interesting problem is posed by the phenomenon of *catch-up growth*. In childhood, disease or malnutrition may slow the rate of growth. When health is restored, it is common to observe a period of rapid catch-up growth until the usual size-for-age is reached within the normal limits of variation.

Loss of certain organs or parts of organs may be followed by compensatory growth or regeneration. This is frequent in plants and lower animals but can occur to a limited extent in humans. For example, removal of part of the liver or of a kidney is followed by hepatic regeneration or compensatory renal hypertrophy. Tissue damage is often healed by the growth of new tissue or of a scar. However, whole limbs cannot be regenerated in mammals in the manner observed in crustacea or newts. No doubt some simpler regenerations such as the mammalian examples quoted above are set in motion by the release of specific growth promoting humoral mediators, akin to the recently characterised nerve and epidermal growth factors, or by mitotic growth regulators such as the chalones, acting in concert with endocrine changes. Regeneration of complex structures such as limbs requires the re-establishment of a population of uncommitted blastema cells in a field coordinate system, as discussed in chapter 8. This type of de-differentiation apparently cannot occur in mammalian tissues.

Human growth and development may be measured in several ways. Regular measurements of height and weight are necessary in infancy and childhood to check that growth, which is rapid at this time, is normal. Naturally there is much variation between individuals: growth must be referred not only to the accepted mean values, but also to the observed variability of these values. For example, values lying outside the 95th percentile are regarded as abnormal, although they do not necessarily indicate pathological disturbance.

Other assessments of growth of clinical importance include measurements of trunk length (sitting height), shoulder and pelvic breadth, X-ray assessment of hand and especially carpal development. Paediatric assessment of child development may be made by measuring functions such as reflex responsiveness, control of bowel and bladder function, posture and walking, motor and feeding ability, speech, growth and eruption of teeth, and so on. These relate to the general, neurological and muscular development of the child, and their

relationship to chronological age is well documented. They may all be considered to reflect aspects of growth, as defined in the broad sense at the beginning of this chapter.

15.2 Puberty

It is not easy to provide a simple but adequate definition of the word 'puberty' although most people intuitively understand that it defines an important part of adolescence during which the child matures physically and psychologically into an adult. One authority on the subject has defined puberty as the phase of bodily development during which the gonads secrete sex hormones in amounts sufficient to cause accelerated growth of the genital organs and appearance of the secondary sexual characteristics. This definition omits to mention that an important landmark in normal puberty is the acquisition of the capacity to produce fertile gametes. However, the onset of fertility does not necessarily mark the finish of puberty, since mature gametes are usually produced before many of the other physical change of puberty are complete. In sum, puberty is an integrated series of anatomical, physiological and psychological changes, many of which are related to or caused by changes in hormonal status, and is a phase linking the immaturity of childhood with the maturity of adulthood.

Before detailing specific changes which occur in each sex during puberty it is appropriate to summarise its main characteristics in broad terms:

(1) A general increase in the growth rate of skeleton, muscles and viscera — the adolescent growth spurt.

(2) Sex-specific increases in the growth rate of particular parts of the body (e.g. the shoulders in boys, and the hips in girls), leading to enhanced physical differences the sexes (*sexual dimorphism*).

(3) Alterations in body composition, such as the change in ratio between muscle and fat, or the changes in distribution of hair.

(4) The development of the reproductive sys-

tem to functional maturity, and acquisition of the secondary sexual characteristics.

The underlying basis for many of these physical changes in both sexes is hormonal. Puberty marks the maturation of the hypothalamo—pituitary—gonadal hormonal axis, and the bodily changes can be understood in terms of the varied metabolic actions of the male and female steroid hormones produced by the maturing gonads. Any lesion in this axis which prevents the adolescent increase in production of androgens in the male or oestrogens in the female prevents many, if not all, of the characteristic changes seen in puberty and results in a permanently immature or eunuchoid individual.

By contrast, there are several types of *sexual precocity* observed in the human on rare occasions. *True precocious puberty* occurs when an apparently normal pubertal state develops abnormally early (that is, before 10 years of age). These conditions are generally caused by some abnormality in the brain, possibly a tumour, or by infection or congenital abnormality, but appear to result from the usual pubertal-type hormonal changes driven by gonadotropins. There is also a type of true precocious puberty which is related to genetically heritable factors, though the exact basis for this condition is not known. *Precocious pseudopuberty* defines those conditions in which the secondary sexual characteristics appear (as in puberty) but are not accompanied by gametogenesis. These diseases result from inappropriate sex-hormone production from the gonads, rather than from stimulation of the gonads by gonadotropins released from the pituitary.

Table 15.1 gives a simplified list of the main changes of puberty in the male and female. Prominent among these are the events concerned with the maturation of the reproductive organs and those changes in the secondary sexual characteristics which create the differences in form between men and women.

In the male, the first visible signs of puberty are the growth of pubic hair, enlargement of the penis and the beginning of a phase of accelerated growth at about 12—13 years of age. However, these are not really the first events of male puberty because the testis has already begun to develop and mature. Up to 5—6 years of age, histological sections of the immature testis show that the seminiferous tubules are solid cord-like structures in which primitive spermatogonia may be recognised. During the gradual testicular growth which proceeds up until puberty, the seminiferous tubules enlarge and acquire a lumen surrounded by characteristic seminiferous epithelium. As yet there are no signs of testosterone-secreting interstitial cells: although these are present at birth, stimulated by hCG from the placenta, they disappear soon after.

At about 11—12 years the testes begin to grow and the seminiferous tubules enlarge with Sertoli cell growth and germ cell meiosis. The interstitial cells become differentiated from fibroblast-like precursors and assume a characteristic clumped distribution between the tubules. Testicular development continues for several years, leading to the production of testosterone and of spermatozoa. Mature spermatozoa are not usually found until the 15th or 16th years.

The early phase of testicular development is the first of a number of other pubertal changes which follow after the first signs mentioned above. Genital growth continues and in mid-puberty there are other visible signs of the maturing man: by about 14—16 years masculine hair growth appears on the face, in the pubic and axillary regions and on the limbs, the growth spurt reaches its maximum and the voice breaks. By this time mature spermatozoa are found and the accessory glands are fully functional. The sequence of these changes is represented diagrammatically in figure 15.5. Puberty ends as gradually as it began with the cessation of growth and the closure of the epiphyses which usually occurs at about 17—19 years. The precise clinical dating and evaluation of puberty in the male is hampered by the absence of any single dramatic landmark comparable to the menarche in the female.

In general, puberty occurs later in boys than in girls as illustrated by figure 15.6. This shows the annual growth rates of boys and girls from childhood until the end of adolescence.

In girls, as in boys, the peak rate of growth

Table 15.1 Changes in the human at puberty

Boys (12–16 years)	*Girls* (10–14 years)
Development of secondary sexual characteristics:	*Development of secondary sexual characteristics:*
(a) GENITAL CHANGES Enlargement of penis, seminal vesicles and prostate glands and onset of secretion from glands; onset of spermatogenesis	(a) GENITAL CHANGES Increase in size of vagina and uterus; establishment of cyclical menstrual activity; enlargement of labia; onset of ovulation and secretion from glands
(b) EXTRAGENITAL CHANGES Deeper voice; increased body hair (pubic hair, male pattern), including on face, axilla, legs and chest; more aggressive behaviour; interest in opposite sex; sebaceous gland secretions increase (acne); body conformation changes with enlargement of muscles and broadening of shoulders	(b) EXTRAGENITAL CHANGES Breasts grow and acquire adult contour; body hair increased (pubic hair, female pattern) but hair on body is less than in male except on scalp; interest in opposite sex; sebaceous gland secretions increase; body conformation changes — hips broaden, fat deposits increase, especially in breast and buttocks; voice remains high pitched
General changes Accelerated rate of growth, especially of muscles and skeleton	*General changes* Accelerated rate of growth but less than in male

Changes common to both sexes initiated at puberty and which continue gradually with age

Age-dependent fall in heart rate, respiratory rate, extracellular fluid volume and basal metabolic rate; increase in respiratory function parameters and in red cell and haemoglobin values

occurs after the first visible signs of the onset of puberty, although it happens earlier in girls as shown in figure 15.6. Puberty usually begins at 10–12 years of age with the development of breast buds, enlargement of the areolar diameter and changes in the vaginal mucosa, and is followed by the growth of sparse downy pubic hair. There follows a stage in which the internal and external genitalia grow considerably. Among the most evident manifestations are the enlargement of the labia, softening of the vulval mucosa and the presence of an acidic vaginal fluid due to bacterial

breakdown of glycogen to lactic acid. Internally, the uterus and uterine tubes enlarge, the endometrium proliferates and the cervical glands acquire secretory activity.

The most sharply defined event in female puberty is the *menarche*, the first menstrual period, which generally occurs around 13 years of age. However, there is considerable variation in its timing. Menarche is generally observed some 6–12 months after the peak of fastest growth. The first menstrual cycles are anovulatory and irregular, and there is normally no endometrial secretory phase

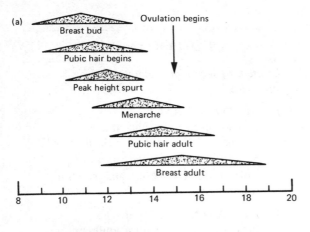

(a)

Breast bud

Ovulation begins

Pubic hair begins

Peak height spurt

Menarche

Pubic hair adult

Breast adult

8   10   12   14   16   18   20

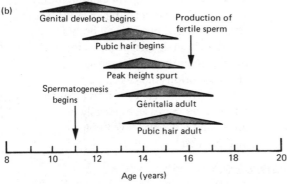

(b)

Genital developt. begins

Production of fertile sperm

Pubic hair begins

Peak height spurt

Spermatogenesis begins

Génitalia adult

Pubic hair adult

8   10   12   14   16   18   20

Age (years)

Figure 15.5 **Approximate sequence of pubertal events in (a) girls and (b) boys. The majority of adolescents undergo the changes illustrated at the time when the triangles are at their maximum height** (Redrawn from Short, R. V. (1976). *Proceedings of the Royal Society of London*, 195, pages 3–24)

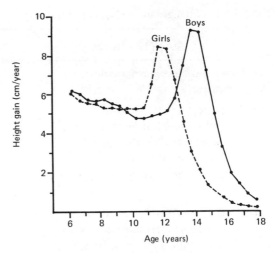

Figure 15.6 **Rate of growth during adolescence, plotted as increment of height gained in each six-month period. This clearly shows that the growth spurt in girls is smaller and occurs sooner than in boys** (Redrawn from Timiras, P. S. (1972). *Developmental Physiology and Aging*, Macmillan, New York)

because no corpora lutea are formed. Menstrual bleeding is thus due to oestrogen withdrawal. At this time the pituitary–ovarian axis is not yet completely functional and the physiological changes of puberty described above are due almost solely to the metabolic effects of oestradiol. Later on the secondary sexual characteristics of the developing woman are shaped additionally by the actions of progesterone on oestrogen-primed tissues.

Female puberty continues after the menarche: axillary hair grows, pubic hair assumes its characteristic female distribution by 14–15 years, and the breasts develop to their mature form. Growth rate slows since high concentrations of oestrogens

cause the fusion of the epiphyses by 16–17 years of age.

It is plain that clinical evaluation of puberty in the female is much easier than in the male since the menarche may be precisely dated, and other events such as breast development and the growth of pubic hair generally follow a well-defined course. However, it is often difficult to be certain just when an adolescent girl becomes fully fertile unless basal body temperature records or steroid production are carefully monitored because the ovary does not become fully functional at the menarche.

Two principal theories have been advanced to explain the mechanism of the onset of puberty. Both are based on the knowledge that puberty is initiated by an increase in the release from the pituitary of gonadotropins, which in turn stimulate development and hormone production in the gonads. At puberty there is an increase of 4–6 times in the plasma levels of FSH and of 10–16 times in LH in girls. Levels of the ovarian sex steroids are very low before puberty and rise in response to the effects of gonadotropins on the ovary. The first theory of the onset of puberty suggests that the brain contains an inhibitory substance which in the immature prepubertal state prevents gonadotropin release by action at either the hypothalamic or pituitary levels. At present there is no sound evidence in favour of this idea as no such substances have been found. However, the concept is compatible with observations that in the prepubertal state the hypothalamus and pituitary contain gonadotropin releasing hormone and gonadotropins respectively and that neither hormone is released. Furthermore, the gonads appear to be responsive to exogenously applied gonadotropins. Therefore in summary it appears that there is no evident deficiency or incompleteness in the hypothalamo–pituitary–gonadal axis, save that it is apparently dormant.

The answer provided by the second and generally accepted theory for the onset of puberty is that in the immature state the hypothalamus is hypersensitive to the negative feedback effects of circulating steroids and that therefore the gonadotropin regulating mechanisms are dormant. It is postulated that in the immature state the low levels of circulating oestrogens and androgens (mainly produced by the adrenals) are sufficient to inhibit secretion of gonadotropin releasing hormone from the hypothalamus, and that consequently pituitary gonadotropin release is low. There is some experimental evidence for this thesis based on work with female laboratory animals. The theory still begs the question of the basis for the mechanism whereby the hypothalamic steroid sensing receptors

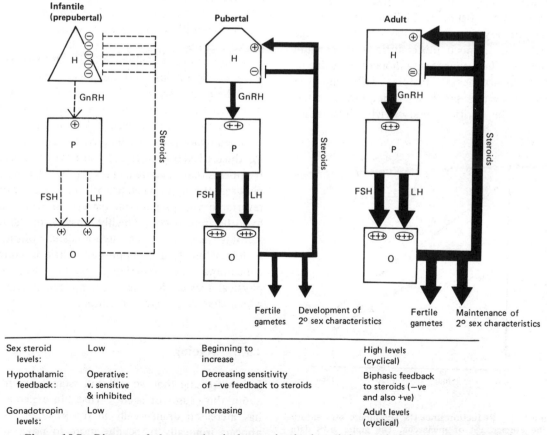

	Infantile (prepubertal)	Pubertal	Adult
Sex steroid levels:	Low	Beginning to increase	High levels (cyclical)
Hypothalamic feedback:	Operative: v. sensitive & inhibited	Decreasing sensitivity of −ve feedback to steroids	Biphasic feedback to steroids (−ve and also +ve)
Gonadotropin levels:	Low	Increasing	Adult levels (cyclical)

Figure 15.7 Diagram of the postulated changes in the hypothalamo–pituitary–ovarian axis during puberty – three different stages in hypothalamic maturation are depicted by changes in shape of the symbol (H, hypothalamus; P, pituitary; O, ovary)

(called the *gonadostat* by several authors) acquire their mature status. Neurophysiological studies have shown that several brain regions, particularly the dorsal hippocampus and the amygdala, influence sexual functions by neural effects on the hypothalamus, and it may be that the maturation of the gonadostat is affected by neural inputs as well as by intrinsic timing or maturational mechanisms. The sum total of a number of changing factors may be required to trigger the events which lead to puberty.

The changes in hormonal release patterns in the female are depicted diagrammatically in figure 15.7 in such a manner as to illustrate the infantile, pubertal and adult states of the hypothalamo–pituitary–ovarian axis.

There is good evidence that the age of menarche has decreased by 3 or 4 years over the past 100 years or more (figure 15.8). It is also true that puberty in boys occurs nowadays at a younger age though this is much more difficult to measure accurately. These changes are thought to be due to several environmental factors, with improved nutrition as the single most important determinant. The 'critical body-weight hypothesis' suggests that puberty occurs when a certain body weight is reached and explains the recent secular trend since better-fed children are reaching this weight sooner. There is evidence that puberty starts earlier in heavier girls and that regression towards a prepubertal amenorrhoeic state occurs in girls who lose weight to excess, for example during the course of the disease anorexia nervosa. Yet this theory is probably a considerable over-simplification and does not provide any satisfactory explanation for the mechanism whereby body-weight influences central nervous system function. Furthermore, there do not appear to be marked differences in the mean age of menarche among wealthy and poor members of a population who presumably differ in their diet. Other variables, such as environmental temperature, altitude, urbanisation, sense of smell and time of year have all been suggested as possible contributing factors.

The condition anorexia nervosa, mentioned above, is a disease in which the individual (usually a young woman) deliberately avoids eating. It leads to weight loss and secondary amenorrhoea and there is reversion to a prepubertal state. Although there is not usually a direct correlation between the degree of weight loss and the onset of amenorrhoea, the events provide some support for the critical body-weight hypothesis of puberty. It appears that in anorexia nervosa the relationship between the hypothalamus, pituitary and ovaries reverts to the prepubertal pattern in which the hypothalamus becomes highly sensitive to the sex steroids so that the hypothalamo–pituitary secretory function is suppressed. Little is known concerning the underlying psychological and physical reasons for the deliberate self-starvation which characterises this condition.

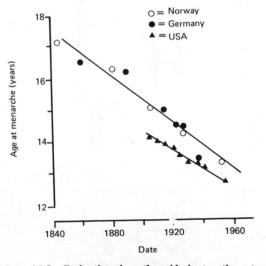

Figure 15.8   Reduction since the mid-nineteenth century in the average age of menarche. The graph gives data showing the same trend in three countries (Redrawn from Short R. V. (1976). *Proceedings of the Royal Society of London*, 195, pages 3–24)

15.3   Ageing

It is surprising that we still understand very little about the causes of ageing. That life expectancy has increased dramatically in the past 200 years appears ironically to be due more to progress in simple hygiene and nutrition than to spectacular advances in medicine or the treatment of disease.

However, the relative frequency of different causes of death has changed dramatically since the advent of chemotherapy. Figure 15.9 shows historical data for life expectancy in different countries, figure 15.10 shows the relationship to age of some of the most common causes of death, and figure 15.11 examines in more detail the important contribution of accidents, cardiovascular diseases and neoplasms (cancer) to age-dependent mortality. Remember in figure 15.11 that absolute mortality at the younger ages is low; thus although accidents account for a high proportion of mortality, the absolute number of fatal accidents is low compared to the absolute number of fatal cardiovascular episodes among older people.

There is unlikely to be one single cause of ageing, since it is improbable that the same processes underlie the gradual ageing and decline in function of, say, the central nervous and cardiovascular systems. Figure 15.12 shows a graph which represents the ageing of several different human physiological functions. Not all functions decline at the same rate in any one individual, and there are wide differences in apparent physiological age between individuals. The sum total in the ageing equation depends upon complex interrelationships between genetic constitution, environmental influences and chance.

Some theorists seek to define ageing in general terms as the gradual breakdown of the homeostatic and adaptive capacities of the body. This is certainly a reasonable definition, and one usually finds marked limitations in the functional capacities of older people, especially when tested under conditions of exercise or stress. However, this broad view of ageing does not explain the under-

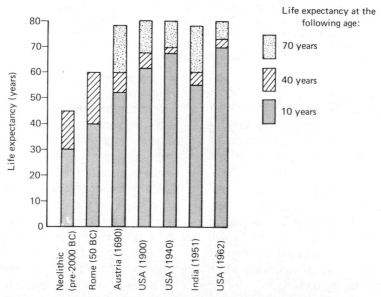

Figure 15.9 Life expectancy as a function of age at different epochs. The histograms show the average total life expectancy at 10, 40 and 70 years of age, and illustrate that life expectancy has increased since prehistoric times. This is indicated by examination of the filled histograms showing life expectancy at 10 years of age, and the increase is due to social and medical advances as well as of hygiene. By contrast, once 70 years of age has been reached there is very little difference in the period 1690–1962 in the total life expectancy, showing that little has been achieved in terms of prevention of disease or mortality in the old

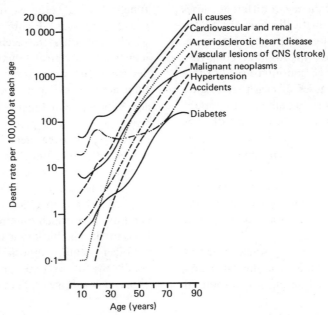

Figure 15.10   Frequency of death due to specific causes as a function of age. The data refer to mortality in the USA in 1955. A similar graph plotted for, say, 1890 would show a very different pattern of causes of death. The total death rate would be higher at all ages, and infectious diseases, especially bronchopneumonia and tuberculosis, would be common causes of death (Modified from Timiras, P. S. (1972). *Developmental Physiology and Aging,* **Macmillan, New York)**

lying cellular causes of the deterioration. Other commentators regard the degree of cellular differentiation as the fundamental determinant of cellular ageing; highly differentiated cells are committed and often cannot reproduce themselves as effectively as more primitive cell types. This means that specialisation of function resulting from elaborate cell differentiation carries with it a penalty — these cells have a finite and limited existence, since they have a reduced capacity for growth and are 'closer to death' than cells which can perpetuate themselves by division.

It is tempting to argue from this thesis that a concept of ageing related to growth and development receives support from the observation that small animals which grow quickly to adult size (i.e. in which the growth *rate* declines rapidly) have brief life spans. However, we might also equally postulate that smaller animals, particu-

larly warm-blooded species, suffer from greater potential homeostatic disequilibrium on account of their larger surface area to volume ratio, and that the higher metabolic rate required to maintain homeostasis wears cells out more quickly. The idea that there might be an inverse relation between ageing and high metabolic rate is reinforced by evidence that certain invertebrate poikilotherms live longer at lower environmental temperatures.

These comments imply that metabolically active cells have a finite life span, and that overall ageing in a complex organism might reflect the intrinsic ageing of certain of its constituent cells. Some interesting support for this concept derives from cultured human fibroblasts. Under optimum culture conditions these cells are only capable of about 50 mitotic divisions, after which they die. The biochemical reason for this apparent inbuilt senescence is not yet clear and the relevance of

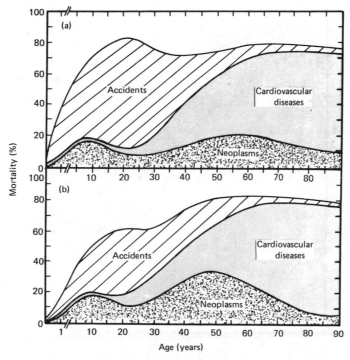

Figure 15.11 Graph showing age-dependent variation in three important causes of death in males (a) and females (b); each cause is plotted as a percentage of the total number of deaths at the given age. The data relate to the USA 1968 (Redrawn from Timiras, P.S. (1972). *Developmental Physiology and Aging*, Macmillan, New York)

these cell culture experiments to the intact animal is uncertain. The 'ageing' could conceivably arise from an accumulation of errors due to defects in the fidelity of nucleic acid replication or transcription.

At this stage the best one can do is to keep an open mind about the causes of ageing since it is probable that there may be several fundamental mechanisms. The concept that metabolic errors may arise spontaneously and accumulate is attractive. Thus it is proposed that accumulated errors of genetic translation may underlie some cancers and the inbuilt senescence of certain cultured cell lines (see above); a similar argument could be used to explain why protective immunological mechanisms may become defective or positively destructive with age, as in the auto-immune diseases. Other workers have suggested that ageing may result from cumulative damage, especially in

biological membranes, caused by spontaneously generated free radicals and lipid peroxides.

15.4 Decline of sexual function with age

Male

Many males retain some degree of sexual activity and fertility into old age and spermatozoa can usually be found in the genital tracts of old men, even in those who are impotent. However, the general trend in men shows a fairly marked decline in sexual function and performance, represented in figure 15.13 which emphasises the increase in impotence among men of above the age of 60. Normal levels of plasma testosterone vary between wide limits (figure 15.13); concentrations of this hormone decline in old age as the number and

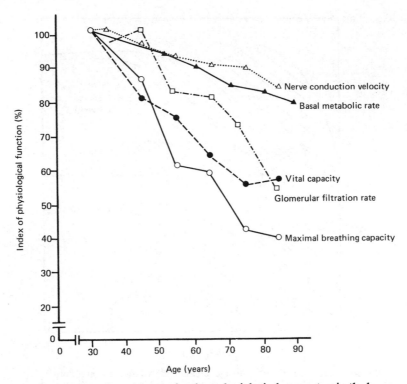

Figure 15.12   Decline with age of various physiological parameters in the human. The data are plotted as a percentage of the average value of the function in healthy 30-year-olds (Modified from Strehler, B.C. (1977). *Time, Cells and Aging,* **Academic Press, New York)**

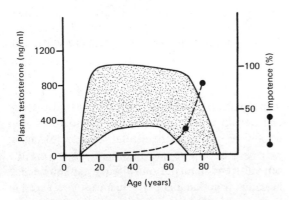

Figure 15.13   Ageing in the male. The graph shows the association in time between impotence and declining levels of circulating testosterone. The graph of the hormone levels shows the wide range of normal values as determined by plasma radioimmunoassay. The curve showing impotence is approximate

secretory function of the interstitial cells decrease. The declining capacity of the testis is also evident from examination of the spermatozoa themselves: with age the proportion of damaged or abnormal forms increases. Libido, ability to achieve erection and frequency of orgasm all diminish with age, accompanied by a decline in the functional activity of the seminal vesicles and prostate gland.

The decline in reproductive potential in the male is essentially a gradual process; the degree of change also varies widely from individual to individual. It appears that many of the events associated with or occurring at the same time as the decline of male reproductive capacity are caused by relative testosterone deficiency which occurs at this time (figure 15.13). Similar changes are seen after castration and it is of interest that eunuchoid or castrated men often age prematurely, suggesting that the ageing process may be affected directly by androgen deficiency.

Female

There is a precipitous decline in fertility of women in the fifth decade as a result of functional changes of the ovaries. These changes culminate in the *menopause*, which defines the transition between the cyclical menstrual activity of the fertile woman and the persistent amenorrhoea which follows. In industrialised nations, the menopause usually occurs in the late forties but it may be precipitated sooner by conditions of poor general health, malnutrition or overwork. In the years preceding the menopause progressive ovarian failure occurs, as evidenced by irregular cycles of bleeding and failure to ovulate. Thus female fertility declines before the menopause is actually reached. Complete cessation of menstruation generally comes 1–2 years after ovulation has stopped.

These changes occur in middle age and indicate that the ovaries age much more rapidly and earlier than other organs of the body. It is believed that ovarian ageing reflects a growing insensitivity to gonadotropins; thus the primordial follicles become unresponsive to FSH and LH and fail to develop in the normal manner. There is also a steep decline with age in the number of primordial follicles in the ovary as determined histologically (figure 15.14). It should be remembered that the follicles are formed during embryological development and exist subsequently in the ovary in a state of arrested meiosis; perhaps it is not surprising then that they should age and lose their function after 40 years or more.

The progressive failure in the development of follicles leads to a decline in ovarian production of oestrogens and progesterone. The absence of a progestational luteal phase explains the menstrual irregularities observed in older women and luteal failure may account for the high frequency of miscarriages which occur when older women become pregnant. The decline in ovarian oestrogen output can be followed by measuring urinary steroid secretion (figure 15.15) and lack of oestrogen accounts for many of the physiological changes

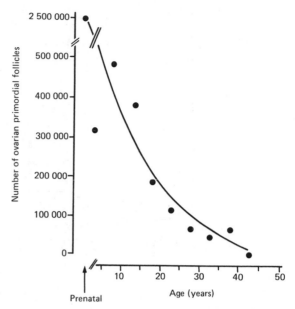

Figure 15.14   Decline of number of primordial follicles in human ovary with age. The data are based on histological inspection of ovaries taken at operation

which accompany the menopause (see below). The pituitary responds by secreting larger amounts of gonadotropins, especially FSH (figure 15.15), because the declining levels of oestrogen release the hypothalamus from negative feedback inhibition. The post-menopausal hormonal relationships of the hypothalamo–pituitary–ovarian axis are shown diagrammatically in figure 15.16. There appears to be an increase in activity of the pituitary gonadotropin-secreting basophil cells and plasma gonadotropin levels are high in post-menopausal women. The urine of these women is one of the richest sources of these hormones (human menopausal gonadotropin) up until very old age when female pituitary function declines sharply.

A number of physiological sequelae involving metabolic, cardiovascular and nervous functions as well as the reproductive system usually follow the decline in oestrogen output, and contribute to the symptoms which occur at the menopause. In some women, these effects are very troublesome and require palliative treatment. There is considerable atrophy of the sexual organs, including shrinkage in size of the uterus and vagina as well as changes

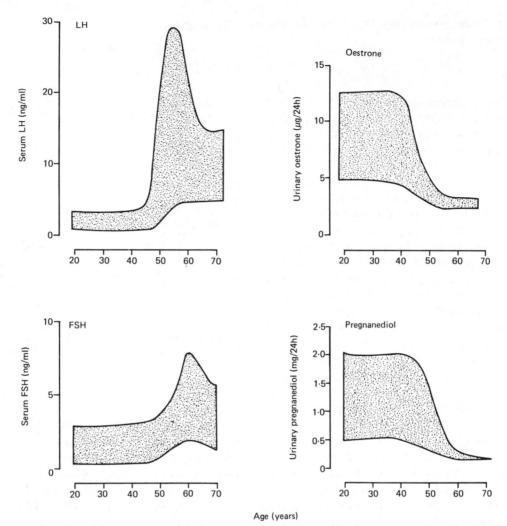

Figure 15.15   Hormonal levels in the female before and after the menopause. The graphs show plasma levels of FSH and LH and urinary excretion of oestrone and pregnanediol. There is considerable variation in the values of all four hormones between women and particularly during the different phases of the menstrual cycle. The graphs show typical values for the maximum and minimum levels achieved during the menstrual cycle in pre-menopausal women

in histology. Secretory activity is reduced; the vagina becomes drier, sometimes causing sexual intercourse to be painful, and there is a reduction in acidity because of decreasing glycogen secretion. The ageing breast becomes flaccid and droops because oestrogen withdrawal is associated with the disappearance of the ramified alveolar structure and shrinkage of the ducts. The skin generally becomes drier and less elastic. Oestrogens promote

skeletal calcification and this explains the gradual decalcification of the skeleton which follows the menopause. These effects, which can be measured radiographically, partly explain the changes in posture of old women, as well as their increased vulnerability to bone fracture if their skeleton has been significantly weakened by osteoporosis.

Many of the symptoms experienced at the menopause are generalised and difficult to measure

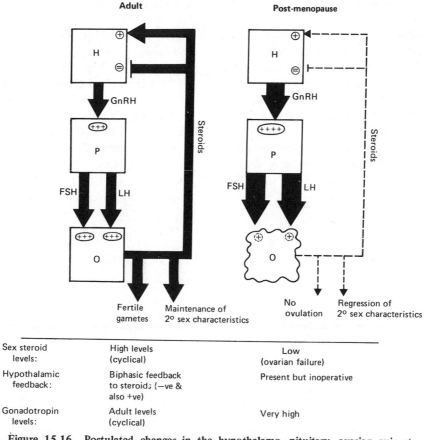

Adult   **Post-menopause**

Sex steroid levels:	High levels (cyclical)	Low (ovarian failure)
Hypothalamic feedback:	Biphasic feedback to steroids (−ve & also +ve)	Present but inoperative
Gonadotropin levels:	Adult levels (cyclical)	Very high

Figure 15.16   Postulated changes in the hypothalamo−pituitary−ovarian axis at the menopause. The ovary is given a wrinkled outline to indicate that it loses its capacity to secrete steroids. Compare this diagram with figure 15.7

with precision. They include neural and psychological components such as depression, hot flushes alternating with chilly sensations, inappropriate sweating, dizziness and fainting, paraesthesias, cramps, pains and neuralgias, anxiety, faintness and lack of vigour. The symptoms are notoriously variable; for some women the menopause brings years of ill-health; for others it is relatively mild. Some of the symptoms mentioned above may result from the actions of elevated plasma FSH and others may be due to oestrogen deficiency. For this reason oestrogen replacement therapy has been promoted vigorously as a suitable treatment for the menopausal woman experiencing distressing

symptoms. Oestrogen therapy is also suitable for ovariectomised women in whom oestrogen deficiency is absolute and immediate.

Oestrogen replacement therapy is certainly very effective as a means of reducing the severity of oestrogen withdrawal symptoms and it slows the rate of skeletal decalcification and atrophy of the reproductive organs. Oestrogens such as ethinyl-oestradiol or mestranol used in the combined contraceptive pill are employed for this purpose. The treatment can be given cyclically with several weeks of tablets plus a break of a week to allow 'withdrawal' bleeding. Addition of a small amount of an androgen is said to enhance physical vigour and libido as well as to reduce the severity of withdrawal bleeding.

The dependence of many women on long-term oestrogen replacement therapy has attracted a good deal of controversy. It is thought that oestrogen therapy carries certain physical risks such as of thromboembolism, as discussed in chapter 6, so it is reasonable to suggest that the aim should be for a gradual reduction in the hormonal dosage rather than constant maintenance at a high level. In short, such maintenance therapy may merely exchange one type of risk or adverse effect for another.

Further reading

Lamb, M. J. (1977). *Biology of Ageing*, Blackie, Glasgow

Sinclair, D. (1978). *Human Growth After Birth*, 3rd edn, Oxford University Press

Strehler, B. L. (1977). *Time, Cells and Aging*, 2nd edn, Academic Press, New York

Tanner, J. M. (1978). *Foetus into Man: Physical Growth from Conception to Maturity*, Open Books, London

Timiras, P. S. (1972). *Developmental Physiology and Aging*, Macmillan, New York

Index